31 : 616.314 /43.50

Design and Analysis in Dental and Oral Research

Design and Analysis in Dental and Oral Research

Second Edition

Neal W. Chilton, BSC, DDS, MPH, FACD

Senior Research Associate in Biostatistics and
Preventive Dentistry, Columbia University;
Diplomate, American Board of Periodontology
Diplomate, American Board of Endodontics;
Research Consultant, School of Dental Medicine,
University of Pennsylvania; Senior Scientist,
Oral Health Research Center, Fairleigh Dickinson
University; Research Professor of Periodontics,
New York University

With a Foreword by
James P. Carlos, DDS, MPH

Director, National Caries Program, National Institute of
Dental Research, National Institutes of Health

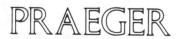

PRAEGER

PRAEGER SPECIAL STUDIES • PRAEGER SCIENTIFIC

Library of Congress Cataloging in Publication Data

Chilton, Neal W.
  Design and analysis in dental and oral research.

  Bibliography: p.
  Includes index.
  1. Dental research—Statistical methods.
2. Experimental design. I. Title.
RK80.C52 1982   617.6'0072   82-591
ISBN 0-03-056157-4   AACR2

Published in 1982 by Praeger Publishers
CBS Educational and Professional Publishing
a Division of CBS Inc.
521 Fifth Avenue, New York, New York 10175 U.S.A.

© 1982 by Praeger Publishers

23456789 145 987654321
Printed in the United States of America

The Second Edition of this book
is DEDICATED to
my wife, Naomi,
and my children,
Peninah and Albert, Jonathan and Ellen,
Abigail, Seth, and Miriam

Foreword

A more widespread application of the principles of good experimental design and analysis to dental research has been the goal of
Dr. Chilton's efforts during much of his professional career. This
book is but one example. Another is his long and fruitful collabora-
tion with Professor Fertig and other biostatisticians at Columbia
University, which has generated a steady stream of publications to
demonstrate the utility of a variety of statistical techniques to tests
of hypotheses with dental data. At the same time Dr. Chilton has
actively encouraged a small but talented group of trained biostatisticians from other laboratories to become interested in dental
research and has seen to it that they talk with each other, and with
dental investigators, freely and frequently. These efforts have had
noticeably positive results.

Even so, there is reason to suspect that an appreciation of the
basics of rigorous research design and the ability to select proper
analytical techniques is not yet universal among dental researchers.
Of course, it is the rare research report these days that does not
include some statement about the statistical significance of results,
and rarer still the editor who does not insist on this. Nevertheless,
contemporary dental literature is still burdened with examples of
poorly controlled experiments and of the application of inappropri-
ate statistical tests. The intent of *Design and Analysis in Dental and
Oral Research* is to help the researcher to minimize these methodolog-
ical lapses.

Design and Analysis is a textbook of the application of basic
statistics to dental data, but a text in which a message is implicit; it
is an attempt to convince the dental researcher that a lack of formal
mathematical training is neither a deterrent to an understanding of

statistical fundamentals, nor an excuse for ignoring them. Those fundamentals are set forth here. Their use is well illustrated and they are adequate to handle many of the design and analytical requirements of dental experiments. When more sophisticated methods are needed, the diligent reader will have learned enough to seek out a practicing biostatistician and to describe the problem with clarity. With luck, the statistician will also have read this book, and will have some insight into the peculiarities of the data we deal with in dental research. In that sense, this book is also a sort of primer of two languages, that of statistics and that of dental research, sufficient to permit a dialogue between specialists in each. Such a dialogue is absolutely essential to high quality research.

So far as I know, that, and nothing more, is what Neal Chilton has been telling us for the past 30 years, and continues to tell us with this second edition of *Design and Analysis in Dental and Oral Research*. The advice is still sound and still necessary for both the experienced and the novice dental scientist, and the more seriously we heed it, the more penetrating and productive our research will be.

James P. Carlos, D.D.S., M.P.H.
Bethesda, Maryland

Preface to the Second Edition

In 1967, *Design and Analysis in Dental and Oral Research* was published by J. B. Lippincott of Philadelphia. It is now out of print. While this was the first edition, it had its origin in Analysis in Dental Research (Office of Technical Services, U.S. Department of Commerce, 1951), written under a contract between the Office of Naval Research and Columbia University. The limited number of copies was out of print by 1953, but through the auspices of the Gies Foundation, a copy was placed in the libraries of the dental schools in the United States and Canada.

Following the completion of that publication, support was provided first, for a short period, by the Office of Naval Research, and later by the National Institute of Dental Research, National Institutes of Health, of the Department of Health and Human Resources through grants to Columbia University, for further development of statistical methods in dental and oral research. Papers dealing with this subject have appeared in dental and statistical journals in the United States and Europe.

As stated in the Preface to the first edition,

Since 1949, there has been a tremendous increase in the application of statistical methods in oral biology, obvious to anyone attending the meetings of the International Association for Dental Research or other scientific meetings in which oral biological research is presented. It was therefore felt that an expanded text would be of great help for classroom teaching of graduate and undergraduate students in dental schools. The use of illustrative examples from studies in oral biology should make the exposition much more applicable to the problems faced by the dental investigator. It is hoped that *Design and Analysis in Dental and Oral Research* will be of great help in improving and furthering research in oral biology at both the basic science and the clinical levels.

In this second edition, extensive revision of the chapters in the first half of the book, particularly of the concepts of estimation of sample size, confidence intervals, multiple comparisons of means, and the introduction of new illustrative examples where appropriate, have been made. The chapters on the Analysis of Variance, Regression and Correlation, and the Analysis of Covariance have been extensively rewritten and expanded and an entirely new chapter, Multiple Regression, has been added. In addition, the ready availability of inexpensive desk-top and hand-held calculators has reduced the need for illustration of detailed arithmetic exposition throughout the text. An Appendix has been provided to illustrate the relation of computer printouts using HP 41C programs, and the widely used, very comprehensive SAS, SPSS, and BMDP software packages (for which thanks are given to Molly Park, Bernard Bollmer, and Robert Lehnhoff). A new section on Ridit Analysis has been added to the chapter on Ranking Tests and a new chapter, Reliability Trials, has been included. The very fine chapter, Epidemiological Data by Professor Robert M. Grainger, which appeared in the first edition, has not been included in the second edition. The addition of much new material in biostatistics in this revised edition has increased the size of the current volume. Revision and expansion of the epidemiology chapter to include the newer developments and indices in this field would have increased the size (and cost) even further.

The reader should feel free to consult other texts which provide general and often more detailed background material in biostatistics, such as: Snedecor, G. W. and Cochrane, W. G.: *Statistical Methods*, 7th ed., Iowa State University Press, Ames, 1980; Steel, R. G. D. and Torre, J. H.: *Principles and Procedures of Statistics*, 2nd ed., McGraw-Hill, New York, 1980; Dixon, W. J. and Massey, F. J.: *Introduction to Statistical Analysis*, 3rd ed., McGraw-Hill, New York, 1969; Armitage, P.: *Statistical Methods in Medical Research*, Blackwell Scientific Publications, Oxford, U.K., 1971. For further detailed background in more specific areas, the reader should consult such other books as: Lehmann, E. I.: *Nonparametrics: Statistical Methods Based on Ranks;* Holden-Day, San Francisco, 1975; Miller, R. G.: *Simultaneous Statistical Inference*, 2nd ed., Springer-Verlag, New York, 1981; Fleiss, J. L.: *Statistical Methods for Rates and Proportions*, 2nd ed., Wiley, New York, 1981; Draper, N. R. and Smith, H.: *Applied Regression Analysis*, 2nd ed., Wiley, New York, 1981; and Feinstein, A. R.: *Clinical Biostatistics*, Mosby, St. Louis, 1977.

The author is indebted to the National Institute of Dental Research, National Institutes of Health, Department of Health and Human Services, for grants to Columbia University for support of our continued activities in Statistical Methods in Dental Research, and for the contract which helped support the writing of this second edition.

He would like to express his sincere thanks to Professor Joseph L. Fleiss, Professor and Chairman of the Division of Biostatistics of the School of Public Health of the Faculty of Medicine of Columbia University for his contributions to the chapters on Ranking Tests and Reliability Trials and who, since 1976, has been the head of the team working on the NIH grants; and to Professor Ralph V. Katz of the Department of Oral Health Ecology of the University of Minnesota, who gave him many valuable suggestions and ideas; to Dean D. Walter Cohen of the University of Pennsylvania for his encouragement and for the use of the technical facilities of the School of Dental Medicine; to Professor Irwin D. Mandel of the School of Dental and Oral Surgery of Columbia University for his friendship and valued support and encouragement of his efforts through these many years; to his wife, Naomi A. Chilton, who has been closely associated with all the activities of the dental biostatistical research program at Columbia and with the writing of this book; to Blanche Agdern and Gerda Cordova for their most valuable help in the administration of the grants; and to Dr. Jerry Stone, Dorothy Breitbart, and Gordon Powell of Praeger Publications for their most valued help and guidance in the editing and publication of this second edition.

Most of all, I want to thank two people: Dr. James P. Carlos, Associate Director of the National Institute of Dental Research and Chief of the National Caries Program, for his enthusiastic support of my efforts over the years and also for the Foreword he has contributed to this second edition; and to Dr. John W. Fertig, Professor Emeritus of Biostatistics and formerly Chairman of the Division of Biostatistics in the School of Public Health of the Faculty of Medicine of Columbia University, my teacher and friend for over 30 years. Professor Fertig has served as constant advisor and resource and editorial consultant through all phases of my biostatistical activities. Without his help and encouragement, this book would not have been possible. Such credit as this new edition earns is to be shared with him; its errors and detractions are my responsibility alone. Finally, to all my colleagues in dental research who have encouraged and supported my efforts in this long and happy task, my gratitude.

Lawrenceville, New Jersey
1 July 1982

Table of Contents

Design and Analysis in Dental and Oral Research

1
Introduction

The first dental college in the United States was established in Baltimore in 1842. In the comparatively short time since then, dental research has advanced to the level of that of other biological sciences. Yet, although the careful, sound scientific training of dental investigators should be the keystone of dental research, often a void has been left in their scientific training — how to use statistical reasoning in planning studies and experiments and in ordering and evaluating the resulting data.

The methods of statistical analysis are essentially techniques used to help solve the problems of basic and applied sciences. The techniques are working tools of science, just as the microscope, the polygraph, and the colorimeter are. The statistical method has wide applicability and usefulness, direct or indirect, in a great variety of problems. No application of statistical methodology, however, can compensate for inadequate study design or poor experimental techniques. Because many of the techniques of statistical analysis are comparatively simple, the mathematics of the analysis may be quite correct, but the data may have been obtained in so unreliable a way that erroneous conclusions can be drawn. This has happened so often in so many fields that the average person has become skeptical of "figures," and the expression "Statistics don't lie but statisticians do" has become a refuge for many professional people.

While it may be true that some discoveries are based on fortuitous circumstances, most research workers have a definite problem in mind when they begin a particular piece of work. The first step in setting up an experiment is to outline clearly a "statement of objectives": Just what does the investigator expect of this study? All too often, an ambitious but unsophisticated worker will attempt to perform an experiment in which he hopes to answer all phases of the problem, whereas a whole series of studies, extending over several years, would be necessary to clarify all his questions.

The statement of objectives should be lucid and specific. It may be in the form of the questions to be answered, the hypotheses to be tested, or the effects to be estimated. Whatever form it takes, the investigator should have clearly in mind what he expects to do, and not perform an experiment merely to see what happens. He should have a pretty good idea of how the experiment is to be performed, including the type of experimental "treatment," the size of the experiment, and the experimental method. Fortunately, such preliminary planning is necessary in many cases to obtain grants to finance the study. This is particularly true of grant applications submitted to the National Institutes of Health for support of extramural research; the reviewing committees carefully examine the research plan and study design. A general knowledge of statistical methods, including an understanding of basic research designs, can be most helpful in this first stage.

Both during the conduct of the study and following its completion, the basic data are usually recorded and preserved in some type of notebook or file, or printout for computer-derived data, in a numerical form with appropriate comments. Statistical techniques, used either consciously or unconsciously, are essential to the organization and ordering of the raw data into a meaningful summary form. Finally, the methods of statistical analysis are a powerful tool in drawing the conclusions and generalizations from the results of the particular study or experiment just completed, i.e., statistical inference.

Not only does the research worker in the basic sciences need statistical orientation; but the clinician as well can make good use of it. When he attempts to evaluate the results of different types of treatment for the same pathosis, statistical considerations are of the greatest importance — not only in preventing incorrect or unwarranted conclusions, but also in evaluating the work of others. This is particularly applicable today, when the public and the profession are being deluged with claims of the effectiveness of different medications and methods advocated for the prevention of disease (e.g., dental caries), which are sometimes based on inadequate studies or incompletely analyzed data.

This book provides the dental research worker and clinician with basic information on statistical techniques and methods of analysis. All its examples are drawn from the oral biological field. The techniques of analysis described are those applied more frequently to this area. If the data are worth statistical analysis at all, they are worth the best type of analysis, . . the type which allows the maximum amount of information to be derived from them. One must remember, however, that the most intricate and highly specialized statistical analysis is not always the best for a particular set of data.

Although the arithmetical aspect of these analyses may at times appear tedious and involved, the methods employed here have been kept as simple as possible. The generally available and relatively inexpensive electronic calculator will be of inestimable help to the researcher. Every year more sophisticated versions are introduced, many of which contain statistical and mathematical functions, obviating the necessity of such formerly necessary tables of squares, square roots, logarithms, and even some tables of statistical functions, such as normal deviates, t-tables, F-tables, etc. Many relatively simple calculators will present means, standard deviations, variances, correlation coefficients, sum of squares, sum of products, etc. literally at the touch of a button.[1] Programmable hand-held or desk-top calculators now available can perform relatively complicated tests and even produce hard copy (printouts).

There are, in general, two methods of calculation used in these pocket calculators, the algebraic and the reverse Polish notation (RPN). The most widely used examples of the former are the models produced by the Texas Instruments Company while the Hewlett Parkard Company produces a diverse line of the latter type. The author prefers the RPN method because of the ease in chain calculations.

Package programs are readily available for use with the larger electronic computers. An investigator can use a standard, or slightly modified, BMDP or SAS software package, for example, and get a "complete solution" to his statistical problem. Unfortunately, these programs may not utilize the proper model and even more importantly may be fed unreliable data or data generated by a poorly designed experiment or a combination of both. The best expression for the dental research worker to remember in this regard, is "Feed in garbage and get out garbage."

Even though preprogrammed and, certainly, programmable pocket calculators will yield final "answers" quite readily, it is most important that the dental investigator understand what, when, and why the appropriate statistical analyses are required, as well as how to push a button and obtain a number. It is the purpose of this book to provide this information to the reader. Since many of the readers may have been away from elementary applied mathematics for too long a time, a refresher text can be most helpful.[2]

REFERENCES

1. Ball, J. A.: Algorithms for RPN Calculators, New York, Wiley, 1978.
2. Walker, H.: Mathematics Essential for Elementary Statistics, New York, Holt, 1951.

2

Organizing, Graphing, and Summarizing Raw Data

The basic raw datum in dental research is an observation (of a characteristic) of an individual, an experimental animal, or a physical or chemical phenomenon. Such an observation may take one of many forms: the patient's ascorbic acid level in saliva is 0.25 mg%; the patient does have at least one DMF tooth; the fluoride concentration of the community's water supply is 1.9 ppm; the patient has 3 DMF teeth; the patient's ascorbic acid level in saliva is low. The background of each such observation has an implied scale of classification or measurement. Any such scale must have at least two divisions or categories. Scales of sex, for example, are male and female; of the number of decayed teeth $0, 1, 2 \ldots 32$.

The scale of classification is either a numerical (*quantitative*) scale or a descriptive or adjectival (*qualitative*) scale. Examples of qualitative scales are sex (dichotomous), race, and cause of tooth extraction. A numerical scale may be *discrete* (number of DMF teeth, number of RBC per milliliter of whole blood) or *continuous* (ascorbic acid level in the saliva in mg%). Many discrete scales are practically continuous — e.g., the RBC counts may be 4,000,000, 4,000,001, 4,000,002 . . . , where the discreteness essentially disappears. On the other hand, because of the limitations of many of the measuring devices, continuous scales appear to be discrete. For example, ascorbic acid is measured, say, to the nearest 0.01 mg%, since finer distinctions cannot be made. Furthermore, a quantitative scale may be so inadequate that often it may be treated as though it were qualitative — e.g., grouping of numerical lactobacillus counts into the four categories, high, medium, low, and none. This scale is actually better than the usual qualitative scale because it involves an ordering

5

of the categories, and might better be called an *ordinal* scale. Some characteristics are presently measurable in qualitative terms only — e.g., fit of oral prostheses — but could be more precisely measured if an appropriate quantitative scale could be found. In general, a good quantitative scale contains more information than a qualitative scale.

Scales are often classified in other terms as well. A *nominal* scale is a primitive type of scale in which the categories are used only as labels, so that it is actually a descriptive qualitative scale, e.g., the number of subjects who are caucasian, black, brown, yellow, etc. The nominal scale leads to the formation of classes. The *ordinal* or ranking scale, mentioned above, is next in the hierarchy of scaling, and brings into account the concept of rank ordering. This type of scale involves the determination of "greater" or "lesser." In clinical studies, patient characteristics are often described in an ordinal scale, and may be ranked as none, mild, moderate, or severe. Numbers are sometimes assigned to these categories, e.g., 0, +, ++, +++, etc., or 0, 1, 2, 3, making the scale appear quantitative. It should be remembered, however, that the differences among the various categories are not uniform. This occurs in the next higher scale in the hierarchy of scales. The first truly quantitative scale is the *interval* scale, in which, in addition to ordering, the distances or intervals between any two numbers on the scale are of a known size. An ordinal scale which ranks temperature as hot, cold, or in-between (warm), can be upgraded to an interval scale by classifying the temperature in degrees. The intervals may not be transferable from one scale to another, e.g., temperature readings are not directly transferable from Centigrade to Fahrenheit and vice versa. Clinical indices utilizing discrete scores, such as the Löe-Silness Gingival Index or the Turesky modification of the Quigley-Hein Plaque Index are sometimes felt to be interval scales, but this interpretation might be considered to be "cheating," since the numbers in these indices are assigned somewhat subjectively. When the scores are averaged over the mouth, however, the scale becomes essentially continuous and an "interval" scale is achieved, thereby allowing for appropriate types of statistical analyses to be performed, i.e., parametric instead of nonparametric or ranking tests. The highest level of scale, the *ratio* scale, is obtained when an interval scale has a true zero point as its origin, e.g., weight as measured in pounds or grams; length in inches or centimeters.

The first step in ordering raw data is to recognize the type of scale present. Often the method of organization and of later statistical analysis depends on the kind of classification employed.

QUALITATIVE SCALES

Tabulating

The records of a university[1] contain the causes for the extraction of 6266 teeth from male patients, and 7,643 from females.

Caries	Periodontoclasia
Caries	Pulp disease
Periodontoclasia	.
Impaction	.
Periodontoclasia	.
Pulp disease	Caries
Periodontoclasia	

    To order the raw data, count the number of teeth that fall into each category on the scale of classification of the characteristic, *cause of extraction*. The most convenient classification in which attention is paid to the most widely understood cause (by the public, at any rate) would be a simple dichotomy: *Caries* and *Other Causes*, as shown in Table 2.1. In this table, the causes of extraction for both sexes, are presented. This very frequent arrangement of data is known as a *fourfold table*, or a *double dichotomy* table, since the classifications are dichotomized for both cause and sex. If the classification or *seriation* includes all the previous enumerated causes of extraction, and the total number of teeth extracted in each category is listed, then the raw data will be grouped and a frequency distribution obtained. The total frequencies of male extraction (6,266 teeth) and of female extractions (7,643 teeth) have been distributed over the scale of the characteristic, cause of extraction. When the divisions of the scale of classification have no natural ordering, the frequencies

TABLE 2.1
Tooth Loss at All Ages by Cause and Sex, 1921–1926, Dental Clinic, University of Minnesota[1]

	Number of Teeth Extracted	
Cause of Extraction	Male	Female
Caries	1,424	2,214
Other causes	4,842	5,429
Total	6,266	7,643

TABLE 2.2

Tooth Loss at All Ages by Cause, and Sex, 1921–1926. Dental Clinic, University of Minnesota[1]

	Number of Teeth Extracted	
Cause of Extraction	Male	Female
Periodontoclasia	2,631	1,846
Caries	1,424	2,214
Pulp disease	1,322	2,193
Prosthetic corrections	706	1,097
Cystic conditions	88	116
Impacted teeth	79	164
Accidents	12	7
Supernumerary teeth	4	6
Total	6,266	7,643

are often listed in ascending or descending order; hence the decreasing frequency in Table 2.2 for both male and female patients. This table represents a simultaneous classification of the teeth by cause of extraction and by sex of the patient. From such data, comparisons can be made, e.g., in this case, between the sexes.

Graphing

A graph of a frequency distribution with a qualitative scale serves to visualize the relative sizes of the categories in the scale. The graph should be made self-explanatory, with appropriate labels and a title. Of the many ways to graph a frequency distribution, one common way is to assign the characteristic to the y-axis (vertical axis or ordinate) and the frequency per category to the x-axis (horizontal axis or abscissa). An arithmetic scale would be used on the x-axis — i.e., equal differences in frequencies are represented by equal distances on the x-axis. A horizontal bar should be drawn directly alongside each category to a length opposite the number on the x-axis equal to the frequency within the category. The bars should be separated to indicate the qualitative nature of the scales.

This graph is given in Figure 2.1, which is a bar graph of the frequency distribution of the teeth extracted for the male patients in Table 2.2. For all the data in Table 2.2, there would be two contiguous bars projected for each category, one for males and one for females, labeled accordingly.

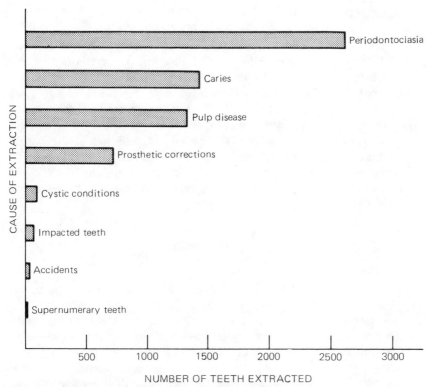

FIG. 2.1 Bar Graph Depicting Number of Teeth Extracted, by Cause, from Male Patients in a University Dental Clinic.

Obviously, the role of x and y may be interchanged at times for convenience. In that case, the graph consists of vertical bars instead of horizontal bars.

The purpose of a graph, in general, is to present the data in a simple and readily understood form so that interrelationships can be appreciated more readily than if the data were in tabular form. If the table itself is very simple — e.g., Table 2.1, nothing would be gained by graphing. Since the data presented in a paper may be of assistance to other investigators, it is often best to present a graph in addition to, not instead of, the table(s) of data, although particular circumstances dictate the final decision. The precise method of graphing used depends, to a large extent on the people who will read the paper and the emphasis to be placed on certain aspects of the data. The graph should not distort the data to bring out unwarranted inferences.[2,3]

Summarizing

A common method of summarizing the frequency distribution with respect to a qualitative scale is to reduce the total frequency to a round number, such as 100 (or 1,000 or 1,000,000), and each partial (category) frequency proportionately, e.g., to percentages. Each resulting relative number is called a *relative frequency*. The round number chosen to replace the total frequency is the "base" and the relative frequencies must sum to the base figure. When the base is 100 (the most frequent choice), the distribution of relative frequencies is called a percentage distribution. From Table 2.2, the percentage of extracted teeth in the caries category for males would be computed as

$$\frac{1,424}{6,266} (100) = 22.7\%$$

The distribution of the 13,909 patients of Table 2.2 could be finally summarized in percentage form as in Table 2.3. The original total frequency should be given, so that the original frequencies in the various categories can be reconstructed and the stability of the relative frequencies evaluated (a problem to be discussed later).

The percentage distribution can be graphed, using the same principles as in graphing the original frequency distribution. Except for the change in the numbers on the x-axis, the graph would be the same as Figure 2.1, with the bars in the various categories having the same relations to each other.

TABLE 2.3
Percentage Distribution of 6266 Teeth Lost for Male Patients and 7643 Teeth Lost for Female Patients by Cause

	% Extracted	
Cause of Extraction	*Male*	*Female*
Periodontoclasia	42.0	24.1
Caries	22.7	29.0
Pulp disease	21.1	28.7
Prosthetic corrections	11.3	14.4
Cystic conditions	1.4	1.5
Impacted teeth	1.2	2.1
Accidents	0.2	0.1
Supernumerary teeth	0.1	0.1
Total	100.0	100.0

TABLE 2.4
Two-year Evaluation of Endodontically Treated Teeth with Positive Cultures Prior to Obturation, According to Prior Periapical Status[4]

Periapical Status	Cases Healed	Cases not Healed	Total Cases	% Cases Healed
With rarefaction	41	20	61	67.2
Without rarefaction	26	4	30	86.7
Total	67	24	91	73.6

The percentage distribution facilitates the evaluation of the relative importance of the various categories of the characteristic. When two or more distributions are involved, the advantages of percentage distributions become more obvious, since all total groups are reduced to the same base — e.g., 100 — and the relative frequencies can be directly compared among the groups — e.g., Table 2.3, with the data for males and females expressed in percentage form.

A common form of presentation of data is the fourfold table, in which each of two groups is distributed over a dichotomous scale of classification. The relative and total frequencies are usually included in the same table. Since each scale has only two categories, it is sufficient to quote the relative frequency in one category only. The relative frequency in the other category is its complement (difference from the base, e.g., 100) e.g., the percentages NOT HEALED are the differences of 67.2% and 86.7% from 100.0%. An example appears in Table 2.4.[4]

In this table, the relative frequencies were computed for each line, i.e., in a horizontal direction since periapical status occurred before healing. It would have been possible, also, to compute the relative frequencies in a vertical direction. For example, of the 67 healed cases, 41 or 61.2% originally had rarefaction, whereas of the 24 cases not healed, 20 or 83.3% originally had rarefaction. This vertical analysis of this table corresponds to a "retrospective" analysis and is not as convenient as the horizontal analysis, which is "prospective" in its approach. Of course, the words "vertical" and "horizontal" are relative, depending upon the way in which the table is constructed.

QUANTITATIVE SCALES

An example of a series of observations of a quantitative nature is given by the following 31 ascorbic acid levels (mg%) of the saliva of noncarious patients[5] : 0.20, 0.11, 0.31, 0.14, 0.19, 0.21, 0.33, 0.25,

0.22, 0.10, 0.28, 0.26, 0.24, 0.36, 0.28, 0.22, 0.37, 0.17, 0.10, 0.13, 0.15, 0.33, 0.31, 0.13, 0.29, 0.10, 0.12, 0.21, 0.08, 0.23, 0.26. (Ascorbic acid level is a continuous, quantitative scale, although the instrumentation distinguishes values to only two decimal places.)

Tabulating

The measurements are listed in order of magnitude from high to low, or low to high, to give an ungrouped frequency distribution, as in Table 2.5. If the total frequency were large enough (say, 50 or more), a regrouping could be superimposed on Table 2.5. Broader intervals of ascorbic acid level could be formed and all of the measurements within these broad intervals grouped together. This process is known as *grouping* or *seriation*. The number of intervals formed depends to a considerable extent on the total frequency. The number of intervals are usually between 8 and 15 (see Tables 2.6 and 2.7).

Ungrouped measurements on percentages of mercury in amalgam restorations are given in Table 2.6. The percentage of mercury in any given amalgam was obtained as a ratio of mercury to amalgam by volumetric analysis and multiplied by 100. Note, therefore, that the numbers in Table 2.6 are ratios that happen to be expressed in percentage form and have no relation to relative frequency percentages as defined previously. The range of measurements is from 28.6 to 61.0, and if intervals of 5% are chosen, the choice results in 8 intervals. The interval should start, preferably, at some multiple of 5, such as 25.0%. All measurements of 25.0 through 29.9 would thus fall in the first interval. Because the measurements are given to the nearest 0.1%, the first interval actually extends from 24.95 to 29.95, the next interval from 29.95 to 34.95, and so on. By counting up the number of measurements in the various intervals, one obtains Table 2.7.

TABLE 2.5
Ascorbic Acid Level to Nearest 0.01 (mg%) in Saliva of 31 Non-carious Patients in Order of Increasing Magnitude[a][5]

0.08	0.11	0.14	0.20	0.22	0.26	0.29	0.33
0.10	0.12	0.15	0.21	0.23	0.26	0.31	0.36
0.10	0.13	0.17	0.21	0.24	0.28	0.31	0.37
0.10	0.13	0.19	0.22	0.25	0.28	0.33	—

[a]The numbers in this table are mg of ascorbic acid per 100 ml of saliva — for convenience, usually referred to as mg%. There is no relation to relative frequency percentages as defined previously.

TABLE 2.6
Percentages of Mercury in 100 Randomly Selected Amalgam Restorations to the Nearest 0.1%[6]

50.2	49.8	54.9	49.6	43.2	49.3	51.0	40.4	36.3	48.4
51.3	43.1	53.8	50.1	48.3	49.9	49.9	38.5	37.9	45.1
49.0	50.5	47.9	50.5	47.5	29.7	41.4	56.0	43.4	41.3
51.1	52.4	46.2	57.7	41.6	52.1	47.7	57.1	38.5	32.4
61.0	42.7	51.3	49.1	37.3	32.7	44.4	48.1	38.7	35.2
44.1	51.3	52.4	47.4	42.0	39.3	51.9	37.1	35.0	37.2
42.6	56.8	53.6	47.7	47.1	47.2	48.2	40.5	34.1	33.5
44.6	56.1	49.4	46.7	54.5	34.2	51.6	34.2	43.5	37.3
39.7	58.8	51.5	41.6	49.7	50.7	43.8	31.2	28.6	40.4
40.9	53.9	44.9	46.9	57.7	47.5	39.5	35.5	41.3	45.4

Graphing

If the total frequency is so small that the measurements are retained in their ungrouped form, there is not much merit in attempting to graph these data. In the grouped frequency distribution with intervals of equal width, as in Table 2.7, the frequencies in the intervals are represented by rectangles standing on the appropriate intervals along the x-axis and of height equal to the corresponding frequency along the y-axis. The rectangles or bars, of course, are contiguous to emphasize the continuity of the scale. The height of the bar really stands for the frequency per interval of 5%, so that the area of the bar also represents the frequency in the interval. This type of graph is often called, accordingly, an *area graph* or *histogram*. The configuration of the graph quickly indicates the most commonly occurring mercury values, their range, and the relative importance of the various mercury levels. No real information will be lost if the bars of the

TABLE 2.7
Distribution of Mercury Percentage in 100 Randomly Selected Amalgam Restorations

% Mercury	Number of Restorations
24.95–29.95	2
29.95–34.95	7
34.95–39.95	15
39.95–44.95	21
44.95–49.95	26
49.95–54.95	21
54.95–59.95	7
59.95–64.95	1
Total	100

histogram are replaced by a line connecting the mid points of the tops of the bars. The graph is then referred to as a *frequency polygon* (Figure 2.2). This is especially useful if the graphs of two or more grouped frequency distributions are to be superimposed for purposes of comparison (Figure 2.2).

Figure 2.2 is typical of many of the graphs of quantitatively scaled frequency distributions occurring in dentistry. There is a single peak, with the peak frequencies occurring near the middle of the range of values tapering downward on either side. The configuration of the graph on one side of the peak approximately duplicates that on the other side. Such a graph is essentially *symmetrical*.

One other curve pattern often occurs with dental data: A asymmetrical curve with one peak. That is, the curve on one side or the other of the maximum height tapers downward but is stretched out over a wide range of values of the characteristic, whereas, on the other side, the curve falls rather abruptly, covering a smaller range of x values. Figures 2.3 and 2.4 are examples of the symmetrical and asymmetrical frequency distributions occurring with oral biological data.

One must realize that the graph of a frequency distribution, whether the scale is qualitative or quantitative, is an abstraction of

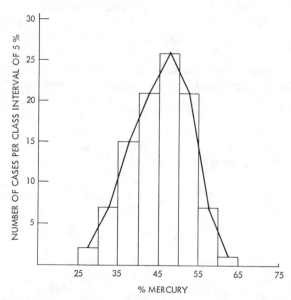

FIG. 2.2 Histogram and Frequency Polygon of Distribution of Mercury in 100 Amalgam Restorations.[6]

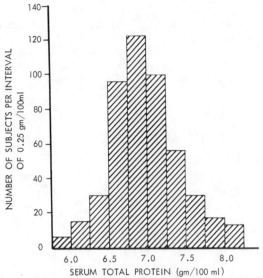

FIG. 2.3 Frequency Distribution for Serum Total Protein Values for 508 Subjects. [Shannon, I. L., and Terry, J. M.: SAM-TR-66-30, *USAF* Schl Aerospace Med, AFSC, Brooks AFB, Texas, March, 1966.]

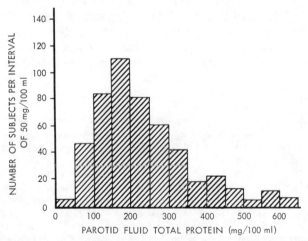

FIG. 2.4 Frequency Distribution for Parotid Fluid Total Protein Values for 508 Subjects. [Shannon, I. L., and Terry, J. M.: SAM-TR-66-30. *USAF* Schl Aerospace Med, AFSC, Brooks AFB, Texas, March, 1966.]

TABLE 2.8
Age Distribution of Dentofacial Injuries to U.S. Army Soldiers
Caused by Sports Accidents[7]

Age at Last Birthday	Number of Cases	Years in Class Interval	Number Cases per 1 Year of Age
17	2	1	2
18	9	1	9
19	17	1	17
20	18	1	18
21	15	1	15
22	14	1	14
23	10	1	10
24	6	1	6
25–29	28	5	5.6
30–39	12	10	1.2
Total	131		

the group of individuals observed. Presumably, each individual can be located on the graph within certain limits. The result is that one looks, in effect, at the total group of individuals at a glance, making all possible comparisons with respect to the characteristics of interest.

Graphing with Unequal Class Intervals.

In most frequency distributions in the dental literature, the size of the various classes is the same. Where the variable is age,* it may be important to make the graph depict the relatively higher frequency in certain age-groups — e.g., deaths caused by accidents or specific diseases. We, therefore, often find such data summarized by intervals of different sizes. When these classes are unequal in size, the fre-

---

*There are two methods which are widely used to record age: age at last birthday and age at nearest birthday. In the first method, the individual is recorded as being say, 19 years old until the very day of the twentieth anniversary of his birthday. In the second method, he is nineteen until the day following six months from the nineteenth anniversary. This latter method is the one usually employed by insurance companies, and is sometimes known as the *insurance age*. The former method is probably more widely used in an individual's statement of age. On the average, age at last birthday is half a year less than age at nearest birthday. The same method must be used consistently throughout the study, particularly in those where age may be related to other important data, e.g., DMF caries prevalence data which are age-related. Furthermore, particular care must be taken when studies in which age is recorded are being compared.

quencies must be expressed in the same basic unit before graphing or making any comparisons.

To illustrate, Table 2.8 presents data on dentofacial injuries to U.S. Army soldiers caused by sports accidents.[7] From the last column of the table where the frequencies are expressed per unit interval (year of age), one may see that there were fewer cases per year of age in the age span 25-29 years, than in any age group 18 and over, and that the span 30-39 had the least number of soldiers per year of age injured of all the age groups. This conveys a different story than that shown by the original frequency appearing in the second column.

The height of the bars in the graph (Figure 2.5) represents the number of soldiers per year of age and the width of the bars represents the number of years in each interval. The area of each rectangle,

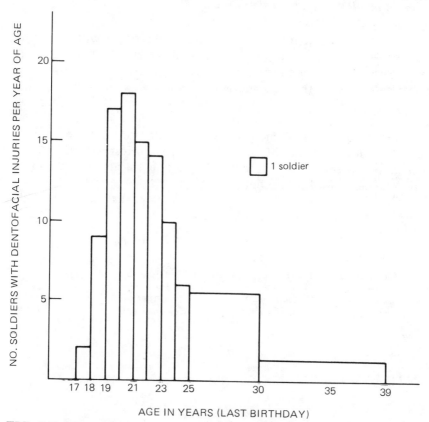

FIG. 2.5 Histogram of the Age Distribution of 131 Soldiers With Dentofacial Injuries Due to Sports Accidents.[7]

therefore, represents the total frequency over the interval. Thus, the area of the bar for the 5-year interval of 25-29 years is 5.6 soldiers per year × 5 years = 28 soldiers and, in the 30-39 years interval, the number of soldiers is 1.2 × 10 = 12. By constructing the graph in this manner, one obtains the same general picture as if the same number of years of age had been maintained for all intervals. If the bars in Figure 2.5 had been constructed without paying attention to the different sizes of the class intervals, the figure would have masked the fact that the older soldiers had experienced less dentofacial injuries from sports accidents than did the younger ones. This area concept is often clarified by including a box of convenient size to denote a unit of area.

Graphing with Discrete Scale

Table 2.9 is an example of a frequency distribution with a discrete quantitative scale. It is customary to graph a distribution of this type as a series of separated (to emphasize the discreteness of the scale) vertical lines with the characteristic on the x-axis and the frequency on the y-axis (Fig. 2.6). When there is a very large difference between the values which would cause the graph to be quite stretched out and awkward looking, the scale and bar(s) can be truncated by making a break in both the line of the scale and the corresponding bar(s) in the graph, as shown in Figure 2.6. This graph is J-shaped, and is thus an extreme example of asymmetry.

Occasionally, distributions have several peaks, i.e., a bimodal curve, as shown in Figure 2.7.

TABLE 2.9
729 Children, Ages 5-18, by Number of Carious Teeth[8]

Number of Carious Teeth	Number of Children	Number of Carious Teeth	Number of Children
0	191	9	16
1	105	10	13
2	99	11	9
3	62	12	3
4	71	13	2
5	57	14	0
6	43	15	2
7	39	16	0
8	17	*Total* (0 to 16)	729

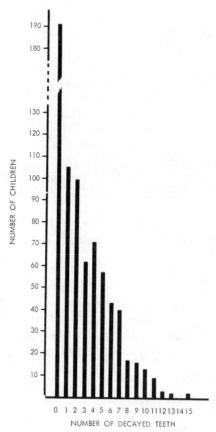

NUMBER OF CHILDREN

NUMBER OF DECAYED TEETH

FIG. 2.6 Distribution of 729 Children According to Number of Decayed Teeth as Seen Without Bitewing Radiographic Examination.[8]

QUANTITATIVE SCALES

Summarizing Data According to Location and Dispersion

Various ways are available to summarize a frequency distribution with a quantitative scale of classification. The preferred method for a given distribution will depend on certain describable features of the data.

If the measurements are in grouped form, the simplest method of summarizing is to convert the original frequency distribution to percentage form, as with qualitative scales. Some other summary form is often chosen, however, because it conveys the same amount

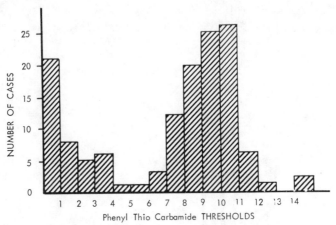

FIG. 2.7 Distribution of PTC Threshold. [Chung, C.S., *et al.:* **Arch Oral Biol 10:645, 1965.]**

of information more concisely and may be more amenable to further analysis and inference. The summary constants utilized fall into two broad categories: (1) constants or measures of location (mean, median, quartiles, percentiles, mode); and (2) constants or measures of dispersion (range, interquartile range, variance, standard deviation).

Measurements of Location

Mean

The arithmetic mean or average of the observed measurements of a group of individuals is simply the sum of the individual measurements divided by the number of measurements. In symbols, if there are N individuals in the group and if the N individuals have, respectively, measurements $x_1, x_2, \ldots x_N$, then the mean of the N measurements is $\dfrac{x_1 + x_2 + \ldots + x_N}{N}$, and is usually written as

$\bar{x} = \sum\limits_{i=1}^{N} x_i \Big/ N$, where $\bar{x}$ (pronounced x bar) is the symbol for the arithmetic mean, Σ is the capital Greek letter sigma, denoting "the sum

of," and $\sum\limits_{i=1}^{N} x_i$ means the sum of all the values of x from x_1 to x_N.

Usually the range of summation is clear, so that the subscripts may be eliminated and the formula may be given simply as $\bar{x} = \Sigma x/N$.

The mean of the data of ascorbic acid salivary levels of Table 2.5 is

$$\bar{x} = \frac{\Sigma x}{\sqrt{N}} = \frac{6.68}{31} = 0.215 \text{ mg\%}.$$

The mean may be carried to one or two more decimal places than the data from which it was obtained, although it is often difficult to interpret more than the number of significant figures originally presented.

Computing the mean of a grouped distribution may seem different, but the principle is the same. It is assumed that the midpoint of each class interval is the average of the readings in each interval. The midpoint of a class interval (known as the class mean) is calculated by taking ½ of the total width and adding it to the beginning of the interval. Alternatively, the midpoint is ½ the sum of the beginning and end values. The sum of the measurements of the individuals within the interval is the number of individuals in the interval multiplied by the midpoint. The addition of these products over all the k intervals is the sum of all N measurements. In symbol form,

$$\bar{x} = \frac{\displaystyle\sum_{i=1}^{k} f_i x_i}{\Sigma f_i} = \frac{\Sigma fx}{N},$$

where f_i = the partial frequency, x_i = the midpoint of the class interval, Σ = the sum over all the class intervals, and N = the total frequency.

The observations of mercury content of amalgam fillings listed in Table 2.6 were initially made to the nearest 0.1, so that the first group in Table 2.7 really includes observations between 24.95 and 29.95, giving a midpoint of 27.45. The subsequent midpoints are 32.45, 37.45. . . .

The data of Table 2.7 are repeated in Table 2.10, which shows the class intervals, the midpoints (x), frequencies (f), and sum of the measurements in each interval (fx). This latter column is needed for the computation of the arithmetic mean as indicated at the bottom of the table.

The mean is most useful as a summary constant when the dis-

Design and Analysis in Dental and Oral Research

TABLE 2.10
Computation of Mean of Data on Mercury Content of Amalgam
Restorations in Table 2.7.

Class Interval	Midpoint x	Frequency f	fx
24.95-29.95	27.45	2	54.90
29.95-34.95	32.45	7	227.15
34.95-39.95	37.45	15	561.75
39.95-44.95	42.45	21	891.45
44.95-49.95	47.45	26	1,233.70
49.95-54.95	52.45	21	1,101.45
54.95-59.95	57.45	7	402.15
59.95-64.95	62.45	1	62.45
Total		100	4,535.00

$$\bar{x} = \frac{\Sigma fx}{N} = \frac{4,535.00}{100} = 45.35\% \text{ Hg}$$

tribution is symmetrical or balanced. It serves as the representative
or typical value of the distribution, and the spread of values below
and above it is about equal with values closer to the mean occurring
relatively more often. If the distribution is asymmetrical, a few extreme measurements can influence the mean unduly, so that it is not
as meaningful a summary constant as it is with symmetry.

Median

The median is the measurement that subdivides the series, when arranged in order of magnitude, into halves. The data of ascorbic acid
salivary levels in Table 2.5 have been arranged in order of increasing
magnitude. Since there are 31 measurements in this series, the 16th
measurement would have 15 lower and 15 higher measurements.
This 16th measurement is 0.22 mg%, which is the median value,
symbolically denoted as Q_2 = 0.22 mg%. If the highest value in the
series, 0.37, were discarded, leaving only 30 measurements, the
median, Q_2, would fall half-way between the 15th (0.21) and the
16th measurement (0.22), and we would state that Q_2 is the mean
of the two, i.e., Q_2 = 0.215 mg%.

The median of the grouped distribution of mercury content of
100 selected amalgam restorations in Table 2.10 is the %Hg value,
below which there are 50 patients. There are 2 + 7 + 15 + 21 = 45 individuals who have values less than 44.95. There are 26 individuals
who have values occurring between 44.95 and 49.95. Five of them

are below the median, which will be, therefore, by linear interpolation, 5/26 of the way from 44.95 to 49.95, i.e.,

$Q_2 = 44.95 + \dfrac{50 - 45}{26} (5.00) = 45.91$. Note that the mean, $\bar{x} = $ 45.35%, showing the symmetry of the distribution.

The median is most apt to be used as a summary constant of location for asymmetric distributions. Regardless of the configuration of the frequency distribution, it has the interpretation that half of the total group have values less than the median value, and the other half of the group have values greater than the median. When the distribution is symmetrical, the median and the mean have the same value, but in that case the mean is usually chosen as the more meaningful centering constant.

Often, the scale of classification of an asymmetric distribution can be arithmetically manipulated or transformed, resulting in a more symmetrical distribution, which can be summarized by a mean in terms of the new scale — e.g., logarithmic, square root, and so forth. Logarithmic transformations are often used in bacterial counts (see Table 7.24).

Quartiles, Percentiles

The first quartile (Q_1) is that value of the characteristic such that 25% of the individuals have measurements less than Q_1, and 75% have measurements above Q_1 value; 75% of the frequency distribution lie below the third quartile (Q_3) and 25% above. The median is actually the second quartile, Q_2. The values of Q_1 and Q_3 are calculated in the same manner as those of Q_2. In Table 2.5, $Q_1 = 0.13$ and $Q_2 = 0.28$ mg% ascorbic acid.

In a very large series of measurements, the series could be subdivided into 100 groups, each with equal frequency, by calculating the percentiles. The first percentile is the value such that 1% of the individuals have readings below it, and 99% have readings above it. The 90th percentile has 90% of the readings below, and 10% above, etc. There are 99 percentiles.

Cumulative Frequency Distribution

When we wish to calculate the median and quartile values from a grouped distribution, we find it helpful to rearrange the original frequencies to form a *cumulative frequency distribution*. In the data on the percentage of mercury in 100 amalgam fillings (Table 2.10), we find that there are 2 cases (f = 2) between 24.95% and 29.95% mercury. Thus, the two cases in the first group have a percentage of mercury less than 29.95%. In the second group, seven cases have between 29.95% and 34.95% mercury, so that these seven amalgams contain less than 34.95% mercury. In addition, the two cases in the first group also contain less than 34.95% mercury so that there are 2 + 7 = 9 amalgams with less than 34.95% mercury. Similarly, 2 + 7 + 15 = 24 cases have less than 39.95% mercury. Finally, all 100 amalgams contain less than 64.95% mercury. Since the total number of cases is 100, these cumulative frequencies are also the cumulative percentages, as shown in Table 2.11.

The median can be obtained easily by interpolating in the last column of Table 2.14 for 50%. Similarly, the Q_1 and Q_3 values can be obtained by interpolating for 25% and 75%, respectively. A graph can be constructed by plotting the cumulative percentages of the last column against the respective end points of the second column. The typical sigmoid curve, going from 0% to 100%, is depicted in Figure 2.8. From this graph, the median and quartiles can readily be estimated graphically as shown.

Such sigmoid curves are frequently seen in lethal (or effective) dose studies, in which the variable represents the lethal, or effective, dose of some drug. The median would then be called the *median lethal dose*, LD50, or *median effective dose*, ED50. These sigmoid curves are examples of cumulative distributions.

Mode

While the arithmetic mean ($\bar{x}$) and the median (Q_2) are very useful values, the clinician examining patients may find the mode (or modal

TABLE 2.11

Cumulative Frequency of 100 Amalgams According to Percentage of Mercury Contained

Class Interval %	Frequency f	Cumulative Frequency	
		Number	%
24.95–29.95	2	2	2.0
29.95–34.95	7	9	9.0
34.95–39.95	15	24	24.0
39.95–44.95	21	45	45.0
44.95–49.95	26	71	71.0
49.95–54.95	21	92	92.0
54.95–59.95	7	99	99.0
59.95–64.95	1	100	100.0
Total	100		

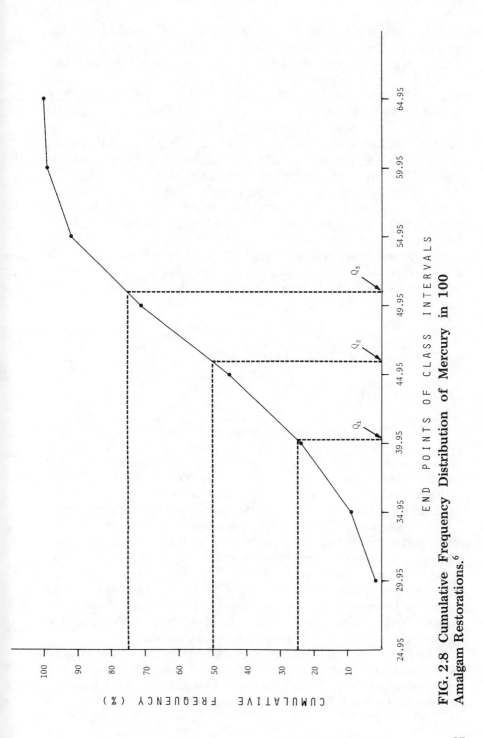

FIG. 2.8 Cumulative Frequency Distribution of Mercury in 100 Amalgam Restorations.[6]

class) of more use to him in markedly unbalanced distributions. For example, in Table 2.9 the mode is 0 decayed teeth, i.e., the value at which the greatest number of children appear. The mean was found to be 3.8 decayed teeth. While this latter number may be of some importance theoretically, the clinician examining the 729 children might be more interested in knowing that the largest number of children he sees in this survey have no carious teeth. In other words, the clinician is often interested in the most frequently occurring value (or class), rather than in any central tendency. While the mode was readily obtained in the preceding example, where the scale was discrete, it is not so readily estimated when the variable is continuous. In such cases, in fact, one must speak of a modal class. Unfortunately, this class is dependent on the particular grouping of the raw data employed. Sometimes the intervals are made unequal in size, and the modal class can then be misleading. The concept of the mode is also of value in describing those distributions that are largely "clumped" into two or more classes, in which case the distribution may be termed a "bimodal," "trimodal," . . . distribution.

Measurements of Variation and Dispersion

Range

Not only is a centering constant employed in summarizing quantitative data, but some idea of the variation or spread of these readings should also be included. In the salivary ascorbic acid values, Table 2.5, the values range in magnitude from 0.08 to 0.37 mg%. The simplest method of measuring the variation would be to find the difference between the highest and lowest readings, in this case, 0.37 - 0.08 = 0.29 mg%, known as the *range*. The difficulty with the range is that it depends on only two outlying values. An additional reading may increase the range tremendously, if this reading is an extreme value. In general, few readings tend to give a small range, many readings a large range. One often finds the "normal range" of a physiologic variable quoted, and is entitled to ask on how many individuals this range is based. For these reasons, the range should seldom be used by itself as a description of variation.

The range from the first to the third quartiles ($Q_3 - Q_1$) is called the *interquartile range* and includes 50% of the cases regardless of the shape of the frequency distribution. It is most apt to be used as a measure of dispersion in asymmetric distributions.

Variance and Standard Deviation

The most useful measurement of dispersion, practically and theoretically, is the *variance* and its square root, the *standard deviation*. In an
ungrouped series (as in Table 2.5), each measurement is first established as a deviation from the mean ($\bar{x} = 0.215$). The number of decimals in the deviations should correspond to the number maintained
in the mean. Those values of x below the mean give negative, and
those above the mean positive, deviations. In any series, these deviations add up to zero, except for errors due to rounding off, $\Sigma(x - \bar{x})$
$= 0$. There is, thus, one restriction on the N values of $(x - \bar{x})$, namely,
that they add to zero. The individual deviations are then squared and
added. The *variance* (s^2) of the sample of measurements is then defined as this sum divided by 1 less than the number of measurements,
i.e.,

$$s^2 = \frac{\Sigma(x - \bar{x})^2}{N - 1}.$$

This divisor (N – 1) is called the number of *degrees of freedom* of
the variance. It is equal to the number of deviations (N) less the number of restrictions (here, one). The older practice was to divide by N.
When the number of observations is large, the difference between the
values obtained by using (N – 1) or N is minor. For a number of theoretical reasons, it is preferable, however, to calculate s^2 using the
number of degrees of freedom in the denominator.

The square root of the variance of the sample is the *standard
deviation*, usually denoted by s. The standard deviation of the sample
is occasionally referred to as SD, and in many older texts as σ (lower
case Greek letter sigma). Specifically, the formula for an ungrouped
series may be written as:

$$s = \sqrt{\frac{\Sigma(x - \bar{x})^2}{N - 1}}.$$

The standard deviation should maintain at least as many decimals as
the mean. Thus, the variance and standard deviation for the 31 measurements of ascorbic acid in saliva can be calculated as in Table
2.12.

The variance and standard deviation measure variation of individual measurements from the mean, as one can see from the fact that
they are based on individual deviations from the mean. If there is

TABLE 2.12
Calculation of Variance, s^2, and Standard Deviations,[a] s, of Salivary
Ascorbic Acid Level (mg%) of 31 Noncarious Patients

		$(\bar{x} = 0.215)$	
x	$(x - \bar{x})$		$(x - \bar{x})^2$
0.20	−0.015		0.000225
0.11	−0.105		0.011025
0.31	+0.095		0.009025
0.14	−0.075		0.005625
0.19	−0.025		0.000625
0.21	−0.005		0.000025
0.33	+0.115		0.013225
0.25	+0.035		0.001225
0.22	+0.005		0.000025
0.10	−0.115		0.013225
0.28	+0.065		0.004225
0.26	+0.045		0.002025
0.24	+0.025		0.001625
0.36	+0.145		0.021025
0.28	+0.065		0.004225
0.22	+0.005		0.000025
0.37	+0.155		0.024025
0.17	−0.045		0.002025
0.10	−0.115		0.013225
0.13	−0.085		0.007225
0.15	−0.065		0.004225
0.33	+0.115		0.013225
0.31	+0.095		0.009025
0.13	−0.085		0.007225
0.29	+0.075		0.005625
0.10	−0.115		0.013225
0.12	−0.095		0.009025
0.21	−0.005		0.000025
0.08	−0.135		0.018225
0.23	+0.015		0.000225
0.26	+0.045		0.002025
Total 6.68 = Σx	+0.015 = $\Sigma(x - \bar{x})$		0.214975 = $\Sigma(x - \bar{x})^2$

$$s^2 = \frac{\Sigma(x - \bar{x})^2}{N - 1} = \frac{0.214975}{30} = 0.007166$$

$$s = \sqrt{0.007166} = 0.085 \text{ mg\%}$$

[a]Note that the method of calculating the standard deviation usually employed utilizes short-cut algebraically-derived formulas, which eliminate the necessity of carrying as many decimals as shown above.

much variation, there will be many large values of $(x - \bar{x})$, so that $\Sigma(x - \bar{x})^2$, which is often called the *Sum of Squares* (SS), will be large, and s^2 and s will be large also. Conversely, if there is little variation, s^2 and s will usually be small.

One often sees a mean written as a certain figure plus or minus ($\pm$) a certain amount. Thus, with the salivary ascorbic acid data, the average for 31 noncarious patients may be listed as 0.215 ± 0.085 mg%. In this case, the figure after the $\pm$ sign refers to the standard deviation of the measurements and denotes that approximately ⅔ of the individuals measured do not deviate more than 0.085 mg% from the average (as in Chapter 3). Unfortunately, this designation of the $\pm$ sign can also refer to the maximum deviation made, such as ½ the range.* Occasionally the $\pm$ refers to the standard deviation of the mean, also known as the standard error of the mean to refer to the stability of the mean. To eliminate confusion, it is preferable to avoid the $\pm$ designation completely. If it is used, it should be labeled as to its meaning.

The computations for the standard deviation of a grouped distribution (mercury content of amalgams) are set out in Table 2.13, which is similar to Table 2.11 except that four extra columns have been added to it. The last three columns present the values for the deviation from the mean $(x - \bar{x})$, the square of each deviation $(x - \bar{x})^2$, and the product of the squared deviation by the frequency (f) in the interval, $f(x - \bar{x})^2$. Each deviation occurs f times. The sum of the values of $f(x - \bar{x})^2$ is calculated and is then divided by $(N - 1)$ to obtain the variance. Thus,

$$s^2 = \frac{\Sigma f(x - \bar{x})^2}{N - 1} = \frac{5,409.0000}{.99} = 54.6364.$$

The standard deviation is then

$$s = \sqrt{54.6364} = 7.39\%Hg.$$

The variance, calculated in the case of grouped data by using the midpoint of each class interval, usually tends to be slightly inflated in comparison with the variance computed from the same data in ungrouped form (52.0050%Hg). This inflation can be corrected by the use of *Sheppard's Adjustment*, which, for the usual type of distribution, consists of subtracting 1/12 the square of the class interval

---

*Sometimes $\pm$ refers to the deviation exceeded no more than 50% of the time, the so-called *Probable Error* (PE, which is 0.6745s).

TABLE 2.13
Computation of Mean and Standard Deviation of Data on Mercury
Content of Amalgam Restorations in Table 2.9

Class Interval	Mid-point (x)	Freq (f)	fx	(x − x̄)	(x − x̄)²	f(x − x̄)²
24.95–29.95	27.45	2	54.90	−17.90	320.4100	640.8200
29.95–34.95	32.45	7	227.15	−12.90	166.4100	1,164.8700
34.95–39.95	37.45	15	561.75	− 7.90	62.4100	936.1500
39.95–44.95	42.45	21	891.45	− 2.90	8.4100	176.6100
44.95–49.95	47.25	26	1,233.70	+ 2.10	4.4100	144.6600
49.95–54.95	52.45	21	1,101.45	+ 7.10	50.4100	1,058.6100
54.95–59.95	57.45	7	402.15	+12.10	146.4100	1,024.8700
59.95–64.95	62.45	1	62.45	+17.10	292.4100	292.4100
Total		100	4,535.00			5,409.0000

$$\bar{x} = \frac{\Sigma fx}{N} = \frac{4,535.00}{100} = 45.35\%Hg$$

$$s = \sqrt{\frac{\Sigma f(x - \bar{x})^2}{N - 1}} = \sqrt{\frac{5,409.0000}{99}} = \sqrt{54.6364} = 7.39\%$$

from the variance. On Table 2.13 the adjustment is $(5)^2/12 = 2.0833$,
making the adjusted variance

$$\text{adj. } s^2 = 54.6364 - 2.0833 = 52.5531$$
$$\text{and adj. } s = \sqrt{52.5531} = 7.25\%Hg.$$

Shortcut Procedures

The methods just presented follow the basic definitions of the mean,
variance, and standard deviation. The constants usually are calculated
by shortcut procedures, however, to reduce the arithmetic effort and
to avoid the errors resulting from the rounding off of the decimals.
The sum of the squared deviations $\Sigma(x - \bar{x})^2$, is often called the sum
of squares (SS) or, more completely, the sum of squares around the
mean, or the corrected sum of squares. Instead of calculating the sum
of squares as $\Sigma(x - \bar{x})^2$, an algebraically equivalent formula is usually
employed. One of the most convenient is

$$\Sigma(x - \bar{x})^2 = \left[\Sigma x^2 - \frac{(\Sigma x)^2}{N}\right].$$

Thus, in the case of the ungrouped ascorbic acid data,

$$\Sigma x^2 - \frac{(\Sigma x)^2}{N} = 1.6544 - \frac{44.6224}{31} = 0.214968,$$

as compared to 0.214975 obtained originally from the defining formula. In the case of grouped data,

$$SS = \Sigma f(x - \bar{x})^2 = \left[\Sigma fx^2 - \frac{(\Sigma fx)^2}{N}\right] = 211,071.25 - \frac{20,566.225}{100}$$

$$= 5,409.0000,$$

which is the same value obtained from the defining formula. The correction for the mean, $\frac{(\Sigma x)^2}{N}$, or, with grouped data, $\frac{(\Sigma fx)^2}{N}$, is often called the *Correction Term* (CT).

In addition, the use in conjunction with this formula of a short-cut method known as *coding* eases the labor even more. Unless the investigator is familiar with the methods illustrated thus far, he should not attempt to utilize short-cut procedures. In coding grouped data, working or coded units are substituted for actual midpoints of class intervals. Thus, the midpoint of a class interval somewhere near the center of the overall distribution can be selected as the origin, or 0. In the case of the mercury data in Table 2.14, 47.45, the midpoint of the interval 44.95–49.95, is chosen. In this manner, 52.45, the

TABLE 2.14
Computation Using Working Units of Percentage Mercury in 100 Amalgam Restorations

| Class Interval | Midpoints | | | | |
	Original Units (x)	Working Units (u)	f	fu	f(u)²
24.95–29.95	27.45	−4	2	− 8	32
29.95–34.95	32.45	−3	7	−21	63
34.95–39.95	37.45	−2	15	−30	60
39.95–44.95	42.45	−1	21	−21	21
44.95–49.95	47.45	0	26	0	0
49.95–54.95	52.45	+1	21	+21	21
54.95–59.95	57.45	+2	7	+14	28
59.95–64.95	62.45	+3	1	+ 3	9
Total				42	234

next midpoint, becomes +1, 57.45 becomes +2, 62.45 becomes +3, and 42.45 becomes -1, 37.45 becomes -2, etc. The use of these working units amounts to using a new variable, u, which represents a linear transformation of the original variable, x. For example,

$$u = (x - a)/b, \text{ where } a = 47.45 \text{ and } b = 5.$$

Using these coded midpoints, u, a computational table can be constructed as in Table 2.14.

The mean can be calculated in working units as:

$$\bar{u} = \frac{\Sigma fu}{N} = \frac{-42}{100} = -0.4200,$$

and the variance and standard deviation as:

$$s_u^2 = \frac{1}{(N-1)} \left[\Sigma fu^2 - \frac{(\Sigma fu)^2}{N} \right] = \frac{1}{99} \left[234 - \frac{(-42)^2}{100} \right] = 2.1855$$

and

$$s_u^2 = \sqrt{2.1855} = 1.4785.$$

u, s_u^2 and s_u must then be translated back into the original units. The mean in working units is -0.42 — that is, 0.42 units below the origin point, which is actually 47.45. Each working unit is equal to 5 original units, so that the real mean must be

$$\bar{x} = a + b\bar{u} = 47.45 - 5(0.42) = 45.35\%.$$

The standard deviation is not affected by subtracting a constant as a, but only by a change of the unit of measurement. Thus,

$$s_x^2 = b^2 s_u^2 \text{ and } s_x = bs_u.$$

To obtain the real variance and standard deviation, the values in working units are multiplied by $(5)^2$ and by 5 respectively — i.e., $s^2 = (5)^2 s_u^2 = (5)^2 (2.1855) = 54.6375$, — and the standard deviation is $5(1.4785) = 7.3925\%$.

Many preprogrammed pocket calculators have the capability of providing values for $\bar{x}$ and s for ungrouped data. These calculators utilize arithmetic shortcuts as described above and the various values, such as Σx, Σx^2, Σy, Σy^2, Σxy, etc., can readily be obtained from memory. Of course, programmable models, such as the Texas Instruments 59, or the very powerful Hewlett Packard 41C, have far more capabilities. Unfortunately, most pocket calculators do not have a built-in program for calculating $\bar{x}$ and s from grouped data.

Coefficient of Variation

One other characteristic of a distribution used in dental research warrants mention here. This is the coefficient of variation or variability (CV), which has been used in anthropometric studies in orthodontics. The CV is the standard deviation divided by the mean, and it is expressed in percentage form. This number thus expresses the variability of measurements in terms of its average, thereby conveying the idea of relative variability. It is a pure number and does not depend on the dimensions used in measurement.

The CV is often used as an indication of the reliability of different indices, so that the investigator would generally prefer to use characteristics that have a lower CV. Thus, in Table 2.15, the measurements of mesiodistal diameter of specific teeth for a group of individuals can be expressed in terms of the range of measurements, mean, standard deviation, and coefficient of variation.[9] The first three are expressed in mm in this example, but the CV is a pure measurement in percentage form. This again serves to point out the usefulness of the CV in anthropometry, since the specific variability

TABLE 2.15
Mesiodistal Diameters of Individual Teeth[a]

	Range (mm)	Mean (mm)	Stand. Dev. (mm)	Coef Var (%)
Upper Teeth				
Central incisor	5.5–11.0	8.91	0.65	7.30
Lateral incisor	3.5– 9.5	7.08	0.64	9.04
Cuspid	6.0–11.0	8.00	0.60	7.50
First bicuspid	6.0– 9.5	7.27	0.50	6.88
Second bicuspid	5.5–10.5	7.14	0.60	8.40
First molar	8.5–13.0	10.98	0.68	6.19
Lower Teeth				
Central incisor	4.5–10.0	5.67	0.48	8.47
Lateral incisor	5.0– 8.5	6.28	0.48	7.64
Cuspid	5.5– 9.0	7.12	0.55	7.72
First bicuspid	5.5– 9.0	7.36	0.52	7.07
Second Bicuspid	5.5–11.5	7.50	0.63	8.40
First molar	7.0–13.0	11.17	0.68	6.09

does not depend on the dimensions employed. As Brodie has stated, the CV "represents ranges of weight, length, rate, capacity and temperature, totally unlike things, yet reveals that oral temperature (CV = 0.49%) would be 100 times more reliable than would weight of the spleen (CV = 50.58%)."[10]

It appears, from Table 2.15, that the mesiodistal diameter measurements of the first molars exhibit the least relative variability for the data in question, in spite of having the maximum standard deviation.

REFERENCES

1. Brekhus, P. J.: Dental disease and its relation to the loss of human teeth, J Amer Dent Ass 16:2237, 1929.

2. Huff, D.: How to Lie with Statistics, New York, Norton, 1954.

3. Myers, J. H.: Statistical Presentation, Totowa (N.J.), Littlefield, 1950.

4. Bender, I. B., Seltzer, S., and Turkenkopf, S.: To culture or not to culture, Oral Surg 18:527, 1964.

5. Hess, W. C., and Smith, B. T.: The ascorbic acid content of the saliva of carious and non-carious individuals, J Dent Res 25:507, 1949.

6. Phillips, R. W., and Swartz, H. L.: Mercury analysis of one hundred amalgam restorations, J Dent Res 28:569, 1949.

7. Katz, R. V., Barnes, G. P., Larson, H. R., Lyon, T. C., and Brunner, D. G.: Epidemiologic survey of accidental dentofacial injuries among U.S. Army personnel, Community Dent Oral Epidemiol 7:30, 1979.

8. Chilton, N. W., and Greenwald, L. E.: Studies in dental public health administration. 2. The role of roentgenograms in public health dental surveys, J Dent Res 26:129, 1947.

9. Ballard, M. L.: Asymmetry in tooth size. A factor in the etiology diagnosis and treatment of malocclusion. Angle Orthodont 14:67, 1944.

10. Brodie, A. G.: Facial patterns, Angle Orthodont 16:75, 1946.

3

The Normal Curve

One mathematical curve is so basic to dental research and analysis that all workers should know its characteristics. It is known by several names — *bell-shaped, Gaussian, normal;*[1] here it will be called the *normal curve*. Many distributions of measurements resemble normal curves. Furthermore, the normal curve plays a central role in the description of chance variation of summary constants computed from samples, such as means and relative frequencies.

The normal curve, completely defined by the mean, μ, and the standard deviation, σ, is regarded as representing the distribution of a universe of measurements. Hence to represent its parameters (true mean and true standard deviation) we shall require symbols different from those used to describe the estimate of these parameters, $\bar{x}$ and s, derived from a sample of N measurements, as used in Chapter 2. An example of a normal curve with $\mu = 45$ and $\sigma = 2$, is given in Figure 3.1.

The normal curve is a symmetrical, one-peaked (unimodal) distribution. The peak occurs immediately above the mean, which, by virtue of symmetry is also the median, Q_2. The two points at which the curve changes from convex to concave upward (the points of inflection) are directly above the x values equal to $\mu - \sigma$ and to $\mu + \sigma$. Any number on the x-axis has a corresponding value on the y-axis, so that theoretically the curve extends over all values of x from $-\infty$ to $+\infty$. Practically speaking, however, the curve covers a range of x values extending from 3 standard deviations below the mean to 3 standard deviations above the mean. Thus, in Figure 3.1 the practical range is from 39 to 51, a total of 6 standard deviations. If the total area under the curve between the configuration is thought of as equal to 100%, then for any normal curve 68.26% of the total area occurs

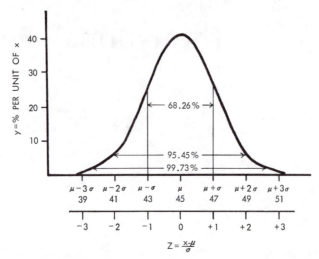

FIG. 3.1 Normal Curve With Mean = 45 and Standard Deviation = 2.

over the range of x values from $\mu - \sigma$ to $\mu + \sigma$. In other words, 68.26% of the area occurs within one standard deviation (σ) of the mean (μ); 95.45% of the area occurs within 2σ of μ and 99.73% within 3σ. Since 50% of the area of a normal curve occurs within 0.6745σ of μ, the first quartile, $Q_1 = \mu - 0.6745\sigma$ and Q_3, the third quartile $= \mu + 0.6745\sigma$ for any normal curve.

The actual shape of the normal curve is standardized, but the scale of plotting the graph will determine how high the peak is or how spread out the base is. Figure 3.2 depicts two normal curves, one with a higher peak and the other with a broader base. Both these curves have the same area and the same mean, but the one with the higher peak has a standard deviation one half that with the broader base. The one with half the standard deviation will have to rise twice as high in order to include the same percentage of the total area or total frequency under the curve. In this way, it will have the same percentage of the area included within 1, 2 or 3 standard deviations of the mean, a characteristic of every normal curve.

The normal curve with a certain μ and σ can be changed to the standard or so-called unit normal curve, whose mean is zero and whose standard deviation is one, by transforming the scale of x. If the measurements, x, are expressed as deviations from μ and these deviations are divided by σ, the resulting new or transformed measurements $(x - \mu)/\sigma$ will have a mean of zero and a standard deviation of one. This new measurement will be denoted by z, so that $z = (x - \mu)/\sigma$; z represents the deviation from the mean in standard deviational

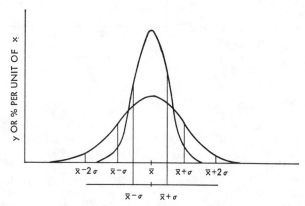

FIG. 3.2 Two Normal Curves, One Having Twice the Standard Deviation of the Other.

units and is often called the *relative deviate* or the *normal deviate*. The values of z are given in Table 3.1. The table of areas of the normal curve, when viewed with respect to the scale of z, becomes the standard normal distribution. The advantage of using z instead of x is that all normal curves with their various μ's and σ's are transformed into the same normal curve. As a result, a single table will suffice to give the areas of the normal curve. Table 3.1 presents, for some z values, the fraction of the total area under the normal curve between $-z$ and $+z$.

To find the portion of the area between the x values 42 and 48 of Figure 3.1, the values of 42 and 48 should be reduced to the corresponding z values: 42 is equivalent to $z = (42 - 45)/2 = -1.5$ and 48 is equivalent to $z = (48 - 45)/2 = +1.5$. Table 3.1 states that $1 - P = 86.64\%$ of the total area under the curve occurs between $z = -1.5$ and $z = +1.5$. This means that 86.45% of the total area occurs between x = 42 and x = 48.

The normal curve is a theoretical curve of great importance in statistical analysis. The exact shape of the normal curve is, in actuality, never duplicated by an observed distribution of measurements. This curve, however, is a good description of many biological distributions so that its properties are invaluable in analyzing these distributions.

The distribution of the ages (last birthday) at which 663 men became edentulous in one or both jaws as recorded at a university dental clinic[2] is given in Table 3.2 and its histogram in Figure 3.3. The mean of the distribution is 45.4 years and the median 45.3 years. The modal class is 40–49, so that the three centering con-

TABLE 3.1
Short Table of Areas (Total Area Under the Normal Curve is 100%)
of the Normal Curve

z	1 – P	z	1 – P	z	1 – P	z	1 – P
0.0	00.00	1.0	68.27	2.0	95.45	3.0	99.73
0.1	07.97	1.1	72.87	2.1	96.43	3.1	99.81
0.2	15.85	1.2	76.99	2.2	97.22	3.2	99.86
0.3	23.58	1.3	80.64	2.3	97.86	3.3	99.90
0.4	31.08	1.4	83.85	2.32	98.00	3.4	99.93
				2.4	98.36		
0.5	38.29	1.5	86.64	2.5	98.36	3.5	99.95
0.6	45.15	1.6	89.04	2.58	98.76	3.6	99.97
0.6745	50.00	1.7	91.09	2.6	99.00	3.7	99.98
0.7	51.61	1.8	92.81	2.7	99.31	3.8	99.99
0.8	57.63	1.9	94.26	2.8	99.49	3.9	99.99
0.9	63.19	1.96	95.00	2.9	99.63		

z = relative deviate or normal deviate, the deviation from the mean
   expressed in standard deviational units.
1 – P = area under the normal curve between –z and +z.
      = probability according to the normal curve of obtaining
      a smaller deviation.
P = area under the normal curve beyond ±z.
  = probability according to the normal curve of obtaining
  an equal or greater deviation.*

*Strictly speaking, the wording *equal or greater* is not quite correct when dealing with a continuous scale, instead, the expressions *greater than* or *less than* should be used, whichever the case may require. When the normal curve is used to approximate a discontinuous distribution, e.g., binomial, then *equal to or greater* would be the correct wording.

stants are very similar, a situation existing in one-peaked, symmetrical distributions. The standard deviation of the distribution (s) is 10.9 years. Taking $\bar{x}$ and s of the distribution as μ and σ, respectively, and 633 as the total area, a normal curve has been superimposed on the histogram. For this purpose, a table of ordinates for the standard normal curve was used.[3]

When a histogram of a distribution resembles a normal curve, the frequency distribution is said to be approximately normally distributed. The mean and standard deviation then afford a very convenient summary of the data. While the frequency distribution of Table 3.2 resembles a normal curve, variations exist between the actual frequencies included within $\bar{x} \pm 1s$, $\bar{x} \pm 2s$, $\bar{x} \pm 3s$ and what would be expected theoretically. For example, $\bar{x} \pm 1s = 45.4 \pm 10.9 = (34.5–56.3$ years). The number of men included in this age span can be found from Table 3.2. The number of men included in the range $\bar{x} - s$ to $\bar{x} + s$, i.e., $\bar{x} \pm 1s$, takes in all those from 34.5 to 40, 40–49,

TABLE 3.2
Age at Which 663 Men Became Edentulous
in One or Both Jaws[2]

Age in Years Last Birthday[a]	Number of Men
10–19	2
20–29	48
30–39	158
40–49	231
50–59	164
60–69	57
70–79	3
Total	663

[a]It would have been advisable to arrange these data into 5-year intervals with 663 cases. They were available only in this grouping; so they are presented in this manner.

and 50–56.3 years of age. To find the number of men in the two incomplete age groups, interpolation must be performed:

$$\frac{34.5 - 40.0}{30 - 40} \times 158 = 87$$

$$\frac{50.0 - 56.3}{50 - 60} \times 164 = 103,$$

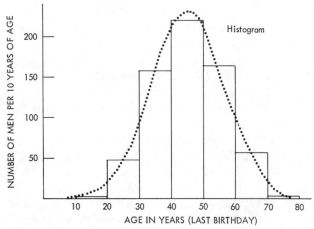

FIG. 3.3 Histogram (and Fitted Normal Curve) of Age Distribution of 663 Men Who Became Edentulous in One or Both Jaws at a University Dental Clinic.[2]

the total number of men included within 1s on either side of the mean is therefore $87 + 231 + 103 = 421$ men. This is 421/663 or 63.50% of the total frequency compared with the theoretical normal curve of 68.26%. Similarly, the interval $\bar{x} \pm 2s$ is found to include 625 men, which is 94.27% of the total frequency compared with the theoretical normal curve value of 95.45%. Included within $\bar{x} \pm 3s$ are 662 men, just about 100% of the total frequency.

In order to be able to interpret the mean and standard deviation effectively, the distribution should resemble a normal curve. No histogram or frequency polygon will ever be a normal curve, since the intervals will not be small enough or the number of readings sufficient. An experienced individual can tell at a glance whether the distribution resembles a normal distribution enough for practical purposes. Probably the first simple check on normality is to note whether it is approximately symmetrical. Then one might check to see whether $\bar{x} \pm 1s$ includes about $\frac{2}{3}$ of the measurements, and finally whether the total range of measurements is roughly included within $\bar{x} \pm 3s$. There are more objective ways of seeing whether the distribution is essentially a normal curve. Although it is impossible to see whether a very small series resembles a normal curve, previous experience with a large series of similar nature might provide a clue.

SOME OTHER TYPES OF FREQUENCY CURVES

Some distributions may be symmetrical and yet not be a normal curve. This can occur when there is excessive central concentration with very long tails at both ends (Fig. 3.4c), in which case the curve is called *leptokurtic*. This situation (symmetry) can also exist when there is a fairly even concentration over a long range, with short tails (Fig. 3.4d), in which case the curve is called *platykurtic*. The normal curve itself is a *mesokurtic* curve. The term *kurtosis* refers to the central clumping and the relative length of the tails of the curve, with mesokurtosis, leptokurtosis, and platykurtosis referring to the different types.

The curve of the frequency distribution can also be lopsided or *skewed*. When the tail of the curve trails off to the right, we refer to the condition as *positive skewness* or positively skewed; when the tail of the curve trails off to the left, *negative skewness* (Fig. 3.4a, b). Curves can have features of kurtosis and skewness at the same time.

If the observed distribution were slightly skewed or exhibited slightly leptokurtotic or platykurtotic tendencies, the true distributions should also present such skewness or kurtosis. Consequently,

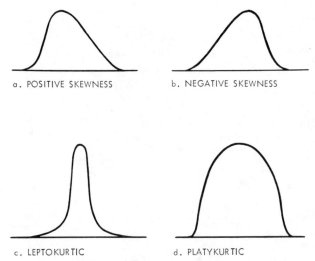

a. POSITIVE SKEWNESS   b. NEGATIVE SKEWNESS

c. LEPTOKURTIC   d. PLATYKURTIC

FIG. 3.4 Some Types of Frequency Curves Other Than the Normal Curve.

parameters other than μ or σ should be estimated. However, in view of the rather slight departures from a normal curve, the constants $\bar{x}$ and s are often used with their customary interpretations. The point at which the statistics ($\bar{x}$, s) will not ordinarily be used will depend on the magnitude of the aberration from the normal curve and what deviations from the normal curve are considered of practical importance in the problem at hand.

REFERENCES

1. The Bell-Shaped Curve: The Sciences, NY Acad Sciences 9:6, 1966.

2. Hall, M. F.: *In* Pelton, W. J., and Wisan, J. M., eds.: Dentistry in Public Health, Philadelphia, Saunders, 1949.

3. Arkin, H., and Colton, R. R.: Tables for Statisticians, 2nd ed., New York, Barnes & Noble, 1963.

4
Concepts of Chance Variation (Means)

The steps in an experimental investigation have been discussed in Chapter 1 and amplified in subsequent pages, but the final step remains, that of drawing conclusions from the data. Drawing proper conclusions is the main purpose of the whole experiment, and may also be the most intricate task. The methods of analysis to be employed to assist the investigator in drawing correct conclusions from the data should be anticipated in planning the experiment. In this way the investigator will be able to generate data in such a way that the statistical analyses and conclusions will proceed as simply and orderly as possible. To understand and apply the methods of analysis described in subsequent chapters, the reader must appreciate the concepts of chance variation presented here.

SAMPLE AND UNIVERSE

The group of individuals, animals, test tubes, or other items actually observed during an experiment is referred to as a sample, and an experiment may deal with one or more samples. The larger group of individuals, animals, etc. from which the sample is conceived of as having been drawn is called the universe or population. The universe of interest will, either consciously or unconsciously, be defined with all of its pertinent characteristics during the planning phase of the experiment. If an investigator were to perform an experiment on germ-free hamsters, the universe under consideration would be the population of germ-free hamsters. This population would be very large and might even be considered infinite in size. If he were to infect the experimental hamsters with a particular strain of *Streptococcus odontolyticus* he would be working with a sample from a universe of hamsters harboring one type of pure organism. If he were working with Golden Syrian hamsters of specified age, weight, and nutritional status and infected with *Streptococcus odontolyticus* then the universe would be all Golden Syrian hamsters harboring the one type of pure organism and of the specified age, weight, and nutritional status. Furthermore, the universe would include all such hamsters existing during the period of time in which all pertinent physiologic conditions and relationships remained stable.

If the universe were actually available, steps could be taken to ensure that the final generalizations and conclusions of the experiment, based on the sample or samples at hand, hold true for the universe. The sample(s) for the experiment must be "representative" of the universe(s) in question. The most elementary type of sample that may be called representative is the *simple* or *unrestricted random sample*, in which the individuals are independently drawn from the totally undifferentiated universe as in a lottery. Each individual in the universe has an equal chance of being included in the lottery.*

Sampling Variation

In investigating characteristics of a universe by drawing samples from it, one must remember that, even if the sample is randomly chosen, the distribution of the members of that sample with respect to a particular variable may differ considerably from the universe distribution. Consequently, although the mean, median, and variance of the sample will give some indication of the corresponding summary values in the universe, they will not necessarily duplicate them. In investigating the possible influence of serum protein level on the prevalence of dental caries in humans, Shannon and Gibson[1] examined (among others) 61 men, age 17–22, with 0 through 10 DMF surfaces. Their serum protein levels (gm%) were:

6.69	7.32	7.35	6.75	7.25	7.14
7.06	6.67	6.45	6.53	7.38	7.19
7.12	6.73	7.46	7.14	6.79	7.42
7.20	7.31	6.86	6.82	6.64	7.24
7.61	7.16	6.45	7.43	7.50	7.24
7.02	7.46	6.70	7.07	6.72	6.63
6.90	6.82	7.46	6.92	7.17	6.66
7.63	6.73	7.40	6.38	7.17	7.24
7.11	7.46	6.33	7.38	7.06	6.90
6.64	6.30	7.70	7.46	7.73	7.06
					6.55

---

*Other types of samples also give the same probability of selection to each individual, e.g., stratified random sampling (see Chapter 18).

Of course, 61 is no magical number and, presumably, the authors could have observed a larger or smaller group of males, age 17 to 22, with 0 to 10 DMFs. If, for example, they had observed a sample of 5 cases, they might have observed the first 5 cases, yielding a mean of 7.14 gm%, or the second 5 cases with a mean of 7.06 gm%, or perhaps cases 1, 3, 8, 9, and 24 with a mean of 7.08 gm%. Assuming that the samples were randomly drawn from the universe, each mean is a reflection of the true mean of the universe of males of the specified type. If repeated random samples of size 5 are drawn from the universe, the means of the samples will sometimes underestimate and sometimes overestimate the true universe mean and may, on occasion, equal this true mean. The variation in sample means is called the chance or sampling variation of means. It is caused by the factor of chance, which determines that some particular individuals rather than others have been included in the sample taken. The argument could be extended to the case of all possible random samples of any specified size. Indeed, the concept also operates with respect to the medians, variances, percentiles, etc. of samples of a designated size and also with respect to differences in means, medians, etc. from two or more samples drawn from one or more universes. The concept also applies to relative frequencies (see Chapter 11).

A Random Sampling Experiment

To develop the concept of sampling variation for classroom exercises, we created a universe of 10,000 chips. In this universe of chips, each chip* was stamped with a number. The numbers were such that the distribution was, for all intents and purposes, a normal curve, whose mean (μ) was 500 and whose standard deviation (σ) was 100. The numbers ranged from $\mu - 3\sigma$ or 200, to $\mu + 3\sigma$ or 800. Provision was made, however, for a few numbers below 200 and a few above 800, since only 99.73% of the area of the normal curve is distributed over the values included within three standard deviations of the mean. The universe of chips was well mixed and repeated samples were drawn from it. In the drawing of a sample, each chip was replaced and the universe again well mixed before the next chip was drawn. The chips of the sample are thus independent of each other.† The

---

*The chips used were flat round cardboard discs with metal perimeters, about $\frac{1}{2}$ inch in diameter.

†Since the total number of chips in the finite universe is very large (10,000) in relation to the size of the sample (10), this step of replacement of each chip is really not necessary. In effect, it renders the universe infinite. Sampling without replacement would, in the present case, have almost identical properties (Chapter 18).

samples may thus be considered randomly drawn and, in addition, independent of each other in the sense that the chips included in one sample in no way determine which chips will be included in any other sample.

In the manner just described, 970 random samples, each of size 10 chips, were drawn from the universe. The resulting frequency distribution of means of samples of size 10 appears in Table 4.1. As expected, the class interval (490–509) containing the true mean ($\mu = 500$) occurs most frequently, but there is considerable variation around it, with means ranging from 390 through 609. Most of the samples (98.5%) have means ranging from 410 to 590.

In general, if all possible independent samples of size N are drawn randomly from a normally distributed universe, the means of the samples will be distributed in a normal curve with a mean equal to $\mu = 500$ and a standard deviation ($\sigma_{\bar{x}}$), also known as the Standard Error of the Mean ($SE_{\bar{x}}$), where

$$\sigma_{\bar{x}} = SE_{\bar{x}} = \sigma/\sqrt{N} = 100/\sqrt{10} = 31.6.$$

We note that the reliability of the mean ($\bar{x}$) depends not only on the sample size (N) but also on the variability of the original measurements (σ).

The mean and standard deviation of the 970 means given in

TABLE 4.1
Chance Distribution of 970 Means
of Samples of Size 10 Drawn From
a Normal Universe of Mean 500
and Standard Deviation 100

Mean ($\bar{x}$)	Number of Samples (f)
390–409	1
410–429	7
430–449	34
450–469	98
470–489	187
490–509	258
510–529	203
530–549	106
550–569	51
570–589	18
590–609	7
Total	970

Table 4.2 as 503.2 and 32.4, respectively, agree very well with the theoretical predictions. Furthermore, the distribution certainly resembles a normal curve. In fact, within one standard deviation of the mean (503.2 ± 32.4 = 470.8 to 535.6) we find 68% and within two standard deviations of the mean (503.2 ± 2 × 32.4 = 438.4 to 568.0) we find 96%. These values are obtained by interpolation within the various intervals and agree very well with what they ought to be according to the normal curve.

When 290 samples, each of size 20 chips, were drawn from the same universe, the resulting distribution of means had a mean of 503.4 and a standard deviation of 22.0 as opposed to a mean of 503.2 and a standard deviation of 32.4 for samples of ten chips each. Of the 290 values, 97.2% were included within the interval 450 to 549, — a narrower interval than in the case of samples of size 10 where we find 96% between 438.4 to 568.0. This illustrates that the means of sample size 20 are more stable, i.e., less variable, than means of samples of size 10.

TABLE 4.2
Computation of Mean and Standard Deviation of Chance Distribution of 970 Means of Samples of 10 Drawn From a Normal Curve Universe of Mean 500 and Standard Deviation 100

Mean $\bar{x}$	Frequency f	Midpoints	Coded Units u	fu	fu^2
390–410	1	400	−5	− 5	25
410–430	7	420	−4	− 28	112
430–450	34	440	−3	−102	306
450–470	98	460	−2	−196	392
470–490	187	480	−1	−187	187
490–510	258	500	0	0	0
510–530	203	520	+1	+203	203
530–550	106	540	+2	+212	424
550–570	51	560	+3	+153	459
570–590	18	580	+4	+ 72	288
590–610	7	600	+5	+ 35	175
Total	970			+157	2,571

$$\bar{u} = \frac{\Sigma fu}{970} = \frac{+157}{970} = 0.162; \text{ or in original units, 503.2.}$$

$$s_u^2 = \frac{1}{970}\left[\Sigma fu^2 - \frac{(\Sigma fu)^2}{970}\right] = \frac{2,545.59}{970} = 2.624.$$

$$s_u = \sqrt{2.624} = 1.62; \text{ or in original units, } s_{\bar{x}} = 32.4.$$

No sharp line separates the samples that could arise from the specified universe and those that could not. For example, if samples of size 10 were drawn from a normal universe of mean 510 and a standard deviation of 100 the chance distribution of means should be centered at 510, with a standard deviation of 31.6. The range of means would be expected to be from about 400 to about 620 ($\mu \pm 3\sigma_{\bar{x}}$). In the absence of other information, a sample of 10 chips with a mean of 467 could not be classified as definitely coming from the universe whose mean is 500 rather than from the universe with a mean of 510. If the second universe has a mean of 1510 rather than 510, then the sampling range of means of size 10 from this universe would be approximately 1400 to 1620. A single sample with a mean of 467 would thus be classified as originating from the first universe (mean of 500) rather than from the second (mean of 1510) unless there are other possible universes in the vicinity of 500.

In a similar manner, using the universe of chips, one could investigate the empirical sampling distribution of medians of samples of a specified size N, the distribution of variances or standard deviations of samples of size N, or the distribution of any other summary constant of interest.

Whenever one draws conclusions from a sample from some universe, it must be emphasized that any summary constant computed for the sample may vary from the corresponding universe value. With simple random sampling, the amount of variation is measurable.* Knowledge of this variation can be used to form inferences about the summary constant in the parent universe.

Sampling fron Non-Normal Universes

When drawing samples of size N from a non-normal universe of x, the sampling distribution of $\bar{x}$ will still be normal if N is large enough (*Central Limit Theorem*).[4] N does not have to be very large if the departure from normality is moderate. For large departures N has to be larger, but then one may not be interested in summarizing the data by $\bar{x}$. The properties that the mean of $\bar{x} = \mu$ and $\sigma_{\bar{x}} = \sigma_x/\sqrt{N}$ hold for any distribution.

---

*Actually, the amount of variation is measurable with any type of probability sampling (see Chapter 18). The simplest type of probability sampling is simple random sampling.

TABLE 4.3
Plasma Inorganic Phosphorus Values (mg%) for 24 Patients With Periodontal Disease[2]

Patient Number	Inorganic Phosphorus	Patient Number	Inorganic Phosphorus
102	4.2	114	3.4
103	3.6	115	3.3
104	4.2	116	3.6
105	3.6	117	3.5
106	3.4	118	3.8
107	3.9	119	3.3
108	3.4	120	3.6
109	4.1	121	3.5
110	3.5	122	3.7
111	3.7	123	3.4
112	3.4	124	3.3
113	4.0	125	3.5

Total (102-125) $\Sigma x = 86.9$

$$\bar{x} = \frac{\Sigma x}{N} = \frac{86.9}{25} = 3.62 \text{ mg\%}$$

COMPARISON OF A SAMPLE MEAN WITH A UNIVERSE MEAN

Normal Curve Test — σ Known

Rose, Kuna, and Kraft[2] obtained values of inorganic phosphorus from the blood plasma of 24 patients with periodontal disease (Table 4.3), with a mean ($\bar{x}$) of 3.62 mg%. Wertheimer et al[3] state the "normal value" of plasma inorganic phosphorus to be, on the average, 3.36 mg% (μ) and the standard deviation (σ) 0.40 mg%. The question is whether the sample of 24 patients could have been drawn as a random sample from the universe of normals whose mean is 3.36, given that the standard deviation is 0.40.

Assuming that Wertheimer's distribution is a normal curve (or not too far from it) independent random samples* of size 24 taken repeatedly from such a universe would have their means normally distributed with a mean (μ) = 3.36 mg% and

---

*It is, of course, always assumed that the x's of the sample are independent of each other. This is a fundamental assumption for statistical inference based on random sampling.

$$\sigma_{\overline{x}} = SE_{\overline{x}} = \sigma/\sqrt{N} = 0.40/\sqrt{24} = 0.08 \text{ mg\%}.$$

A sample mean of 3.62 mg% corresponds to a normal deviate (the *test statistic*) of

$$z = \frac{3.62 - 3.36}{0.08} = +3.25.$$

From Table 3.1 it is found that 99.88% of all means of samples of size 24 will fall within 3.25 $SE_{\overline{x}}$'s of μ = 3.36 mg%. The probability is therefore only (100.00% − 99.88%) = 0.12% of drawing a sample with a mean farther removed from the μ value in one direction or the other as the one observed (that is, of drawing a sample as rare as or rarer than the one observed).

With such a small probability and an alternative possibility that the sample could have been drawn from another universe, the decision is that there is a difference between the universe from which the 24 patients were drawn and Wertheimer's universe, with respect to the mean. Thus, the two universes in question are considered to be different from each other.

STATISTICAL SIGNIFICANCE
AND NONSIGNIFICANCE

The usual terminology employed when the sample is considered as coming from a universe with a different mean (the *alternative hypothesis*, H_1) than the one of reference (the *null hypothesis*, H_0) is that the difference between the sample mean (3.62) and the hypothetical mean (3.36) is "statistically significant." "Statistically significant" means that although it is possible that the sample was drawn from the universe in question, it is improbable. Consequently, without any other evidence, it is assumed that the sample came from some alternative universe. The opposite decision of "statistically not significant" means that the deviation of the sample value from the universe value could be explained as part of the random process and so no alternative need be embraced. Note that the decision "statistically not significant" is not a declaration that the sample came from the hypothesized universe, but is rather a statement that evidence is insufficient to take the bold stand that the sample did not come from the hypothesized universe.

A decision of "statistical significance" is made whenever the sample value is such that samples are rare or rarer occur only a small proportion of the time, say 1%. The critical value of 1% (P, the probability of a sample as rare or rarer, = .01) is somewhat arbitrary and depends on the concept and meaning of the terms "unusual," "improbable," "of rare occurrence," etc. If something is declared improbable — i.e., statistically significant — and action is taken accordingly, a possibility always exists that it did occur by chance and that no action was necessary. On the other hand, if it is declared statistically not significant, the possibility always exists that it did not occur by chance and that some action should have been taken. Where the line is drawn will depend on the consequences of making a wrong decision. It certainly is important to guard against taking action when none is necessary, and it is also important to guard against inaction when action is indeed necessary. Any small probability could serve as the critical value, although customarily P = .01, as mentioned or perhaps more frequently, P = .05. Another value used fairly often is P = .02. The choice should be made during the planning phase of the experiment, keeping in mind that the smaller the critical value of P chosen, the more difficult it is to attribute the observed fluctuation to something other than chance. This critical value of P, often expressed as α (Greek lower case letter alpha), is known as the "level of significance."

We note here that rejection of the hypothesized mean can take place in either tail of the normal curve, i.e., P is allocated in the two tails, e.g., .005 in each tail if α = .01. We are thus using what is called a *two-tailed test*. If α is taken as .05, then .025 is allocated in each tail. If α is taken as .02, then .01 is allocated in each tail. We thus note that a one-tailed significance test at the 1% level is equivalent to a two-tailed significance test at the 2% level. The significance test on page 61 was a two-tailed test. It is far more common to find a significance test as two-tailed rather than one-tailed. For further discussion, see Chapter 6.

One commonly used variation in the above procedure is worth a special mention. This involves an a posteriori level of significance, usually termed the *P-value*. In this procedure, the investigator does not choose a level of significance at the outset. He indicates the probability that a test statistic, e.g., z, value "as excessive" as the one observed would occur if the null hypothesis, H_0, were true. If this approach is used, it is left up to the investigator, or to the reader of his paper, to judge whether the value of P is so small as to rule out chance as the cause of the discrepancy between H_0 and the observed result. If he considers P small enough, he rejects H_0 in favor of one of the alternatives in H_1.

In the illustration above, the sample was compared with some reference universe by means of a significance test. Frequently, we do not have in mind doing a significance test against a reference universe. Rather, we are taking our sample in order to estimate the characteristics of the universe from which that sample is drawn. For further elaboration of this point, see the discussion of confidence intervals in Chapter 6.

Type I and Type II Errors

In any test of statistical significance, i.e., significance test, two kinds of universes are under consideration — the reference one (the *null universe* or *null hypothesis*, H_0) and a set of possible *alternative universes* or *alternative hypotheses*, H_1. No matter what decision is made, an error is always possible. If significance is declared, thereby rejecting the null universe, H_0, and embracing an alternative, H_1, there is always the possibility that the sample actually did come from H_0. The error thus committed is known as an "error of the first kind" or a *Type I error*; the probability of committing this error is controlled by the choice of α. In diagnostic tests, this first type of error is often referred to as a false positive error. If the deviation is declared not significant, thereby not rejecting H_0, there is the possibility that the sample actually did come from another universe. The error thus committed is known as an "error of the second kind" or a *Type II error*. The probability of committing this type of error depends on what universe the sample actually came from and on the size of the sample. The probability of this type of error is often referred to as β. In diagnostic tests, this is often referred to as a false negative error. $(1 - \beta)$ is generally referred to as the *power of the test*, the probability of detecting the falseness of the null hypothesis, when the specific alternative is true. It must be emphasized that β and $(1 - \beta)$ are a function of the alternative, i.e., of the distance between μ_0 and μ_1. The "power of the test" has no meaning except in terms of a specific alternative.[4]

The first kind of error is usually more important than the second kind of error, so that every attempt is usually made to guard against it strongly by insisting that the deviation be quite rare before calling it statistically significant (i.e., P = .05 or P = .01). Unfortunately, it is a fact of life that the more the first type of error is guarded against, the wider the door is opened to the second. Thus, the place where the line is drawn between significance and nonsignificance depends on the consideration given to the consequence of committing one or the other type of error. Again, this depends on the particular problem being considered.

If the 1% level of significance is used (α = 1%), then in standard deviational units the zone of significance lies outside the range of values of z between -2.58 and +2.58. Wertheimer's reference universe is considered normal with a mean (μ = 3.36 mg%) and a standard deviation (σ = 0.40 mg%). Repeat random samples of size 24 drawn from this universe will be centered at μ = 3.36 mg% with a standard deviation of $\sigma_{\bar{x}}/\sqrt{24}$ = 0.08 mg%. In this normal curve of means, the zone of nonsignificance (with α = .01) will extend from 3.15 to 3.57 mg% (3.36 ± 2.58 × 0.08). To obtain statistical significance, the $\bar{x}$ value must be less than or equal to 3.15 or greater than or equal to 3.57 mg%. The observed $\bar{x}$ of Rose, Kuna, and Kraft of 3.62 falls outside of this zone and is thus adjudged to be statistically significant at the 1% level.

If the sample size were reduced, the $SE_{\bar{x}}$ would be increased. Thus, if the sample were only of size 12, assuming the same mean value, $\bar{x}$ = 3.62,

$$\sigma_{\bar{x}} = SE_{\bar{x}} = \frac{0.40}{\sqrt{12}} = 0.12$$

$$z = \frac{\bar{x} - \mu}{SE_{\bar{x}}} = \frac{3.62 - 3.36}{0.12} = 2.17,$$

falling into the zone of nonsignificance if α = .01. In general, the smaller the sample size, the larger the variability of the means ($SE_{\bar{x}}$), and the more difficult it is to assert statistical significance with the same difference between the sample and the hypothesized universe mean.

Even though an experimenter may show that one procedure is significantly different from another statistically, one must also consider whether it is significantly different (i.e., sufficiently different) from a practical point of view. Thus, a new denture base may prove to be "better" than another when measured quantitatively, the difference being statistically significant. If, however, the cost of this new material is much greater than that of the older denture base, and it is difficult to work with, the difference may be relatively unimportant and hence of no practical significance. But if, on the other hand, this new material is tolerated by tissue to a markedly greater extent than previously available denture bases, any improvement between denture bases is certainly of great practical significance to those patients who are prone to neoplastic disease.

t-Test for a Single Sample — σ Unknown

In the story of the 24 patients with periodontal disease, the standard deviation of the hypothesized universe was specified as 0.40 mg%. It is unusual to have a known value for the universe standard deviation, and, even were one available, it is not necessary or wise, if the main interest is in the universe average, to make the assumption that the universe generating the sample in hand has the same standard deviation as the universe whose mean is given. There could be a difference between the means of two universes with or without a change in their standard deviations. The verdict of statistical significance in the analysis of the data of Rose et al. could be due to the fact that the μ value of the universe of individuals with periodontal disease is not 3.36 mg%, or to the fact that the value of σ is not 0.40 mg%, or to both. A wiser course would be to use a statistical test which just investigates whether μ could be some specific value without making any assumptions about the value of the standard deviation of the universe in question. A resultant decision of statistical significance can then be attributed to the fact that μ is not the value hypothesized.

The main question in the study of Rose et al. is whether the sample of 24 patients could have been drawn from a normally distributed universe with a mean plasma inorganic phosphorus value of $\mu = 3.36$ mg%. The mean for the sample of 24 patients is 3.62 mg%. The estimate of the standard deviation of the universe is given by the sample standard deviation,

$$s = \sqrt{\frac{\Sigma(x - \bar{x})^2}{N - 1}} = \sqrt{\frac{1}{N - 1}\left[\Sigma x^2 - \frac{(\Sigma x)^2}{N}\right]}$$

$$= \sqrt{\frac{1}{23}\left[316.43 - \frac{7551.61}{24}\right]} = 0.28 \text{ mg\%}.$$

If all possible independent random samples, each of size N, are drawn from a normally distributed universe, and if for each sample the value $\dfrac{\bar{x} - \mu}{s/\sqrt{N}}$ is computed, then the sampling distribution of these ratios is a t-distribution with (N - 1) degrees of freedom (df). The

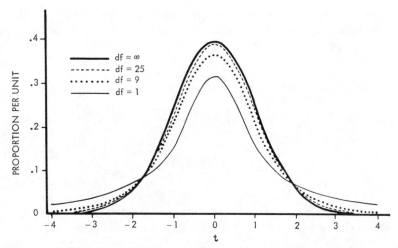

FIG. 4.1 t-Curves for Different Degrees of Freedom. [From Lewis, D., Quantitative Methods in Psychology, New York, McGraw-Hill, 1960].

ratio is not distributed in the standard normal curve as is z. The customary designation for such a ratio is

$$t_{df} = \frac{\bar{x} - \mu}{s/\sqrt{N}}.$$

It will be noted that t is computed precisely like the normal deviate, z, except that s is used instead of σ. In fact, z is often denoted as t_∞ to indicate that σ is merely an s based on an infinite number of degrees of freedom.

The t-curve is very much like the standard normal curve except that it has to reflect the fact that the denominator uses a sample estimate, s, instead of the universe parameter, σ. The denominator, $\sigma_{\bar{x}} = \sigma/\sqrt{N}$ or $SE_{\bar{x}}$ in z is replaced by $s_{\bar{x}}$ = est. $SE_{\bar{x}}$* = $s/\sqrt{N}$. The t-curve is symmetrical and centered at 0. However, its effective range is wider than that of the standard normal curve, in fact, it is leptokurtic. There is a whole family of t-curves, one for each number of degrees of freedom (Figure 4.1). It is not possible to transform the t-curves to a single t-curve as in the case of the normal curve.

---

*$s_{\bar{x}}$ or est. $\sigma_{\bar{x}}$ or est. $SE_{\bar{x}}$ is frequently written as SE_x. Often, the caret ("hat") is omitted.

Tables of the t-distribution usually list only some of the t-values corresponding to certain tail areas under the curves (P), as shown in Table 4.4. The first column labeled df refers to the degrees of freedom. Any one row contains values on the t-curve with df degrees of freedom. The t-values given are those values, positive and negative, so that P% of the area of the t-curve lies in the tails beyond this point. $\frac{1}{2}$ P is the portion of the area in each tail. Thus, for the t-curve with 15 degrees of freedom, 1% of the area of the t-curve lies in the tails beyond the t-values +2.95 and –2.95. These values of t are larger than the corresponding z of 2.58; 10% of the area lies beyond the values of +1.75 and –1.75. The corresponding value of z is 1.64. For any t-curve with degrees of freedom about 30 or more, the t-values for the various values of P do not differ very much from the corresponding z values of the standard normal curve. These z values are given in the last row (df = ∞) of the t-table.

If there are a large number of degrees of freedom, t can be interpreted as z. The same statistical decision will usually result. Exceptions will occur only when the t-value is in the immediate vicinity of the critical value. It is in the case of small sample sizes that the t-test is particularly necessary.

To illustrate, the t-value computed from the data of Rose et al., is

$$t_{23} = \frac{\bar{x} - \mu}{s/\sqrt{N}} = \frac{3.62 - 3.36}{0.28/\sqrt{24}} = \frac{0.26}{0.06} = 4.33,$$

with (N – 1) = 24 – 1 = 23 degrees of freedom. From the t-table at 23 degrees of freedom, 1% of the area of the curve lies beyond the values –2.81 and +2.81. The zone of nonsignificance for α = .01 thus extends from –2.81 to +2.81 inclusive, and the zone of significance lies below –2.81 and above +2.81. A t-value of 4.33 with 23 degrees of freedom is, therefore judged to be statistically significant at the 1% level (α = .01). Therefore, the plasma inorganic phosphorus level of periodontal patients of the type in this study is, on the average, different from the mean inorganic phosphorus level of "normals," as cited by Wertheimer et al.

From more extensive t-tables,[5] it could be found that the probability, P, of a sampling deviation larger than the observed in either direction is actually less than .001. Actually, however, this is not an important point since once the significance level has been set at α = .01 or .05 the only t-values needed are those corresponding to those probability levels.

TABLE 4.4
Table of t Probability in the Two Tails Beyond $\pm t$[9]

Degrees of Freedom (df)	0.50	0.10	0.05	0.02	0.01
1	1.000	6.34	12.71	31.82	63.66
2	0.816	2.92	4.30	6.96	9.92
3	.765	2.35	3.18	4.54	5.84
4	.741	2.13	2.78	3.75	4.60
5	.727	2.02	2.57	3.36	4.03
6	.718	1.94	2.45	3.14	3.71
7	.711	1.90	2.36	3.00	3.50
8	.706	1.86	2.31	2.90	3.36
9	.703	1.83	2.26	2.82	3.25
10	.700	1.81	2.23	2.76	3.17
11	.697	1.80	2.20	2.72	3.11
12	.695	1.78	2.18	2.68	3.06
13	.694	1.77	2.16	2.65	3.01
14	.692	1.76	2.14	2.62	2.98
15	.691	1.75	2.13	2.60	2.95
16	.690	1.75	2.12	2.58	2.92
17	.689	1.74	2.11	2.57	2.90
18	.688	1.73	2.10	2.55	2.88
19	.688	1.73	2.09	2.54	2.86
20	.687	1.72	2.09	2.53	2.84
21	.686	1.72	2.08	2.52	2.83
22	.686	1.72	2.07	2.51	2.82
23	.685	1.71	2.07	2.50	2.81
24	.685	1.71	2.06	2.49	2.80
25	.684	1.71	2.06	2.48	2.79
26	.684	1.71	2.06	2.48	2.78
27	.684	1.70	2.05	2.47	2.77
28	.683	1.70	2.05	2.47	2.76
29	.683	1.70	2.04	2.46	2.76
30	.683	1.70	2.04	2.46	2.75
35	.682	1.69	2.03	2.44	2.72
40	.681	1.68	2.02	2.42	2.71
45	.680	1.68	2.02	2.41	2.69
50	.679	1.68	2.01	2.40	2.68
60	.678	1.67	2.00	2.39	2.66
70	.678	1.67	2.00	2.38	2.65
80	.677	1.66	1.99	2.38	2.64
90	.677	1.66	1.99	2.37	2.63
100	.677	1.66	1.98	2.36	2.63
125	.676	1.66	1.98	2.36	2.62
150	.676	1.66	1.98	2.35	2.61
200	.675	1.65	1.97	2.35	2.60
300	.675	1.65	1.97	2.34	2.59
400	.675	1.65	1.97	2.34	2.59
500	.674	1.65	1.96	2.33	2.59
1,000	.674	1.65	1.96	2.33	2.58
∞	.674	1.64	1.96	2.33	2.58

[a]The probability in one tail is half that shown in the table.

CONFIDENCE LIMITS

A sample is usually taken to estimate a characteristic of the universe from which it was drawn and not merely to compare with a reference universe where available. It is possible to use the sample of the 24 individuals with periodontal disease, presumably randomly drawn from the universe of all such individuals, to set up a range of values that can be stated, with a measurable degree of certainty, to include the mean of the parent universe. Here it will be assumed that this parent universe is normally distributed. Since a sample t with 23 degrees of freedom occurs within the range from -2.81 to $+2.81$ in 99% of the samples, the "minimum" value of the true mean may be taken as $\bar{x} - 2.81$ est. $SE_{\bar{x}}$ where est. $SE_{\bar{x}} = s/\sqrt{N}$ and the "maximum" value as $\bar{x} + 2.81$ est. $SE_{\bar{x}}$. Consequently, the range from $\bar{x} - t$ est. $SE_{\bar{x}}$ to $\bar{x} + t$ est. $SE_{\bar{x}}$, where t is the positive value on the t curve with 23 degrees of freedom at $P = .01$ (both tails), is fairly certain to include the true unknown mean, unless, of course, this sample is the rare kind that occurs only 1% or less of the time.

When the numerical values are substituted, these limits are called the 99% *confidence limits*, and the range the 99% *confidence range or interval*. Since est. $SE_{\bar{x}} = \dfrac{0.28}{\sqrt{24}} = 0.06$, the confidence range is $3.62 \pm 2.81(0.06)$, or 3.45 to 3.79 mg%. The statement that the confidence range covers the true mean is apt to be true since 99% of such statements are true. The fact that the confidence range does not include the value of 3.36 is another way of demonstrating that the observed mean of 3.62 differs significantly from the hypothesized universe mean of 3.36 at the 1% level. The confidence interval includes all those values of μ from which $\bar{x}$ does not differ significantly, i.e., all hypothetical values of μ not disputed by the data. The confidence range can be calculated for any degree of confidence although usually either the 95% or the 99% confidence limits are chosen.

When one has available a reference universe and does a significance test, it is still frequent practice to give the confidence interval in addition to the significance test. The confidence interval should be the $(1 - \alpha)$ confidence interval, i.e., corresponding to the level of significance. The significance test is a reject-not reject test, whereas the confidence interval gives a whole range of possibilities for μ of the universe from which the sample came. Even if the null hypothesis is not rejected, it is, of course, possible that the sample came from some other universe and the whole battery of other possible universes is contained within the confidence interval. Thus, one might say, to quote Freiman et al., "the exact location and width of the confidence interval suggest a good deal about the direction in which the truth lies and the adequacy of the sample size to pin it down."[6]

ONE-TAILED AND TWO-TAILED TESTS

Sometimes during the planning phase of the experiment it is possible or desirable to specify that the universe alternative to the null universe is larger (or smaller), in terms of the parameter of interest, than the null universe value. The zone of significance would then be in the upper (or lower) tail only, corresponding to 1%, 5% or some other small percent of the area of the curve. Such a significance test is a "one-tailed test".

The critical value of z for a one-tailed significance test at the 1% level is 2.33 instead of 2.58 for the two-tailed version. For the 5% one-tailed version, the critical value of z is 1.64 instead of 1.96 for the two-tailed version. Similarly, for t, the values of P at the top of the table should be halved for one-tailed tests.

Imagine that the context of the experiment of Rose et al. enabled them to hypothesize that if the μ of the universe from which the 24 patients were drawn is different from 3.36 mg%, it is larger than 3.36 mg%. Then, the one-tailed critical value of t with 23 degrees of freedom at P = .01 is +2.50. This corresponds to α = .02 for a two-tailed test. The observed value, $t_{23} = \dfrac{3.62 - 3.36}{0.06} = +4.33$, is, therefore, statistically significant also at the 1% level, using a one-tailed test. Obviously, if a two-tailed test asserts statistical significance at a certain α level, a one-tailed test will also assert significance at that level.

If a one-tailed or one-sided test is used, we can state the result of hypothesis testing as "significantly greater than," or "significantly lesser than" instead of "significantly different from" when the two-sided or two-tailed test has been used. Sometimes the investigator decides to employ the one-tailed criterion after the data have been generated in order to assert statistical significance or nonsignificance at a higher level. This is improper procedure. The two-sided test is the one usually performed and is more stringent in terms of the error of the first kind.

It must be emphasized that the decision to utilize a one-tailed test must be made in planning the experiment and certainly before viewing the data. If Rose et al. had observed in their experiment an $\bar{x}$ smaller than 3.36, even considerably smaller, it would have had to be classified as due to sampling fluctuation, under the terms of the one-tailed test. In the majority of experiments, it is advisable to specify a two-tailed test, i.e., $\frac{1}{2}$ P in the lower tail and $\frac{1}{2}$ P in the upper tail of the sampling curve (assuming the curve to be symmetrical).

Both one- and two-sided tests are legitimate tests, but reviewers and purists often look askance at the one-sided test. This is because of the suspicion that the investigator may have decided to employ the one-tailed criterion for significance *after* the data have been generated in order to assert significance at a lesser critical ratio (z or t), thereby increasing the power of his comparison. By performing a one-tailed test, he is only interested in the alternative hypothesis that one "treatment" is better (worse) than the other treatment. This is in contrast to the two-tailed test that yields the inference that one treatment differs significantly (for better or for worse) from the other treatment.

The two-sided test is the more frequent test and is more conservative. It has been accepted more readily than the one-sided test because there is often the suspicion that the choice was not made before the start of the study. If, however, the protocol specifies and with good reason, a one-tailed test, this objection is no longer valid. There are good reasons for the use of the one-sided test: First, there is the ethical question of testing a new treatment against an established one. Is it ethical to test a treatment that may very well be worse than the standard treatment when the condition being treated is a serious or life-threatening one? Second, the sample size required to assert a statistically significant difference is smaller using a one-sided test; and third, two-tailed tests based on asymmetrical sampling distributions are difficult to interpret, especially for discrete asymmetrical sampling distributions.

It should be noted that the confidence interval is typically two-sided (with very few exceptions), so that a $(1 - \alpha)$ confidence interval in essence puts $\alpha/2$ in each of the two tails of a sampling distribution. Thus, a two-sided significance test is consistent with the two-sided confidence interval.

Considerations of Normality

As indicated in Chapter 2, if the distribution represents a moderate amount of non-normality in terms of skewness or kurtosis, as might be evidenced by past experience or a preliminary study, the data will still be summarized by the mean and standard deviation. As has been indicated before (page 48), the distribution of means in repeated samples from such universes will follow the normal curve unless N is very small (*Central Limit Theorem*). If σ were known, the z test for comparing x̄ with μ would evidently be correct. If σ is unknown and t is used, there would be no particular problem with the moderately non-normal distributions, which is why the t-test is called "robust." Of course, if N is large, s is essentially σ so that the z test can be used.

If the distributions were very non-normal, the mean and standard deviation would not be the summary constants of choice in the first place. The fact that for a large N the x's would follow the normal curve is therefore of little interest since x̄ would not be used at any rate. In such instances, some non-linear transformation such as logarithms might make the distributions more normal. The comparison of medians, or some other distribution-free or nonparametric method might be used (Chapter 15, Ranking Tests), in particular, the Wilcoxon Signed Rank Test.

REFERENCES

1. Shannon, I. L., and Gibson, W. A.: Serum Proteins in Relation to Periodontal Status and Caries Experience, Tech. Doc. Rep. No. SAM–TDR–63–81, USAF Schl. Aerospace Med., 1963.

2. Rose, H. P., Kuna, A. and Kraft, E.: Systemic manifestations of periodontal disease, J Periodont 34:253, 1963.

3. Wertheimer, A. R., Eurman, G. H., and Kalinsky, H. J.: J Clin Invest 33: 565, in Documenta Geigy Scientific Tables, 5th ed. Ardsley (NY), 1962, p. 567.

4. Mood, A. M., Graybill, F. A., and Boes, D. C.: Introduction to the Theory of Statistics, New York, McGraw-Hill, 3rd ed., 1974.

5. Pearson, E. S., and Hartley, H. O.: Biometrika Tables for Statisticians, Vol. I, Table 9, London, Cambridge University Press, 1956.

6. Freiman, J. A., Chalmers, T. C., Smith, H., Jr., and Kuebler, R. R.: The importance of beta, the type II error and sample size in the design and interpretation of the randomized control trial, New Engl J Med 299:690, 1978.

5

Comparison of Means of Two Samples

When an investigator obtains an average of a sample of measurements, he usually does not know the average of an appropriate universe or population with which to compare his sample mean. For this situation various reasons may exist: (1) He lacks experience with the variable under consideration; (2) his data might have been obtained from individuals whose measurements refer only to some specific part or stratum of the universe; or (3) his past experience may have to be discarded, since the characteristics of the universe have changed from the time when its mean was established to the time when the sample was drawn.

INDEPENDENT SAMPLES

To illustrate, the experiment may be concerned with the effect of a supplementary dietary intake on the mandible ash content of the marmoset, the experimental animal. The mean of the sample of a specified number of animals, with weight, lineage, etc. specified, is to be compared with similar marmosets that are not on the supplementary diet. The mean of the latter measurements is obviously not known for an appropriate universe of marmosets. Information about the latter universe can be obtained by withholding the supplement from a limited number of marmosets similar in all ways to those receiving the supplement. In other words, a *control* or *comparative group* is formed.

Frequently, the experiment is (and often *should be*) set up so that the sizes of the experimental and control groups are equal, although this is not a prerequisite. Since the mean of the control group is subject to chance or sampling fluctuations to an extent similar to the mean of the experimental group, it cannot be regarded as a stable point of reference for the mean of the experimental group, as was the case where a control universe was available (Chapter 4). The procedure for comparing the two means is therefore not the same as that illustrated in the previous chapter for the comparison of a sample mean with the mean of a known universe.

Although both the experimental and control groups will usually have been very carefully selected, in that certain specific conditions are met, they must be similarly selected, so that they will be comparable with respect to all factors, both ponderable (weight, dietary intake, etc.) and imponderable (heredity, etc.). If this is not so, the difference obtained may be referable not to the experimental "treatment" but to other uncontrolled factors. In other words, the treatment effect is *confounded* with uncontrolled factors.

A common method for obtaining comparability is to divide the available marmosets at random into two groups. Let it be supposed that 20 animals are available and 10 are to be assigned to each of the two groups. A number is assigned to each of the 20 marmosets, and 10 numbers are picked at random (for example, from a table of random numbers; see Chap. 17) from these 20 so that each group has 10 animals. This type of unrestricted random design corresponds to an unrestricted random sample from a universe. This selection procedure ensures that the two groups are alike within chance variation, and the investigator will know how to measure and take account of chance.

A Random Sampling Experiment

To illustrate the chance variation of differences between two means, a hypothetical situation can be set up. The mean blood level of a particular chemical ($\bar{x}_1$) in a sample of 10 patients is 475 units, with a standard deviation of approximately 100. The mean ($\bar{x}_2$) for another group of 10 similar patients is 525, with a standard deviation of approximately 100. The question is whether the two samples are derived from the same universe (the null hypothesis). In order to answer the question, the frequency of obtaining a difference of 50 or more units (525 – 475) when samples of size 10 are drawn from the same universe must be found.

From a normal curve universe with a mean of 500 and a standard deviation of 100, the universe of chips described in Chapter 4, 970 pairs of samples of size 10 were drawn. Since the chips were well mixed, the measurements in the sample are independent of each other, a basic prerequisite for the usual significance tests. For each pair the difference in means was computed. The distribution of these differences appears in Table 5.1. As expected, the class interval containing zero occurs with the greatest frequency, but there is considerable variation. Most of the differences are included in the range from –110 to +110. In the absence of information that the two samples arose from a common universe, differences greater than these would suggest that they originate from different universes.

Actually, there are two universes involved, one in the background for the first sample, and the second in the background for the second sample. If these two universes have the same mean but different standard deviations, then the null hypothesis just refers to the difference between means, i.e., $(\mu_1 - \mu_2) = 0$.

Among 485 pairs of samples, a difference of –50 was exceeded in $40 + 20 + 7 + 0 + 1$, or 68 pairs, while a difference of +50 was exceeded in $39 + 21 + 8 + 2 + 3$, or 73 pairs. Thus, a difference of 50 is exceeded 141 times out of 485, or 29% of the time. This probability (P) is too large to postulate that the samples arose from two different universes. In order to postulate the presence of two sepa-

TABLE 5.1
Chance Distribution of Difference in Means for 485 Pairs of Samples of 10 Drawn from a Normal Universe of Mean 500 and Standard Deviation 100

Difference in Means $(\bar{x}_1 - \bar{x}_2)$	Number of Pairs of Samples
–150 to –130	1
–130 to –110	0
–110 to – 90	7
– 90 to – 70	20
– 70 to – 50	40
– 50 to – 30	52
– 30 to – 10	77
– 10 to + 10	83
+ 10 to + 30	76
+ 30 to + 30	56
+ 50 to + 70	39
+ 70 to + 90	21
+ 90 to +110	8
+110 to +130	2
+130 to +150	3
Total	485

rate universes (the alternative hypothesis), the probability of exceeding the difference should be quite small — say, less than 5% or less than 1%, the same criteria of significance used previously (Chapter 4).

COMPARISON OF TWO SAMPLE MEANS
BY THE NORMAL CURVE TEST

The chance distribution of differences in means for pairs of samples from the same normal curve universe is a normal curve with a mean of zero, and a standard deviation

$$\sigma_{\bar{x}_1 - \bar{x}_2} = SE_{\bar{x}_2 - \bar{x}_2} = \sqrt{SE_{\bar{x}_1}{}^2 + SE_{\bar{x}_2}{}^2},$$

where

$$SE_{\bar{x}_1} = \sigma/\sqrt{N_1} ; SE_{\bar{x}_2} = \sigma/\sqrt{N_2}.$$

$SE_{\bar{x}_1}$ measures the chance variation of the means ($\bar{x}_1$) of samples of size N_1 while $SE_{\bar{x}_2}$ is a measure of the chance variation of the means ($\bar{x}_2$) of samples of size N_2:

$$SE_{\bar{x}_1} = 100/\sqrt{10} = 31.6 ; SE_{\bar{x}_2} = 100/\sqrt{10} = 31.6$$
$$SE_{\bar{x}_1 - \bar{x}_2} = \sqrt{(31.6)^2 + (31.6)^2} = 44.7.$$

Actually, calculating the mean and standard deviation of the distribution of $\bar{x}_1 - \bar{x}_2$ of Table 5.1 by conventional methods yields +1.6 and a standard deviation of 45.9.

The probability of exceeding a difference of 50 units in means can be obtained by reference to the normal curve. Thus,

$$z = \frac{(\bar{x}_1 - \bar{x}_2) - 0}{SE_{\bar{x}_1 - \bar{x}_2}} = \frac{-50}{44.7} = -1.1.$$

The tails of the normal curve beyond ± 1.1, comprise 27% (P) of the total area under the curve, almost the same as the probability obtained from the empirical sampling distribution. Since this probability is larger than 1% (or 5%), the difference ($\bar{x}_1 - \bar{x}_2$) is statistically not significant at the 1% (or 5%) level. We thus conclude that the two samples might have been drawn from the same universe.

We note, that under the alternative hypothesis that $\mu_1 - \mu_2 \neq 0$, the sampling distribution of $(\bar{x}_1 - \bar{x}_2)$ would be distributed in a normal curve centered at $\mu_1 - \mu_2$, as could be verified by setting up two boxes of chips with one box with μ_1 and the other with μ_2, both having a standard deviation of σ. A sampling experiment also could have been set up for two universes of chips having different standard deviations, σ_1 and σ_2, and having either the same means (null hypothesis) or different means (alternative hypothesis). With this sampling experiment, the difference $(\bar{x}_1 - \bar{x}_2)$ would still be a normal curve centered at zero, but the standard error of the difference $(SE_{\bar{x}_1 - \bar{x}_2})$ would have involved σ_1 and σ_2, namely,

$$SE_{\bar{x}_1} = \sigma_1 / \sqrt{N_1} \text{ and } SE_{\bar{x}_2} = \sigma_2 / \sqrt{N_2}.$$

The use of the above normal curve significance test would still be perfectly correct.

COMPARISON OF TWO SAMPLE MEANS BY THE t-TEST

Usually, σ is not available to enable us to perform the normal curve test on the difference between means. We have to use an estimate of σ based on the two respective samples. Hence, we have a ratio of the difference to the estimated standard error which does not follow the normal curve distribution.

Table 5.2 presents the plasma ascorbic acid levels (AAPL) in mg% of two samples of size 13 each. One sample was of indoor workers in Antarctica, the other of an independent group of outdoor workers in the same locale. These two groups may be considered independent random samples from two universes of healthy men working indoors and outdoors in the polar region, and may be called a *parallel group* study. The question is whether the difference among the average AAPL for the two groups is due to sampling variation (the null hypothesis) or a real difference in universe means (the alternative hypothesis). The null hypothesis is that $(\mu_1 - \mu_2) = 0$ and the alternative hypothesis is that $(\mu_1 - \mu_2) \neq 0$. A two-tailed test is evidently called for because, according to the statement of the alternative hypothesis, a difference in either direction is of interest.

If the universes are at least approximately normal, differences between the means of repeated pairs of samples would be distributed in a normal curve centered at 0. Furthermore, if both universes have

TABLE 5.2

Ascorbic Acid Plasma Level (AAPL) Determination in mg% of 26
Individuals[1]

Individual Number	Indoor Group (x_1)	Individual Number	Outdoor Group (x_2)
1	0.60	14	0.60
2	0.90	15	0.65
3	0.92	16	0.68
4	0.88	17	0.70
5	0.87	18	0.70
6	0.91	19	0.70
7	0.87	20	0.65
8	0.90	21	0.75
9	0.95	22	0.80
10	0.95	23	0.75
11	0.97	24	0.70
12	0.95	25	0.75
13	1.10	26	0.84

Summary Values

	Indoor Group	Outdoor Group
Σx	11.77	9.27
Σx^2	10.8011	6.6605
N	13	13
$\bar{x}$	0.905	0.713
$SS = \Sigma(x - \bar{x})^2 = \Sigma x^2 - (\Sigma x)^2/N$	0.1447	0.0503
$MS = s^2$	0.0121	0.0042
s	0.110	0.065

the same standard deviation, σ, then the ratio of the difference in
means to the standard error of the difference in means is

$$z = \frac{(\bar{x}_1 - \bar{x}_2) - 0}{\sigma^2 \sqrt{\dfrac{1}{N_1} + \dfrac{1}{N_2}}}.$$

For fixed N_1 and N_2, the factor $(1/N_1 + 1/N_2)$ in the standard
error is a minimum when $N_1 = N_2$. Thus, the efficiency (power) of
a comparison is greater for equal sample sizes. Since σ^2 is unknown,
however, it will be estimated from $s_1{}^2$ and $s_2{}^2$, as s^2 (MS). This s^2 is
a weighted average of $s_1{}^2$ and $s_2{}^2$, and is considered the best sample
estimate of the universe σ^2. It is obtained as

$$s^2 = \frac{\Sigma(x_1 - \bar{x}_1)^2 + (x_2 - \bar{x}_2)^2}{(N_1 - 1) + (N_2 - 1)} = \frac{0.1447 + 0.0503}{24} = \frac{0.1950}{24} = 0.0081.$$

Instead of forming the ratio z, we then form the ratio

$$t = \frac{(\bar{x}_1 - \bar{x}_2) - 0}{\sqrt{s^2 \left(\frac{1}{N_1} + \frac{1}{N_2}\right)}} = \frac{(0.905 - 0.713) - 0}{\sqrt{0.0081 \left(\frac{1}{13} + \frac{1}{13}\right)}} = \frac{0.192}{0.0353} = 5.44.$$

Under the null hypothesis, this ratio is distributed in the t-distribution with $(N_1 - 1) + (N_2 - 1) = 12 + 12 = 24$ degrees of freedom since s is based on 24 degrees of freedom.

The critical t-value with 24 degrees of freedom for $P = .01$ is 2.80, so that a $t = 5.$ is judged to be statistically significant at the 1% level. Thus, the null hypothesis, that the mean AAPL for the indoor and outdoor groups is the same, is rejected. In other words, it can be concluded that the means of the AAPL of the two groups are different from each other.

Frequently, because of the large sizes of N_1 and N_2, small differences of no practical importance attain statistical significance. Whether such differences merit interpretation depends on the investigator or the reader.

CONFIDENCE INTERVAL ON THE TRUE DIFFERENCE $(\mu_1 - \mu_2)$

Whether the null hypothesis $(\mu_1 - \mu_2 = 0)$ is rejected or not, one very often would like to know what the true difference $(\mu_1 - \mu_2)$ is. In view of the chance distribution of $(\bar{x}_1 - \bar{x}_2)$, one can use the same methods elaborated in Chapter 4 for pinning down the parameter $(\mu_1 - \mu_2)$. In other words, the 99% confidence interval,

$$(\bar{x}_1 - \bar{x}_2) - t \left(s \sqrt{\frac{1}{N_1} + \frac{1}{N_2}}\right) \text{ to } (\bar{x}_1 - \bar{x}_2) + t \left(s \sqrt{\frac{1}{N_1} + \frac{1}{N_2}}\right),$$

should cover the true value $(\mu_1 - \mu_2)$ with a confidence of 99%. The value of t involved is the value corresponding to df $= (N_1 + N_2) - 2$ which cuts off 1% in the tails. In our case, the interval is

$$(0.905 - 0.713) - 2.80(0.09)\sqrt{\frac{1}{13} + \frac{1}{13}} \text{ to } (0.905 - 0.713)$$

$$+ 2.80(0.09)\sqrt{\frac{1}{13} + \frac{1}{13}} = 0.093 \text{ to } 0.291.$$

We note that this interval does not include zero, which is consistent with our test of the null hypothesis. This confidence interval includes all the values of $(\mu_1 - \mu_2)$ against which $(\bar{x}_1 - \bar{x}_2)$ does not test as statistically significant at the 1% level. In our particular case, zero is not included since $(\bar{x}_1 - \bar{x}_2)$ differs significantly from zero. Even if $(\bar{x}_1 - \bar{x}_2)$ does not differ significantly from zero, so that the null hypothesis $(\mu_1 - \mu_2)$ is not disputed, the interval will still include a whole spectrum of values that is not disputed either. So, in this sense, the confidence interval is much more informative than the significance test which is just a yes or no proposition, as discussed in Chapter 4.

Of course, if one prefers to make significance tests at the 5% level, then one would use the 95% confidence interval. Parenthetically, before the actual values are filled in, the word "probability" may be used for the coverage of the interval. As soon as the actual values are filled in, for semantic reasons, the word "probability" is no longer correct.

ASSUMPTIONS UNDERLYING THE t-TEST FOR TWO INDEPENDENT SAMPLES

The use of the t-distribution for the testing of hypotheses about a difference of means assumes first of all that the x's of each sample, as well as the samples themselves, are independent of each other. A second assumption is that the universes or populations from which the samples were presumably drawn are normal distributions. Past experience with the variable or characteristic under examination will sometimes clue us about the underlying distributions, but on occasion one has to depend on the features of the samples themselves. Fortunately, the t-test is quite "robust," and the use of this test is not vitiated for moderate departures from normality.

If there is judged to be a considerable departure from normality, then the means are not very descriptive statistics in the first place, and the "robustness" of the t-test is of no particular consequence. Of course, with large departures from normality there may be some question as to just how robust the t-test is anyway. With such large degrees of non-normality, other techniques for testing hypotheses about centering constants can be utilized — e.g., distribution-free or nonparametric methods (Chapter 15, Ranking Tests) or, if possible, a transformation of the data to make the t-test more valid might be performed.

In addition to the assumption of normality of the parent populations, the t-test for two independent samples also assumes equality of the variances (σ_1^2 and σ_2^2) of the two universes (homoscedasticity).* The t-test is quite robust in this connection, too, particularly when the samples are of equal size, so that slight departures from equality of the variances do not rule out the t-test. If the variances are quite different, one would be inclined to calculate the ratio

$$\frac{(\bar{x}_1 - \bar{x}_2) - 0}{\sqrt{s_1^2/N_1 + s_2^2/N_2}}.$$

This ratio follows the t-distribution only approximately, with degrees of freedom somewhere between $(N_1 + N_2) - 2$ and the smaller of $(N_1 - 1)$ and $(N_2 - 1)$. If N_1 and N_2 are large, however, the ratio follows the standard normal curve — i.e., follows the distribution of z. This is, in fact, a better solution to the problem than to refer the ratio to the t-distribution. The same transformation or nonparametric method suggested for easing the problem of non-normality may ease the problem of heteroscedasticity.

Alternative Computation of t

The t-test just illustrated can be computed in a different manner using the analysis of variance approach. The results will be the same. The variation about the mean is measured in the indoor group (sample 1) as

$$SS_1 = \Sigma(x_1 - \bar{x}_1)^2 = \Sigma x_1^2 - (\Sigma x_1)^2/N_1 = 0.1447,$$

and in the outdoor group (sample 2) as

$$SS_2 = \Sigma(x_2 - \bar{x}_2)^2 = \Sigma x_2^2 - (\Sigma x_2)^2/N_2 = 0.0503.$$

The total sum of the squared deviations about the respective means of the two samples, called Sum of Squares or better, Sum of Squares Within Groups, is

$$SS = SS_1 + SS_2 = \Sigma(x_1 - \bar{x}_1)^2 + \Sigma(x_2 - \bar{x}_2)^2 = 0.1447 + 0.0503$$
$$= 0.1950.$$

---

*There is a test of the null hypothesis, $(\sigma_1^2 = \sigma_2^2)$, namely the F-test, where $F = s_1^2/s_2^2$. This ratio must be referred to the distribution of F under the null hypothesis (Chapter 7).

The Mean Square Within Groups is

$$s^2 = MS = \frac{\Sigma(x_1 - \bar{x}_1)^2 + \Sigma(x_2 - \bar{x}_2)^2}{N_1 + N_2 - 2} = \frac{0.1950}{24} = 0.0081,$$

as was previously calculated. This Mean Square, the pooled variance s^2, is also the sample estimate of the assumed common σ^2 of the two universes sampled. It is referred to as the Mean Square Within Groups (or samples) to indicate that it is the sample estimate of the fluctuation of observed experimental items about their respective means.

A measure of the difference between the two means is the SS Between Groups which is calculated

$$N_1(\bar{x}_1 - \bar{x}_0)^2 + N_2(\bar{x}_2 - \bar{x}_0)^2 = 13(0.91 - 0.81)^2 + 13(0.71 - 0.81)^2$$
$$= 0.2600,$$

where $\bar{x}_0 = 0.81 = $ the mean of all 26 readings. Since there are only two groups, i.e., only two means, $\bar{x}_1$ and $\bar{x}_2$, there is only one degree of freedom for this Sum of Squares. There is one restriction on the sum of the two squared deviations since

$$N_1(\bar{x}_1 - \bar{x}_0) + N_2(\bar{x}_2 - \bar{x}_0) = 0.$$

The Mean Square Between Groups is the Sum of Squares divided by the number of degrees of freedom, or $0.2197/1$. If there is no difference between the means of the populations μ_1 and μ_2, this Mean Square is an estimate of σ^2, just as is the Mean Square Within Groups. The final figures are summarized in Table 5.3, in which the Total Sum of Squares represents the variation of the 26 values of x about their mean, $\bar{x}_0$, without regard to group distinction. That is,

$$\text{Total SS} = \Sigma(x - \bar{x}_0)^2 = \Sigma x^2 - (\Sigma x)^2/(N_1 + N_2) = 0.4147.$$

Under the null hypothesis ($\mu_1 = \mu_2$), 0.2197 and 0.0081 represent two independent estimates of the same value, σ^2. If there is a real difference between the universe means (the null hypothesis is false), the Mean Square Between Groups tends to be inflated and will, on the average, be larger than the Mean Square Within Groups. The ratio

$$\sqrt{\frac{\text{Mean Square Between Groups}}{\text{Mean Square Within Groups}}} = \sqrt{\frac{0.2197}{0.0081}} = \sqrt{27.1235} = 5.21$$

TABLE 5.3
Analysis of Variance Table of AAPL Data in Table 5.2

Source of Variance	Degrees of Freedom (df)	Sum of Squares (SS)	Mean Square
Between Groups	1	0.2197	0.2197
Within Groups	24	0.1950	0.0081
Total	25	0.4147	

is precisely equal to the t-value calculated by the previous method, and obviously has 24 degrees of freedom.

The advantage of this alternative method of calculation is that it can be extended to more than two samples (groups) as well as to more complex experimental designs. This will be illustrated in Chapter 7 where shortcut formulas are also presented to facilitate the arithmetic.

RELATED OR PAIRED SAMPLES

In another type of experimental design, instead of the available experimental material being divided into two groups and the mean of the two groups (i.e., treated and control) then compared, the same group is subjected to two different situations. This assumes that an individual can be used for both situations. The individual is then said to serve as his own control, the *cross-over design*. The two situations (treatments) should be assigned in random order. The data are then obtained as two series of measurements, for the same groups of individuals, so that the measurements in the two series are not independent of, but, in fact, are correlated with each other. Such correlated or paired samples also occur when the subjects are twins, litter mates, or bilateral parts of the same individual, where one member of the pair is assigned one treatment and the second member is assigned the other treatment. The pairs may also be formed by stratifying on some underlying relevant characteristic, such as weight, or age.

Such types of experimental design are preferred to those employing two independent samples, since the use of correlated samples serves to reduce experimental errors more than is possible in the former case, because of the correlation produced by the pairing. One of the more frequently employed examples of the paired-sample design occurs in the so-called "before and after" experiment. Unfortunately, the experimental design dictates the order of assignment of treatments, so that randomization is generally not possible with the result that the treatment effect may be confounded with a time effect.

For example, Dorman and Bishop[2] studied the oxygen tension of dog gingiva by varying the total body metabolic demand. They measured the metabolic rates of eight mongrel dogs by the use of a Benedict-Roth metabolator before and after injection of 130 mg/100 cc of saturated dinitrophenol solution into the femoral artery. The data appear in Table 5.4, measured in Cal/M^2/hr.

In these data, the before measurement for each animal is paired with the after measurement, and the increase in metabolic rate (after minus before) calculated as the difference, d. These eight values of d are then treated as a series of eight measurements. If the injection of dinitrophenol has no effect on the metabolic rate of the dogs, then in a universe of such animals the average increase would be zero (the null hypothesis). The question is whether the observed average increase for the eight dogs differs significantly from zero — a two-tailed test. The appropriate test would be the one sample t-test (Chapter 4), assuming that the distribution of d is normal.

The ratio of the average difference to the standard error of the average difference is

$$t = \frac{(\bar{d} - 0)}{\text{est. SE}_{\bar{d}}} = \frac{(\bar{d} - 0)}{s_d/\sqrt{N}}.$$

This ratio is distributed in the t-curve with $(N - 1) = 8 - 1 = 7$ degrees of freedom.

$$\bar{d}^2 = \Sigma d/N = 724/8 = 90.50 \text{ Cal/M}^2/\text{hr}.$$

$$s_d{}^2 = \Sigma d^2 - (\Sigma d)^2/N = 79,078 - (724)^2/8 = 1,936.571$$

$$\text{est. SE}_{\bar{d}} = \sqrt{s_d{}^2/N} = \sqrt{(1,936.5714)} = 15.56$$

$$t = \text{est.}\frac{\bar{d} - 0}{\text{SE}_{\bar{d}}} = \frac{90.50}{15.56} = 5.82 \text{ with df} = 7.$$

The critical t-value with 7 degrees of freedom for $P = .01$ is 3.50, so that a t of 5.82 is statistically significant at the 1% level. The null hypothesis that dinitrophenol has no effect on the metabolic rate of these dogs, is therefore rejected. We are assuming, of course, that the act of injection, per se, as well as the lapse of time between the

TABLE 5.4
Gingival Oxygen Tension Following Dinitrophenol*

Dog Number	Before Dinitrophenol	After Dinitrophenol	(d) After – Before
1	47	73	26
2	47	208	161
3	60	183	123
4	55	157	102
5	58	95	37
6	47	154	107
7	60	147	87
8	37	118	81
Total			724

*$Cal/M^2/hr$.

before and after measurements does not produce any changes in the metabolic rate.

If we are not satisfied with these assumptions, we need a control group, another group, obtained by randomization in which we repeat all the maneuvers of the experimental group except for the actual drug (treatment) itself. The d's of the two groups are then compared by the method of independent samples.

The confidence interval on the true difference in a universe of dogs is obtained as described in Chapter 4 for the one sample case, namely, $\bar{d} \pm t(est. SE_{\bar{d}})$. The 99% confidence interval is 13.68 – 167.33.

For the analysis of paired samples to apply, the pairing must be an integral part of the structure of the experiment from the beginning. If, in a fully randomized arrangement with two independent samples and $N_1 = N_2$, measurements were grouped at random into pairs before analysis, no advantage would be gained (since, on the average, there would be no correlation between the two samples and the variance of the difference would be unaffected), and degrees of freedom would be unnecessarily lost, i.e., $(N - 1)$ as opposed to $2(N - 1)$. On the other hand, if pairs were formed in accordance with some property of the measurements themselves (e.g., highest of the controls with highest of the treatments, second highest with second highest, and so on), the analysis using pairs would be biased.[3]

The computations of the t-test for paired samples can also be carried out by an analysis of variance procedure, although more complicated than in the case of two independent samples. Again, this has the advantage that it can be extended to more than two treatments (see Chapter 7).

TABLE 5.5

Caries Activity Measured as New Carious Surfaces Per 100 Intact Surfaces Per Year for Individuals Using Zephiran or Urea as a Dentifrice[4]

	Zephiran Group				Urea Group		
Patient	Control Period (C)	Expt. Period (E)	$C - E$ (d_1)	Patient	Control Period (C)	Expt. Period (E)	$C - E$ (d_2)
EB	15.0	5.1	+ 9.9	EB	13.0	2.6	+10.4
RB	7.3	0.7	+ 6.6	DB	8.8	0.5	+ 8.3
TC	12.0	5.3	+ 6.7	RD	29.0	0.0	+29.0
GH	6.1	0.8	+ 5.3	JJ	25.0	0.0	+25.0
CH	8.3	3.1	+ 5.2	AM	9.0	0.0	+ 9.0
ER	18.0	3.2	+14.8	ET	11.0	1.4	+ 9.6

Summary Values

	Zephiran Group	Urea Group
Σd	48.5	91.3
Σd^2	460.63	1,816.21
N	6	6
$\bar{d}$	+8.08	15.22
$SS = \Sigma(d - \bar{d})^2$	68.59	426.93
$MS = s^2$	13.72	71.16
s	3.70	8.44

TWO INDEPENDENT SAMPLES OF DIFFERENCES

Stephan and Miller[4] performed a pilot study in which the results of brushing with a 1:1000 flavored solution of a synthetic detergent, Zephiran, twice a day, were compared with the results obtained with a similar group of patients brushing similarly with a saturated solution of urea. Since it was realized that individual caries susceptibility varies greatly, all the patients were studied for about 18 months prior to the experimental period. In that way, the "normal" caries attack-rate for each individual was obtained. Because the periods of observation during the control and experimental phases varied somewhat for each individual, the caries attack-rate was calculated for each subject for each phase as new carious surfaces per year per 100 intact surfaces. These attack-rates and their differences appear in Table 5.5.

The average difference in the caries attack-rate of one group is then compared with the corresponding average difference for the other group by the t-test for independent samples. It is assumed that the difference in caries attack-rates is approximately normal. Thus,

$$s^2 = \frac{\Sigma (d_1 - \bar{d}_1)^2 + (d_2 - \bar{d}_2)^2}{(N_1 - 1) + (N_2 - 1)} = \frac{68.59 + 426.93}{5 + 5} = 49.552$$

and

$$t = \frac{(\bar{d}_1 - \bar{d}_2) - 0}{\sqrt{s^2 \left(\frac{1}{N_1} + \frac{1}{N_2} \right)}} = \frac{8.08 - 15.22}{\sqrt{49.552 \left(\frac{1}{6} + \frac{1}{6} \right)}} = \frac{-7.14}{4.06} = -1.76.$$

In this problem, there are $N_1 + N_2 - 2 = 10$ df. From Table 4.4, for $P = .01$, $t = 3.17$, so that the average difference in the caries attack-rate of the group using Zephiran does not differ significantly at the 1% level from the average difference in caries attack-rate for the group using urea.

The confidence interval on the true difference between the two groups would be calculated as in the case of two independent samples already described.

For further reading on the background and application of the t-test, the reader is referred to recent papers by Feinstein.[5,6]

REFERENCES

1. Perlitsch, M. J., Neilsen, A. G., and Stanmyer, W. R.: Ascorbic acid plasma levels and gingival health in personnel wintering over in Antarctica. J Dent Res 40:789, 1961.

2. Dorman, H. L., and Bishop, J. G.: Effect of increased metabolism on oxygen tension of gingival tissue, J Dent Res 44:57, 1965.

3. Finney, D. J.: Experimental Design and Its Statistical Basis, Chicago, Univ. of Chicago Press, 1955, p. 41.

4. Stephan, R. M., and Miller, B. F.: Effectiveness of urea and synthetic detergents in reducing activity of human dental caries, Proc Soc Exp Biol Med 55:101, 1944.

5. Feinstein, A. R.: Clinical Biostatistics. LV. The t test and the basic ethos of parametric statistical inference (Part I), Clin Pharm and Thera 29:548, 1981.

6. Feinstein, A. R.: Clinical Biostatistics, LVI. The t test and the basic ethos of parametric statistical inference (conclusion), Clin Pharm and Thera 30:133, 1981.

6
Estimation of Sample Size (Means)

How large a sample is necessary to estimate adequately a population parameter or to test adequately a particular hypothesis? Every investigator who employs inductive reasoning confronts this question. And it is more than theoretical, because the size of the sample to be used will determine, to some extent, the funds requested in a grant, the experimental model to be used, and, in some cases, the type of experiment to be performed.[1]

Many investigators have recognized the need for consultation with someone to assist them in determining how many cases or animals or patients (size of sample) are necessary in the contemplated survey or experiment. The investigator will often phrase the question, "How many cases do I need to make my experiment mean something?" This question has no answer. A more careful phrasing, "How many cases do I need to have a significant result?" still has no answer. What is needed is information as to what precision of the estimate is desired or what contemplated result is considered important. Often, a certain amount of preliminary data is essential. Such information may have been gained through previous experience with the problem under investigation, either by the individual or others, or as a result of a preliminary or pilot study.

In other words, before a definite answer can be given about the necessary sample size of a survey or an experiment, some clue as to how the results are going to run must be available. As a matter of fact, this is the usual sequence in most laboratories: Some preliminary studies are performed before the larger, more definitive experiment is set up.

The estimations of sample size discussed in this chapter are concerned only with the simple problems of estimating a mean of a population, estimating the difference between the means of two populations, comparing a sample mean with a population mean, and comparing the means of two independent or two correlated samples. Since these are problems involving only a single comparison, they may be referred to as *one degree of freedom* problems. They are problems that can be typically solved by the t-test, or, in the case of large samples, by the normal curve test. Problems involving more than one degree of freedom, such as many in the analysis of variance, are much more complicated and are not amenable to the simple solutions offered here, except insofar as they can be broken up into 1 df problems.

SAMPLE SIZE FOR
SPECIFIED CONFIDENCE INTERVAL

One-Sample Problem

The confidence interval problem for the one-sample case is simpler than the significance test, since one merely specifies the desired precision, $D = |\bar{x} - \mu|$, and the probability or confidence coefficient, $(1 - \alpha)$, that this discrepancy will not be exceeded. In the hypothesis test, a null hypothesis, μ_0, and a suitable alternative hypothesis, μ_1, are specified, as well as the two probabilities: α, that μ_0 will be rejected when it is the true mean and $(1 - \beta)$, that μ_0 will be rejected when μ_1 is the true mean. Discrimination between μ_0 and μ_1 will require a larger sample size than pinning down the parameter μ with the desired precision.

An idea of the variability of the material should be available, i.e., σ_x, in order to specify any meaningful interval. Suppose, for example, on the basis of a preliminary study, or a past study, it is known that the standard deviation of plasma inorganic phosphorus is 0.40 mg%. A sample of size N is taken under somewhat different conditions and we would like to pin down the μ of the universe from which the sample is regarded as being drawn. What sample size is required so that $\bar{x}$ will be within 0.10 units of μ, so that $D = |\bar{x} - \mu|$ i.e., half the confidence interval, does not exceed 0.10? If a 95% confidence interval is desired, then half the width of the confidence interval corresponds to 1.96 standard errors. That is

$$0.10 = 1.96[(0.40)/\sqrt{N}].$$

Solving,

$$N = 61.5.$$

A sample of approximately 62 would be required in order to have the universe mean covered by the interval $\bar{x}$ -0.10 to $\bar{x}$ +0.10 with the desired probability. It is assumed here that σ is known to be 0.40 so that the normal distribution (z) would be appropriate. Ordinarily, what happens is that only a vague idea of the value of σ is available, so that once the sample is obtained, the estimated standard error of the mean, using s, is employed. The value of 1.96 would then not be appropriate for the 95% confidence interval, but rather the value obtained from the t-table. The value of N obtained by the above procedure is thus a slight underestimate. Of course, once the sample of N is taken, $\bar{x}$, s_x, and est. $SE_{\bar{x}}$ are computed and the confidence interval established is $\bar{x} \pm t$ est. $SE_{\bar{x}}$ as in Chapter 4.

Perhaps a more frequent approach is to specify the precision as a certain fraction of the standard deviation, say

$$\Delta = \frac{|\bar{x} - \mu|}{\sigma} = \frac{D}{\sigma}.$$

While this procedure seems to avoid the need for some preliminary knowledge of σ, such knowledge is essential if the specified fraction Δ is to be meaningful. It is true, of course, that the importance of a given discrepancy $D = |\bar{x} - \mu|$ should depend upon the variability of x. A discrepancy of 0.10 when $\sigma = 0.4$ is quite different than if σ were 1.

If the precision is specified as $\frac{1}{4}$ of the standard deviation to correspond to the above example, then, using the normal curve procedure, $\Delta = \frac{1}{4} = 1.96/\sqrt{N}$. Solving, N = 61.5, as found previously.

In general, $N = (1.96)^2\sigma^2/D^2 = (1.96)^2/\Delta^2$. Of course, the 1.96 is changed if some other confidence interval is desired, e.g., 2.58 for a 99% confidence interval.

Paired Sample Problem

The procedure just given is also sufficient for paired or correlated samples, since problems of this nature are transformed into a one-sample type involving a difference between the two samples. The sample of differences is summarized by $\bar{d}$ and s_d. One either specifies a desired precision $D = |\bar{d} - \mu_d|$ and has some idea of σ_d, or else one specifies $\Delta = |\bar{d} - \mu_d|/\sigma_d$. For example, in a small study, the change in the erythrocyte sedimentation rate of patients with periodontal disease subsequent to surgical eradication of the periodontal pockets, varies with $s_d = 5$ units. What should the N of a large definitive study be so that $|\bar{d} - \mu_d|$ does not exceed 2, with a probability $(1 - \alpha)$ of .99? Taking

$$\Delta \text{ as } |\bar{d} - \mu_d|/\sigma_d = 2/5 = 0.4,$$
$$N = (2.58)^2/(0.4)^2 = 41.6.$$

we find that 42 cases are evidently required. Again, this is a slight underestimate since s_d of the sample and the critical value of t would be used.

Case of Two Independent Samples

In this case, we wish to estimate $(\mu_1 - \mu_2)$ with a precision

$$D = |(\bar{x}_1 - \bar{x}_2) - (\mu_1 - \mu_2)|.$$

From some preliminary observations or past experience, some knowledge of $\sigma_1 = \sigma_2 = \sigma$, is available. D is expressed in terms of σ as $\Delta = D/\sigma$. If we take $N_1 = N_2$,* so that $SE_{\bar{x}_1 - \bar{x}_2} = \sigma\sqrt{2/N}$, then for the 95% confidence interval,

$$D = 1.96\sigma\sqrt{2/N}, \text{ or } \Delta = 1.96\sqrt{2/N}.$$
$$N = 2(1.96)^2\sigma^2/D^2 \quad = 2(1.96)^2/\Delta^2.$$

Suppose that in a small group of caries-free patients and in caries-active patients, σ is estimated as approximately 5. Question: What N is required in each group to pin down $(\mu_1 - \mu_2)$ with a precision, i.e., half confidence interval, of 3 units, with a probability of $(1 - \alpha) = .95$? Using our estimate of σ as stable,

$$\Delta = 3/5 = 0.6, N = 2(1.96)^2/(0.6)^2 = 21.3,$$

22 cases would evidently be needed in each group. Of course, after samples of this size have been taken, $\bar{x}_1, \bar{x}_2,$ s, and est. $SE_{\bar{x}_1 - \bar{x}_2}$ will

---

*If it assumed that N_1 is a certain multiple, k, of N_2, i.e., $N_1 = kN_2$, then the sample size problem can be solved for unequal N's.

be calculated in the usual manner, and the confidence interval established as $(\bar{x}_1 - \bar{x}_2) \pm$ est. $SE_{\bar{x}_1 - \bar{x}_2}$, as in Chapter 4.

SAMPLE SIZE FOR SIGNIFICANCE TESTS

One-Sample Case

One-Tailed Test

A standard mean for plasma inorganic phosphorus is given as $\mu_0 = 4$ units. It is known that the standard deviation is 0.4 units. In patients with generalized osteoporosis, it is suspected that the mean organic phosphorus, μ_1, differs from the standard, being larger than μ_0. If the difference is as large as 0.20, i.e., $\mu_1 - \mu_0 = 0.2$, it is desirable to reject the null hypothesis that the mean is μ_0 and to declare statistical significance, stating that $\mu_1 > \mu_0$. The test is to be made at the α level. In addition, one has to specify the desired probability of rejecting the null hypothesis if, in fact, $(\mu_1 - \mu_0) = 0.2$ is the true difference, i.e., the power $(1 - \beta)$ has to be specified. The question, as phrased, called for a one-sided (one-tailed) test.

Using the standard deviation of 0.40 as σ, the problem amounts to determining N so that two sampling distributions of $\bar{x}$ do not overlap more than a stated amount. One of the distributions is centered at $\mu_0 = 4$, and the other at $\mu_1 = 4.2$. Using a 1% significance level ($z = 2.33$) and a power of 95% ($z = -1.64$), the overlap is shown in Figure 6.1.

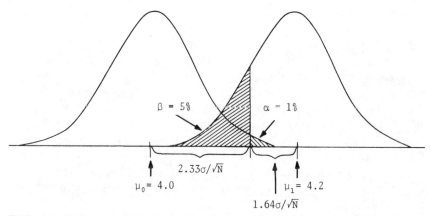

FIG. 6.1 Estimate of Sample Size for Distinguishing Between $\mu_0 = 4.0$ and $\mu_1 = 4.2$ in a One-Tailed Significance Test.

The point cutting off $\alpha = 1\%$ in the upper tail of the curve centered at μ_0 is $\mu_0 + 2.33\sigma/\sqrt{N}$ and must coincide with the point cutting off 5% in the lower tail of the curve centered at 4.2, which is $\mu_1 - 1.64\sigma/\sqrt{N}$. Evidently, the distance from μ_0 to μ_1 must equal $2.33\sigma/\sqrt{N} + 1.64\sigma/\sqrt{N}$.

That is, $(\mu_0 - \mu_1) = (2.33 + 1.64)\sigma/\sqrt{N}$

$$0.2 = (2.33 + 1.64)(0.4)/\sqrt{N}$$

Solving for N, $N = 63.$

In general, $N = (2.33 + 1.64)^2 \sigma^2/(\mu_1 - \mu_\varrho)^2.$

The specification of $(\mu_1 - \mu_0)$ is often expressed as a multiple (Δ) of σ. While the use of Δ seems to make an idea of σ unnecessary, Δ cannot be translated into a meaningful $(\mu_1 - \mu_0)$ without knowledge of σ. In our example,

$$\Delta = (\mu_1 - \mu_2)/\sigma = 0.2/0.4 = 0.5.$$

The size of Δ tells us the amount of overlap of the two distributions of x's, e.g., $\Delta = 1$ implies that 16% of each curve lies beyond the mean of the other curve. $N = (2.33 + 1.64)^2/\Delta^2 = 63$, as before. Actually, the significance test will be performed using s and the t-distribution, so that the required sample size is slightly larger (66, by using the *noncentral t-distribution*).[2]

Two-Tailed Test

The more usual significance test is two-tailed. In that case, the difference is specified as $|\mu_1 - \mu_2| = 0.2$. The specified α, say .01, is put into two tails of the curve centered at μ_0, with .005 in each tail. The alternative curve is centered at 4.2 or at 3.8, (the same solution results) with 5% of the area in the lower tail of the curve centered at 4.2 (or 5% in the upper tail centered at 3.8). With the usual choices of α and β, rejection cannot be made in both tails, i.e., if $\mu_1 = 3.8$, $\bar{x}$ cannot fall into the upper tail of the curve centered at 4.0. Similarly, if $\mu_1 = 4.2$, $\bar{x}$ cannot fall into the lower tail of the curve centered at 4.0. The indicated solution is given in Figure 6.2 for a power $(1 - \beta)$ of 0.95. In essence, we have two distributions of $\bar{x}$, one centered at μ_0 and one at μ_1.

The distance from μ_0 to μ_1 must equal $(\mu_1 - \mu_0) = (2.58 + 1.64)\sigma/\sqrt{N}$. In our case,

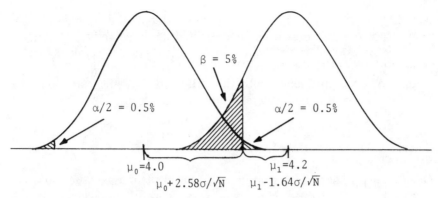

FIG. 6.2 Estimate of Sample Size for Distinguishing Between μ_0 = 4.0 and μ_1 = 4.2 in a Two-Tailed Test.

$0.2 = (2.58 + 1.64)(0.4)/\sqrt{N}$. Solving, N = 71.2, or 72. (Using the noncentral t-distribution, N = 75.)

The solution amounts to the following: If the true mean is 4.2 (or 3.8), we want the smallest (or largest) $\bar{x}$ still to be significantly different from 4.0 at the α level, where the smallest (or largest) value is determined by β.

We note that if one were solving for N for a 99% confidence interval (see page 81), one would not speak of power $(1 - \beta)$, and the factor 1.64 does not enter into the solution, and

$0.2 = (2.58)(0.4)/\sqrt{N}$, giving N = 26.6 or 27, a great deal smaller than when a discrimination is to be made between two parameters (N = 72).

In essence, the confidence interval solution corresponds to centering a second curve at 4.2, but using a power $(1 - \beta)$ of 0.5. Indeed, the question often posed is: "If I get a difference of 0.2, what must N be to make this difference statistically significant at the particular α level?"; instead of "If the true difference is 0.2, what must N be to have a high probability $(1 - \beta)$ of saying that it is not 0, i.e., of finding statistical significance"?

Obviously, the N required depends on the quantities $\Delta - (\mu_1 - \mu_0)/\sigma$, α, and β. In the example described above, if Δ is taken as 0.1, just half the previous value, N is quadrupled to 285. If a very high power is specified, e.g., $(1 - \beta)$ = .99, with α = .01, Δ = 0.2, N = $(2.58 + 2.33)^2/\Delta^2$ = 96. A frequent choice for α is .05 and for β is .80, particularly in clinical trials. With these values for Δ = 0.2, N becomes N = $(1.96 + 0.84)^2/\Delta^2$ = 31.

Sometimes the size of N determined by the procedure is said to be the N necessary to detect the alternative mean μ_1 when it is true.

Actually, it is only the size necessary to detect the falseness of μ_0 when μ_1 is the true mean. When statistical significance is declared, all that can be said is that the mean is not μ_0. Its possible values can be given by a confidence interval and will not include μ_0. Likewise, a finding of nonsignificance with the indicated N means that the mean is not μ_1. A confidence interval would not cover μ_1.

Selecting Alpha and Beta Levels

One of the problems facing an investigator in planning a study is what levels of α and β to use. He can be very "careful" and select $\alpha = .01$ and $\beta = .99$, but this may indeed be too conservative and require very large samples, also incurring great expense. If the consequences of declaring statistical significance when the null hypothesis is true are extremely important, such as the replacing of a standard treatment or diagnostic method with a new one, then a Type I error may be quite serious and α should be kept small, say, .01. If previous studies, which are part of the published literature, have tended to establish certain conclusions and the current study would merely confirm these concepts, the consequences of making this Type I error are less grave, and $\alpha = .05$ would usually be acceptable, particularly in clinical trials.

The power of the test $(1 - \beta)$ is usually selected after the level of α has been determined. Cohen[3] has suggested that in many instances, the Type I error is about four times as serious as the Type II error, so that, as Fleiss[4] has stated, "This implies that one should set β, the probability of a Type II error, approximately equal to 4α, so that the power becomes approximately $1 - \beta = 1 - 4\alpha$. Thus, when $\alpha = .01$, $1 - \beta$ may be set at .95; for $\alpha = .02$, set $\beta = .90$; and for $\alpha = .05$, set $1 - \beta = .80$."

CORRELATED SAMPLES

Since the data from the two paired samples are converted into a single sample of differences d, the question of sample size (number of pairs) has already been answered in the previous section on the one-sample problem. Because this design has wide application in dental and oral research, however, another example will be given: Two different techniques may be used to measure the same characteristic of one sample of individuals, or the same characteristics may be measured in one group at two different times. A frequent application of this is the so-called *before-and-after design*, in which a sample is studied for the same characteristic before and after a certain treatment is applied. Thus, for example, we can take the problem of comparing the erythrocyte sedimentation rate in a group of individuals with periodontal disease, before and after surgical eradication of the periodontal pockets. The results of a preliminary study using a small group of nine patients are presented in Table 6.1.[5]

The t-test for statistical significance then proceeds as follows:

$$s_d^2 = \left[\Sigma d^2 - \frac{(\Sigma d)^2}{N} \right] / (N-1)$$

$$= \frac{N \Sigma d^2 - (\Sigma d)^2}{N(N-1)} = \frac{9(349) - (27)^2}{9(9-1)} = 33.50,$$

$$\text{est. SE}_{\bar{d}}^2 = \frac{s_d^2}{N} = \frac{33.50}{9} = 3.72,$$

$$\text{est. } t = \frac{\bar{d}}{SE_{\bar{d}}} = \frac{3.00}{1.93} = 1.55.$$

From the standard tables of t at N - 1 = 8 df (Table 4.4), we find that t_8 = 1.86 at the 10% level and 1.40 at the 20% level of P. Thus,

TABLE 6.1
Erythrocyte Sedimentation Rates (mm/hr) of Nine Patients With Periodontal Disease, Before and After Surgical Eradication of the Periodontal Pockets*

Patient Number	Before Surgery (x_1)	After Surgery (x_2)	Difference $(x_1 - x_2)$ (d)
1	10	15	− 5
2	8	3	+ 5
3	6	2	+ 4
4	9	5	+ 1
5	11	4	+ 7
6	23	15	+ 8
7	13	4	+ 9
8	11	8	+ 3
9	2	10	− 8
	Σx_1 = 93	Σx_2 = 66	Σd = +27
	$\bar{x}_1$ = 10.3	$\bar{x}_2$ = 7.3	$\bar{d}$ = + 3.0

*These data have been taken for illustrative purposes only; any conclusions drawn do not necessarily pertain to the results of the original study.

the value of $t = 1.55$ which we have found, can be exceeded by chance factors alone between 10% and 20% of the time, so that the average difference in ESR before and after periodontal surgery is statistically not significant.

The investigator might feel, however, that there is a real difference in means, μ_d, but that more extensive data are needed to establish this fact. The question then arises: If further experimentation were to produce a sizable difference in the ESR after periodontal surgery, how many cases would be needed to demonstrate the statistical significance of this difference?

We may set up confidence limits on μ_d to guide us as to what average difference it is feasible to expect. For 8 df we find that a value of t of 2.31 will be exceeded 5% of the time through the action of chance factors alone. Accordingly, the 95% confidence range on μ_d is $3.00 - 2.31$ est. SE_d to $3.00 + 2.31$ est. SE_d, or from -1.46 to 7.46.

The investigator may feel that it is worthwhile to detect a true average reduction of 3.00 mm/hr. If the true average reduction $D = (\mu_d - 0)$ were 3.00 mm/hr., how many cases would be necessary for there to be a 95% probability that the observed average reduction would be significantly greater than zero at the 1% level? The question as asked calls for a one-tailed significance test. The upper 1% of the area of the normal curve centered at zero difference (the null hypothesis corresponding to μ_0 in the one-sample test in the previous section) falls to the right of $0 + 2.33(s_d/\sqrt{N})$; 5% of the area of the curve centered at 3.00 falls to the left of $3.00 - 1.64(s_d/\sqrt{N})$. Thus,

$$2.33(s_d/\sqrt{N} + 1.64(s_d/\sqrt{N}) = 3.00$$

(s_d will be used as if it were σ_d). Solving, we find N to be about 56 cases, i.e., pairs. Of course, the 9 cases do not form a part of the 59! Frequently, D is expressed as a multiple of σ as $\Delta = D/\sigma_d$. Of course, the same N results using a one-sided significance test.

Table 6.2 presents the approximate size of the sample necessary for significance to be asserted in this experiment for selected values of the true average reduction corresponding to various significance levels and powers of the test.

Note that while the problem can be solved by the normal curve (or more accurately, by the noncentral t-distribution) in terms of Δ without knowing σ, one does not know what μ_d is implied by a certain Δ unless one has some knowledge of σ. Taking $\Delta = 3.00/5.79 = 0.52$, for $\alpha = 1$, $\beta = 5$, the noncentral t-distribution gives N = 62 for a one-sided test and 70 for a two-sided test.

TABLE 6.2
Approximate Size of the Sample Necessary to Assert Significance, Assuming s_a = 5.79 mm per hour.

True Average Difference to Be Detected	1% Level of Significance, 99% Power of Test	1% Level of Significance, 95% Power of Test	5% Level of Significance, 95% Power of Test
3.00	80(90)*	59(66)	40(48)
4.00	45(50)	33(37)	23(27)
5.00	29(32)	21(24)	14(17)

*Numbers in parentheses refer to two-sided tests which always require larger samples.

INDEPENDENT SAMPLES

Hess and Smith performed salivary ascorbic acid determinations on two small groups of individuals with and without dental caries.[6] They presumably were comparable in all pertinent characteristics, for example, age, sex, general health status, except their caries susceptibility. The data presented in Table 6.3 were taken from the overall observations and are employed here for illustrative purposes,

TABLE 6.3
Ascorbic Acid Content of Saliva (mg/10,000 cc) of Nine Caries-Free and Nine Caries-Active Patients

Caries-Free Patients (x_1)	Caries-Active Patients (x_2)
20	19
31	9
14	13
19	20
21	21
17	15
13	12
24	19
22	18

Summary Values

$\Sigma x_1 = 181$	$\Sigma x_2 = 146$
$\Sigma x_1^2 = 3{,}877$	$\Sigma x_2^2 = 2{,}506$
$N_1 = 9$	$N_2 = 9$
$\bar{x}_1 = 20.1$	$\bar{x}_2 = 16.2$
$SS_1 = 236.99$	$SS_2 = 137.56$

so that any conclusions drawn do not necessarily pertain to the results of the original study as a whole.

The pooled variance, s^2, is obtained as the weighted average of the two variances, as

$$s^2 = \frac{SS_1 + SS_2}{(N_1 - 1) + (N_2 - 1)} = \frac{236.99 + 137.56}{8 + 8} = 23.41.$$

The t-test for comparing the means of two independent samples is

$$t = \frac{(\bar{x}_1 - \bar{x}_2) - 0}{SE_{\bar{x}_1 - \bar{x}_2}} = \frac{20.1 - 16.2}{\sqrt{23.1 \left(\frac{1}{9} + \frac{1}{9}\right)}} = \frac{3.9}{2.3},$$

and

$$t = 1.70, \text{ at } df = (N_1 - 1) + (N_2 - 1) = 16.$$

Referring to standard tables of t (Table 4.4), the values of t for 16 df exceeded by chance alone 10% and 5% of the time are found to be 1.75 and 2.12, respectively. The difference between the average ascorbic acid level in the two groups (3.9 mg) thus can be exceeded more than 10% of the time through the action of chance factors alone, and it is termed "statistically not significant." The null hypothesis being tested, that there is no difference between the average salivary ascorbic acid level of caries-free and caries-active individuals, therefore cannot be rejected.

The investigator may examine his results and feel that, while the difference in average salivary ascorbic acid is not significant, it is suggestive. Further, he may feel that if he were to conduct a larger experiment with more cases in each group, the difference in salivary ascorbic acid would become statistically significant. The question to be answered, then, is: How many patients are needed for the definitive experiment.[2]

This question can be answered now, since we have some preliminary information about the way in which the results occur. What is first needed, however, is a clear statement of what difference in average salivary ascorbic acid is considered to be statistically significant. The investigator must realize that in the two new groups to be selected, the average difference may not be 3.9 mg. From the preliminary study, it is known that the variability of the difference in means, est. $(SE_{\bar{x}_1 - \bar{x}_2})$ for groups of nine each is 2.3 mg. Therefore, confidence limits can be set up around the average difference (3.9

mg), which will cover the true difference in means $(\mu_1 - \mu_2)$. The 95% confidence interval on $(\mu_1 - \mu_2)$, extending from

$$(\bar{x}_1 - \bar{x}_2) - 2.12 \text{ est. } SE_{\bar{x}_1 - \bar{x}_2} \text{ to } (\bar{x}_1 - \bar{x}_2) + 2.12 \text{ est. } SE_{\bar{x}_1 - \bar{x}_2};$$

in this case, from

$$3.9 - (2.12)(2.3) \text{ to } 3.9 + (2.12)(2.3), \text{ or from } -1.0 \text{ to } 8.8.*$$

Although the observed difference in means of 3.9 mg was not significantly different from zero, it can be noted from the confidence limits that the true difference in means could be as large as 8.8 mg in favor of the caries-free group. The investigator may use this confidence range to guide him to what true difference might be feasible or possible in a future, more definitive experiment. For example, the investigator may decide that a difference of 4.0 mg in salivary ascorbic acid in favor of the caries-free group is important and, from the confidence range given previously, evidently feasible. Once he decides what true difference to focus on, he can start to answer the question regarding sample size. An approximate solution to this question is given in the following discussion.

One-tailed Test

If the investigator is interested in "detecting a true difference" of at least 4.0 mg in favor of the caries-free group, he can determine how many cases the new study must include so that the observed difference between the means of the caries-free and caries-active groups $(\bar{x}_1 - \bar{x}_2)$ is significantly greater than zero. If the true difference were zero, the normal curve of differences in means would be centered at zero with an estimated standard deviation given by

$$\text{est. } SE_{\bar{x}_1 - \bar{x}_2} = s \sqrt{\frac{1}{N_1} + \frac{1}{N_2}}.$$

Since it is always simpler and, generally, more efficient to have the sizes of both samples the same, we shall put $N_1 = N_2$, so that

$$\text{est. } SE_{\bar{x}_1 - \bar{x}_2} = s \sqrt{\frac{2}{N}}.$$

---

*Without reference to the t-tables, we often say that the true value should fall within 2 standard errors of the observed value, i.e., $3.9 \pm 2(2.3) = -0.7$ to 8.5.

It is assumed that the value of s, determined in the preliminary experiment, will continue to be the average standard deviation of the readings in the two groups in the second, larger experiment. It is further assumed that the second experiment will be large enough for the normal curve to be used instead of the t-curve.

The investigator must next decide whether he should use the 5% or 1% level of significance. He chooses 5% if he is willing to take a chance five times out of 100 of saying that the true difference in means is greater than zero when, in fact, it is zero. Let us assume that he chooses 1% because he would like to take this chance only once in 100 times (α).

If 40 mg were the true difference, then of course the normal curve of differences in means would be centered at 4.0 mg with a standard deviation

$$SE_{\bar{x}_1 - \bar{x}_2} = s \sqrt{\frac{2}{N}}.$$

The investigator must decide how large a chance he wants to take of having the observed difference be not significantly greater than zero, when, in fact, the true difference is 4.0 mg. He may want to take this chance only five times in 100. This would insure that if the true difference is 4.0 mg, the observed difference will be significantly greater than zero 95% of the time. The power of the test, $(1 - \beta)$, is 0.95.

The specific question then can be framed: "If the true difference (in favor of the caries-free group) between the mean values of salivary ascorbic acid in the caries-free and caries-active groups is really 4.0 mg, how many cases should be studied in the new experiment so that the probability is 95% that the observed difference in means ($\bar{x}_1 - \bar{x}_2$) will be significantly greater than zero at the 1% level?"

In the normal curve of differences in means centered at zero, the upper 1% of the area of the curve (one-tailed test) is found to the right of $0 + 2.33SE_{\bar{x}_1 - \bar{x}_2}$. In the normal curve of differences in means centered at 4.0 mg, the lower 5% of the area is found to the left of $4.0 - 1.64SE_{\bar{x}_1 - \bar{x}_2}$. The total distance between 4.0 mg and 0 mg thus must equal the sum of $2.33SE_{\bar{x}_1 - \bar{x}_2}$ and $1.64SE_{\bar{x}_1 - \bar{x}_2}$ (Figure 6.3). Remembering that est. $SE_{\bar{x}_1 - \bar{x}_2}$ equals $s \sqrt{\frac{2}{N}}$, we then have:

$$2.33s \sqrt{\frac{2}{N}} + 1.64s \sqrt{\frac{2}{N}} = 4.0$$

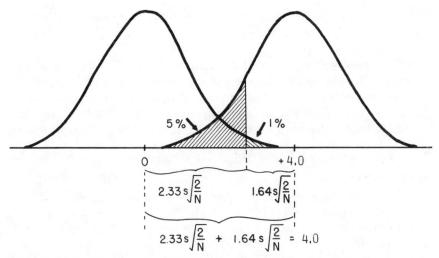

FIG. 6.3 **Estimation of Sample Size (Means). True Difference = 4.0;** $\alpha = 1\%; \beta = 5\%;$ **One-Tailed Significance Test.**

$$3.97s\sqrt{\frac{2}{N}} = 4.0,$$

but s is taken to be 4.8 mg.

$$(3.97)(4.8)\sqrt{\frac{2}{N}} = 4.0.$$

Solving this equation for N,

$$\sqrt{N} = \frac{(3.97)(4.8)\sqrt{2}}{4.0} = 6.74.$$

N equals about 45 cases in each group would be necessary to show a statistically significant difference between the means under the circumstances stated. The cases available in the pilot study do not form a part of this definitive experiment.

Two-tailed Test

In the more common two-tailed test for $\alpha = .01$, $\alpha/2 = .005$ is put into each tail of the curve centered at 0. If the power $(1 - \beta)$ is 95%, then

$$\sqrt{N} = \frac{(2.58 + 1.64)(4.8)\sqrt{2}}{4.0} = 51.3 \text{ or } 52.$$

The specified $(\mu_1 - \mu_2)$ of 4.0 expressed as a multiple of σ gives $\Delta = 0.83$. Referring to the table of the noncentral t-distribution for the two-tailed test, gives 54 as the size of each group.

If the investigator wished to use the 5% level of significance in a two-tailed test (Figure 6.4), rather than the 1% level, the equation to be solved would be: $1.96s \sqrt{\frac{2}{N}} + 1.64s \sqrt{\frac{2}{N}} = 4.0$, and, solving for N, we find N = about 37 cases in each group.

If one were merely putting a confidence interval on $\mu_1 - \mu_2$, then the consideration of β disappears. Thus, for a 95% confidence interval (half-confidence interval of 4), the sample size required is $\frac{(2.58)(4.8)\sqrt{2}}{4.0} = 19$, which is much smaller than the N required for a significance test (52). Again, the calculation of N for the confidence interval corresponds to a β of 0.50.

It can be seen readily that the more conservative the level of significance chosen and the greater the power of the test, the more cases are necessary. If the value of the true difference desired were increased, one can see from the preceding equations that N would be smaller and, similarly, if the value of the desired true difference were decreased, N would be larger. Table 6.4 presents the approximate

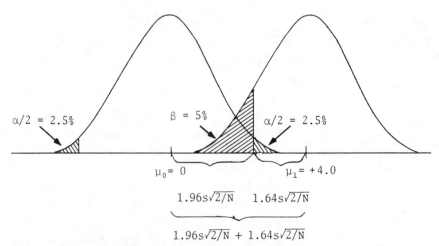

FIG. 6.4 Estimation of Sample Size (Means). True Difference = 4.0; $\alpha = 5\%$; $\beta = 5\%$; Two-Tailed Significance Test.

TABLE 6.4
Approximate Size of Each Sample Necessary to Assert Significance,[a]

True Difference in Means To Be Detected	Number of Cases in Each Group		
	1% Level of Significance, 99% Power of Test	1% Level of Significance, 95% Power of Test	5% Level of Significance, 95% Power of Test
3.0	123	91	66
4.0	69	51	37
5.0	44	33	24

[a] Assuming s = 4.8 mg, two-sided test.

size of the sample necessary in each group for significance to be asserted, corresponding to various levels of the true difference in means at selected significance levels and powers of the test.

The method just described for one- or two-sided tests affords a convenient way of approximating the sample size necessary for significance. It is approximate for two reasons: (1) The normal curve is the curve of reference instead of the t-curve; and (2) the average standard deviation obtained in the preliminary study is assumed to remain the same for the second, larger experiment. The effect of the approximation is generally to make the estimated sample size somewhat too small. The noncentral t-distribution gives values of N corresponding to Δ which are only slightly larger than the values obtained by the approximate procedure. Of course, Δ should be translatable to a $(\mu_1 - \mu_2)$, and this requires some knowledge of σ.

FURTHER CONSIDERATIONS

A very common way in which investigators select a sample size for their study for either the problem of estimation or significance testing, is to select a convenient size, or a size determined by financial consideration related to experimental animals or supplies, or by considerations of the amount of time available. The size of the samples in such cases is therefore determined without regard to any precision of the estimate or without regard to any alternative hypothesis of interest (H_1). In testing the null hypothesis (H_0), insufficient power may be available to rule out such an alternative hypothesis.

With this method of selecting the sample size in advance, suppose that a sample of size 100 were chosen. The measurements are then made on this whole sample and a significance test performed. If this test demonstrates significance at a predetermined level, say $\alpha = 1\%$ or 5%, then sufficient doubt is cast on the tenability of the null hypothesis to reject it. The verdict of significance is always meaningful regardless of sample size, because some hypothesis is ruled out as being untenable. If, however, the significance test showed that the "probability of chance occurrence" was too great to reject the null hypothesis, then the verdict of nonsignificance is stated, i.e., the null hypothesis is "accepted," or rather, "not rejected." This does not necessarily signify that the null hypothesis is true, however, nor does it necessarily mean that some alternative hypothesis of interest is untenable. Indeed, it is only when the sample size is sufficiently large — i.e., there is enough power to reject or rule out some alternative hypothesis of interest — that nonsignificance or "acceptance" of the null hypothesis is particularly meaningful.

When the size N of the sample is small, the confidence range on the unknown parameter is usually large. This wide confidence range may cover both the null (H_0) and the suitable alternative hypothesis (H_1) and thereby fails to distinguish between them. As N increases in size, the confidence range becomes narrower. If the sample size is sufficiently great, the confidence range becomes so narrow that H_0 and H_1 cannot both be covered. A suitable sample size is that which gives a narrow enough confidence range so that not both H_0 and H_1 can be covered. In this manner, the null hypothesis can be "accepted" only by rejecting the alternative hypothesis. The probability of rejecting the alternative when it is true is taken as β. Thus it is only by giving consideration to both the errors of the first and second kind, rather than to the first kind alone, that the verdict of nonsignificance is particularly meaningful.

In some instances, instead of continuing the investigation up to the originally agreed on sample size, the experimenter decides to "peek" at the results after, say, about half the sample has been obtained. Such peeking may involve examining the data, analyzing them, and making a significance test. If the test shows significance at the α level, the null hypothesis is rejected and the alternative hypothesis, which has meanwhile been waiting in the wings, advanced. If the test does not reach the conventional level but the probability (P) of equaling or exceeding the difference obtained is found to be promisingly low, for example 15%, the investigator may well feel that he should continue with his experiment, possibly up to the number of cases originally agreed on and again perform a test. If the experimenter originally had planned to work at say, a 5% level of significance, the "peeking" procedure described above is, in effect, changing that level. The effective level amounts to more than 5%, since this peeking is giving him more than one opportunity to reject a true null hypothesis. Actually, the second type of error is also "decontrolled" by this procedure. When peeking at the data has occurred and the investigator has been influenced by the results of the peeking in determining whether to continue the investigation or not, then he must "penalize" himself in some way, possibly by using criteria of significance more stringent than those he would ordinarily use.

There are ways of repeatedly peeking at the data and using decisions to stop or proceed with the experiment based on the results of these peekings — with proper validity, i.e., "controlled peeking." Special rules of procedure are necessary in these instances, and these are embodied in the method of Sequential Analysis, discussed in Chapter 16.

REFERENCES

1. Chilton, N. W., and Fertig, J. W.: The estimation of sample size in experiments. 1. Using comparisons of averages, J Dent Res 32:530, 1953.

2. Beyer, W. H., ed.: Basic Statistical Tables, Cleveland, Ohio, Chemical Rubber Co., 1971, pp. 85–88.

3. Cohen, J.: Statistical Power Analysis for the Behavioral Sciences, New York, Academic Press, 1969.

4. Fleiss, J. L.: Statistical Methods for Rates and Proportions, 2nd ed., New York, Wiley, 1981.

5. Veatch, H., and Young, J.: Sedimentation rates in periodontal disease and changes in sedimentation rates following the surgical treatment of periodontal disease, J Amer Dent Assn 36:580, 1948.

6. Hess, W. C., and Smith, B. T.: The ascorbic acid content of the saliva of carious and noncarious individuals, J Dent Res 28:507, 1949.

7

Analysis of Variance

ONE-WAY ANALYSIS OF VARIANCE (INDEPENDENT GROUPS, ONE-WAY LAYOUT)

Fixed Effects Model

Much of the language of experimental design in modern statistical usage has derived from agricultural science, in which different types of experimental treatments (fertilizers, varieties, methods, etc.) were applied to different experimental units (plots of ground, animals, patients). Thus a useful experimental design in oral biological research is one in which patients are allocated at random to a number of different treatment categories. This type of design is often called a completely randomized design and results in a *one-way classification* or a *one-way layout* of the observations. The purpose of the experiment is to compare the means of the various treatments. Since the treatments are fixed and not regarded as a sample from a universe of treatments, this one-way layout is often called a *fixed effects* model, or, more succinctly, a *fixed model*. If the experiment were to be repeated, the same treatments would be used.

Many one-way layouts also occur with naturally existing groups, i.e., the investigator either cannot or does not randomly subdivide the patients into groups. This does not actually constitute an experiment but rather corresponds to observational data. The analysis of such data, however, proceeds in the same way as does that of experimental data.

An example of such nonexperimental data is presented in Table 7.1 of the fasting blood glucose levels (glucose oxidase enzyme method) of 136 healthy young men who were classified according to

TABLE 7.1
Fasting Blood Glucose Levels (mg%) of 136 Normal Males, Classified
According to Periodontal Index Group[1]

Group 1	Group 2	Group 3	Group 4	Group 1	Group 2	Group 3	Group 4
89.8	84.2	89.0	85.0	96.0	86.0	90.0	81.0
97.8	91.0	85.5	88.0	85.8	82.3	86.5	74.8
75.9	78.8	86.5	90.5	96.9	86.5	90.0	88.9
86.0	89.8	89.9	97.5	77.5	92.0	85.0	75.0
79.0	84.0	98.0	80.0	92.5	92.2	99.8	62.0
93.5	84.0	93.0	76.2	87.6	81.0	91.5	88.0
84.0	92.0	94.8	92.2	88.0	82.0	97.5	79.9
85.5	87.8	82.9	92.2	84.8	92.9	93.5	91.9
74.5	92.0	83.5	81.5	84.2	83.2	90.5	78.0
93.0	85.0	87.1	95.5	86.5	88.1	68.5	93.7
98.5	89.5	94.8	79.5	89.5	97.0	92.2	87.1
86.5	86.8	85.2	78.9	95.5	86.2	94.0	
75.6	92.4	86.6	93.0	99.5	79.2	86.0	
88.2	81.6	85.5	93.2	86.5	81.5	83.8	
81.0	90.5	90.5	102.5		89.5	85.5	
93.0	93.0	85.5	97.0		91.0	78.5	
82.5	93.5	93.0	87.0		89.0		
77.0	89.5	83.5	102.5		87.5		
94.0	89.8	106.0	90.1		81.8		

the Periodontal Index, into four (symbolized, in general, by k) PI
groups (1.00–1.80, 1.81–2.17, 2.18–2.83, and over 2.83). The original study[1] utilized 300 individuals, but 136 were selected randomly from the study for illustrative purposes. It is assumed that the
various measurements of the different individuals are independent of
each other. It is also assumed that the distribution of measurements
from each PI group is at least approximately normal.

The various summary constants and indices of dispersion have
been calculated for the individuals in these four groups, and appear
in Table 7.2. A typical calculation, for Group 1, would be:

$$\bar{x}_1 = \frac{\Sigma x_1}{N_1} = \frac{2{,}886.1}{33} = 87.46 \text{ mg\%}$$

$$s_1^2 = \frac{\Sigma(x_1 - \bar{x}_1)^2}{N_1 - 1} = \left[\Sigma x_1^2 - \frac{(\Sigma x_1)^2}{N_1} \right] \Big/ (N_1 - 1)$$

$$= \left[254{,}018.23 - \frac{(2{,}886.1)^2}{33} \right] \Big/ 32 = \frac{1{,}606.92}{32} = 50.2163.$$

In the terminology developed previously, $\Sigma(x_1 - \bar{x}_1)^2$, which is
the numerator of s_1^2, is also known as the Sum of Squares or SS for

TABLE 7.2
Summary Values for Individuals in Table 7.1

	Group 1	Group 2	Group 3	Group 4	All Groups
$N_i =$	33	38	35	30	$136 \quad = N$
$\Sigma x_i =$	2,886.10	3,324.10	3,113.60	2,602.60	$11,926.40 = \overset{N}{\Sigma} x$
$\bar{x}_i =$	87.46	87.48	88.96	86.75	$87.69 = \bar{x}_0$
$\Sigma x_i^2 =$	254,018.23	291,544.27	278,478.58	228,177.30	$1,052,218.38 = \overset{N}{\Sigma} x^2$
$CT_i = (\Sigma x_i)^2/N_i =$	252,411.31	290,780.02	276,985.86	225,784.23	$1,045,961.42 = \overset{k}{\Sigma} CT_i$
$SS_i =$	1,606.92	764.25	1,492.72	2,393.07	$6,256.96 = \overset{k}{\Sigma} SS_i$
$MS_i = s_i^2 =$	50.2163	20.6554	43.9035	82.5197	

Group 1, i.e., Within Group 1, or SS_1. This is the sum of the squared scores (Σx_1^2) for Group 1 less $(\Sigma x_1^2)/N_1$. This latter term is often called the *correction for the mean* or, more simply, the *Correction Term* or *CT*, in this case CT_1, for Group 1. This CT is an allowance for the fact that the average for all the measurements is not zero.

The variances or MS for the four groups in Table 7.2 do not seem to differ very much. In fact, it seems reasonable to assume that the various values of s^2 are estimates of the same variance σ^2.* This assumption of equality of variances (homoscedasticity) is, in fact, necessary for the significance test conducted by means of the analysis of variance. A pooled estimate of σ^2 can be obtained from the Within Groups Mean Square which is an average of the various values of s^2.

The basic question is whether the four PI groups were derived from universes with different mean fasting blood glucose values, or whether all four universes have the same μ value. Since the σ's are presumed to be the same, the equality of the μ's implies equality of the universes, provided, of course, that the universes are distributed as the normal curve. Thus, the null hypothesis, H_0, is that $\mu_1 = \mu_2 = \mu_3 = \mu_4$; and the alternative hypothesis, H_1, that there is at least one inequality among the μ's. This null hypothesis can be tested by the ANOVA and its associated significance tests.

A pooled estimate of σ^2 can be obtained from the Within Groups Mean Square which is a weighted average of the various values of s^2, the weights being the respective degrees of freedom. The degrees of freedom for the pooled s^2 is the sum of the respective degrees of freedom. The Within Groups MS measures the uncontrolled variation, in this case, the fact that different individuals with their imprecise measurements appear in each group. In a sense, one could say that individuals are *nested* within groups, so that Within Groups MS could be labeled as Between Individuals (Within Groups) MS.

$$s^2 = \text{Within Groups MS} = (\text{Within Groups SS})/(N - k)$$

$$= \overset{k}{\Sigma} SS_i/(N - 4) = 6{,}256.96/132 = 47.40.$$

$\overset{k}{\Sigma} SS_i$ can also be calculated as the sum of all the squared observations minus the sum of the various correction terms for the various groups, i.e.,

---

*A test is available for the hypothesis that $\sigma_1^2 = \sigma_2^2 = \ldots = \sigma_k^2$, where k is the number of groups. This is known as Bartlett's Test[2] and is beyond the scope of this book.

$$\overset{k}{\underset{i}{\Sigma}} SS_i = \overset{N}{\Sigma} x^2 - \overset{k}{\underset{i}{\Sigma}} CT_i = 1{,}052{,}218.38 - 1{,}045{,}961.42 = 6{,}256.96.$$

A total or overall sum of squares can be calculated about the overall mean of the $N = 136$ measurements, $\bar{x}_0 = 87.69$, as $\overset{N}{\Sigma}(x - \bar{x}_0)^2$. This Total SS is generally calculated as the $\overset{N}{\Sigma} x^2$ for all the measurements in the four groups, less the overall Correction Term (CT_0), which is the squared grand total of all the measurements divided by the total number of measurements (N). Thus, from the last column of Table 7.2,

$$\text{Total SS} = 1{,}052{,}218.38 - (11{,}926.4)^2/136 = 6{,}342.87.$$

The Total SS is always greater than the Within Groups SS, unless the group means are equal. The difference is $6{,}342.87 - 6{,}256.96 = 85.91$. This difference is the Between Groups SS and reflects differences between the means of the four groups. It may be computed directly as:

$$\text{Between Groups SS} = \overset{k}{\underset{i}{\Sigma}} N_i (\bar{x}_i - \bar{x}_0)^2$$
$$= 33(87.46 - 87.69)^2 + 38(87.48 - 87.69)^2$$
$$+ 35(88.96 - 87.69)^2 + 30(86.75 - 87.69)^2$$
$$= 85.91, \text{ and has 3 degrees of freedom, i.e.,}$$
$$(k - 1).$$

A much more convenient computing method is to subtract from the sum of the correction terms of the various groups the overall correction term. Thus, from the last column in Table 7.2,

$$\text{Between Groups SS} = \overset{k}{\underset{i}{\Sigma}} CT_i - CT_0 = 1{,}045{,}960.92 - (11{,}926.4)^2/136$$
$$= 85.91.$$

The fundamental identity of the one-way ANOVA is:

$$\text{Total SS} = \text{Between Groups SS} + \text{Within Groups SS}$$
$$\overset{N}{\Sigma} x^2 - CT_0 = (\overset{k}{\underset{i}{\Sigma}} CT_i - CT_0) + (\overset{N}{\Sigma} x^2 - \overset{k}{\underset{i}{\Sigma}} CT_i)$$
$$\text{df: } (N - 1) = (k - 1) + (N - k).$$

Thus one sees that the Total SS is composed of two parts, Within Groups SS and Between Groups SS. While the Total SS was based on

136 individual measurements, there was one restriction on it, due to the correction for the position of the overall mean, $\bar{x}_0$, so that the 136 deviations $(x - \bar{x}_0)$ add to zero. Consequently there are N - 1 or 135 *degrees of freedom* for the Total SS. When the variance, s_i^2, for each group was calculated, each separate group SS_i was divided by $N_i - 1$, its respective degrees of freedom, so that the total number of degrees of freedom for the Within Groups SS is the total number of measurements (N), less the number of groups (k), or (N - k) = (136 - 4) = 132. The Between Groups SS has degrees of freedom equal to the number of groups less one, or k - 1 = 4 - 1 = 3. The single restriction here occurs because $\bar{x}_0$ is the weighted mean of the four group means, $\bar{x}_i$, so that $\Sigma N_1 (\bar{x}_i - \bar{x}_0) = 0$.

The various values obtained thus far can be summarized in an analysis of variance table (Table 7.3). The values for Mean Square are obtained by dividing the Sum of Squares by its degrees of freedom. Thus Between Groups MS = 85.91/3 = 28.61, and Within Groups MS = 6,256.96/132 = 47.40. The Total MS is not calculated since it does not serve any useful purpose here.

Test of Significance, F-Test

In this one-way analysis of variance, the null hypothesis to be tested is that there is no difference between the mean values of fasting blood glucose of the four parent universes. The Total SS has been divided into two parts: one part derived from differences between the groups and the other from differences among individual measurements within the groups. The MS Within Groups is an estimate of σ^2 of the measurements, which was assumed to be the same for all four PI groups. The MS Between Groups is an estimate of this same σ^2 only if all the universe means (μ's) are the same, i.e., if the null hypothesis is true. If the μ's are not the same, i.e., if the null hypothesis is false, then the MS Between Groups tends to be inflated in that it is estimating σ^2 *plus* a term measuring differences among the

TABLE 7.3.
Analysis of Variance Table for Data of Table 7.1

Source of Variation	Degrees of Freedom (df)	Sum of Squares (SS)	Mean Square (MS)
Between Groups	3	85.91	28.64
Within Groups	132	6,256.96	47.40
Total	135	6,342.87	

μ's. The ratio of the MS Between Groups to the MS Within Groups follows the F-distribution if the null hypothesis is true. F is often called the *Variance Ratio*.

The F-distribution is an asymmetrical distribution extending from zero to large values of F. The exact shape of the distribution depends on the degrees of freedom of the numerator of the ratio, df_1, and the degrees of freedom of the denominator, df_2. The mean value of F is equal to $df_2/(df_2 - 2)$, which is close to one. The null hypothesis of equality of the μ's is rejected only for ratios considerably larger than one, i.e., in the upper tail of the F-distribution. Ratios less than one do not lead to rejection of the null hypothesis in the use of the F-distribution for the Analysis of Variance (ANOVA). In this ANOVA, F is always formed as Between Groups MS/Within Groups MS. In general, the numerator of the F ratio is the MS which is sensitive to the falseness of the null hypothesis.*

Critical values of F corresponding to 1% and 5% probabilities in the upper tail for various combinations of df_1 and df_2 appear in Table 7.4. The table is entered at the appropriate df_1 for the numerator of the ratio and df_2 for the denominator of the ratio. From Table 7.3.:

$$F = \frac{\text{Between Groups MS}}{\text{Within Groups MS}} = \frac{28.64}{47.40} = 0.60, df_1 = 3 \text{ and } df_2 = 132.$$

Since the ratio is less than one, there is no statistical significance. The population or universe means, from which all four group means are derived, may very well be the same. If this ratio were quite large, so that there is much greater variation among the means of the various groups than among the measurements within each group, doubt could be cast on the tenability of the null hypothesis. If this ratio were large enough (from Table 7.4. F = 2.67 at the 5% level) the null hypothesis could be rejected and the alternative hypothesis, that the four universe means differ from each other because of some association with the Periodontal Indices, might be embraced.

---

*F is also used to compare the variances of two samples, i.e., s_1^2 and s_2^2. Here the null hypothesis is that $\sigma_1^2 = \sigma_2^2$ and the alternative hypothesis usually is that $\sigma_1^2 \neq \sigma_2^2$. In this case, F is formed so that it is larger than 1, i.e., by putting the larger variance in the numerator. Then the value of F exceeded 5% of the time really corresponds to 10% in the two tails of the distribution, corresponding to a test at the 10% level. To make the significance test at the 5% level, more detailed tables of the F-distribution are required, giving the value of F exceeded 2.5% of the time.[3]

TABLE 7.4
Table of F

Values of df_1 (Degrees of Freedom of Numerator)

$P =$	1		2		3		4		5		6		7	
	5%	1%	5%	1%	5%	1%	5%	1%	5%	1%	5%	1%	5%	1%
1	161	4,052	200	4,999	216	5,403	225	5,625	230	5,764	234	5,859	237	5,928
2	18.51	98.49	19.00	99.01	19.16	99.17	19.25	99.25	19.30	99.30	19.33	99.33	19.36	99.34
3	10.13	34.12	9.55	30.81	9.28	29.46	9.12	28.71	9.01	28.24	8.94	27.91	8.88	27.67
4	7.71	21.20	6.94	18.00	6.59	16.69	6.39	15.98	6.26	15.52	6.16	15.21	6.09	14.98
5	6.61	16.26	5.79	13.27	5.41	12.06	5.19	11.39	5.05	10.97	4.95	10.67	4.88	10.45
6	5.99	13.74	5.14	10.92	4.76	9.78	4.53	9.15	4.39	8.75	4.28	8.47	4.21	8.26
7	5.59	12.25	4.74	9.55	4.35	8.45	4.12	7.85	3.97	7.46	3.87	7.19	3.79	7.00
8	5.32	11.26	4.46	8.65	4.07	7.59	3.84	7.01	3.69	6.63	3.58	6.37	3.50	6.19
9	5.12	10.56	4.26	8.02	3.86	6.99	3.63	6.42	3.48	6.06	3.37	5.80	3.29	5.62
10	4.96	10.04	4.10	7.56	3.71	6.55	3.48	5.99	3.33	5.64	3.22	5.39	3.14	5.21
11	4.84	9.65	3.98	7.20	3.59	6.22	3.36	5.67	3.20	5.32	3.09	5.07	3.01	4.88
12	4.75	9.33	3.88	6.93	3.49	5.95	3.26	5.41	3.11	5.06	3.00	4.82	2.92	4.65
13	4.67	9.07	3.80	6.70	3.41	5.74	3.18	5.20	3.02	4.86	2.92	4.62	2.84	4.44
14	4.60	8.86	3.74	6.51	3.34	5.56	3.11	5.03	2.96	4.69	2.85	4.46	2.77	4.28
15	4.54	8.68	3.68	6.36	3.29	5.42	3.06	4.89	2.90	4.56	2.79	4.32	2.70	4.14
20	4.35	8.10	3.49	5.85	3.10	4.94	2.87	4.43	2.71	4.10	2.60	3.87	2.52	3.71
25	4.24	7.77	3.38	5.57	2.99	4.68	2.76	4.18	2.60	3.86	2.49	3.63	2.41	3.46
30	4.17	7.56	3.32	5.39	2.92	4.51	2.69	4.02	2.53	3.70	2.42	3.47	2.34	3.30
40	4.08	7.31	3.23	5.18	2.84	4.31	2.61	3.83	2.45	3.51	2.34	3.29	2.25	3.12
50	4.03	7.17	3.18	5.06	2.79	4.20	2.56	3.72	2.40	3.41	2.29	3.18	2.20	3.02
70	3.98	7.01	3.13	4.92	2.74	4.08	2.50	3.60	2.35	3.29	2.23	3.07	2.14	2.91
100	3.94	6.90	3.09	4.82	2.70	3.98	2.46	3.51	2.30	3.20	2.19	2.99	2.10	2.82
150	3.91	6.81	3.06	4.75	2.67	3.91	2.43	3.44	2.27	3.14	2.16	2.92	2.07	2.76
200	3.89	6.76	3.04	4.71	2.65	3.88	2.41	3.41	2.26	3.11	2.14	2.90	2.05	2.73
400	3.86	6.70	3.02	4.66	2.62	3.83	2.39	3.36	2.23	3.06	2.12	2.85	2.03	2.69
1,000	3.85	6.66	3.00	4.62	2.61	3.80	2.38	3.34	2.22	3.04	2.10	2.82	2.02	2.66

Values of df_2 (Degrees of Freedom of Denominator)

TABLE 7.4
Table of F

Values of df_1 (Degrees of Freedom of Numerator)

P =	8 5%	8 1%	9 5%	9 1%	10 5%	10 1%	20 5%	20 1%	50 5%	50 1%	100 5%	100 1%	500 5%	500 1%
1	239	5,981	241	6,022	242	6,056	248	6,208	252	6,302	253	6,334	254	6,361
2	19.37	99.36	19.38	99.38	19.39	99.40	19.44	99.45	19.47	99.48	19.49	99.49	19.50	99.50
3	8.84	27.49	8.81	27.34	8.78	27.23	8.66	26.69	8.58	26.35	8.56	26.23	8.54	26.14
4	6.04	14.80	6.00	14.66	5.96	14.54	5.80	14.02	5.70	13.69	5.66	13.57	5.64	13.48
5	4.82	10.27	4.78	10.15	4.74	10.05	4.56	9.55	4.44	9.24	4.40	9.13	4.37	9.04
6	4.15	8.10	4.10	7.98	4.06	7.87	3.87	7.39	3.75	7.09	3.71	6.99	3.68	6.90
7	3.73	6.84	3.68	6.71	3.63	6.62	3.44	6.15	3.32	5.85	3.28	5.75	3.24	5.67
8	3.44	6.03	3.39	5.91	3.34	5.82	3.15	5.36	3.03	5.06	2.98	4.96	2.94	4.88
9	3.23	5.47	3.18	5.35	3.13	5.26	2.93	4.80	2.80	4.51	2.76	4.41	2.72	4.33
10	3.07	5.06	3.02	4.95	2.97	4.85	2.77	4.41	2.64	4.12	2.59	4.01	2.55	3.93
11	2.95	4.74	2.90	4.63	2.86	4.54	2.65	4.10	2.50	3.80	2.45	3.70	2.41	3.62
12	2.85	4.50	2.80	4.39	2.76	4.30	2.54	3.86	2.40	3.56	2.35	3.46	2.31	3.38
13	2.77	4.30	2.72	4.19	2.67	4.10	2.46	3.67	2.32	3.37	2.26	3.27	2.22	3.18
14	2.70	4.14	2.65	4.03	2.60	3.94	2.39	3.51	2.24	3.21	2.19	3.11	2.14	3.02
15	2.64	4.00	2.59	3.89	2.55	3.80	2.33	3.36	2.18	3.07	2.12	2.97	2.08	2.89
20	2.45	3.56	2.40	3.45	2.35	3.37	2.12	2.94	1.96	2.63	1.90	2.53	1.85	2.44
25	2.34	3.32	2.28	3.21	2.24	3.13	2.00	2.70	1.84	2.40	1.77	2.29	1.72	2.19
30	2.27	3.17	2.21	3.06	2.16	2.98	1.93	2.55	1.76	2.24	1.69	2.13	1.64	2.03
40	2.18	2.99	2.12	2.88	2.07	2.80	1.84	2.37	1.66	2.05	1.59	1.94	1.53	1.84
50	2.13	2.88	2.07	2.78	2.02	2.70	1.78	2.26	1.60	1.94	1.52	1.82	1.46	1.71
70	2.07	2.77	2.01	2.67	1.97	2.59	1.72	2.15	1.53	1.82	1.45	1.69	1.37	1.56
100	2.03	2.69	1.97	2.59	1.92	2.51	1.68	2.06	1.48	1.73	1.39	1.59	1.30	1.46
150	2.00	2.62	1.94	2.53	1.89	2.44	1.64	2.00	1.44	1.66	1.34	1.51	1.25	1.37
200	1.98	2.60	1.92	2.50	1.87	2.41	1.62	1.97	1.42	1.62	1.32	1.48	1.22	1.33
400	1.96	2.55	1.90	2.46	1.85	2.37	1.60	1.92	1.38	1.57	1.28	1.42	1.16	1.24
1,000	1.95	2.53	1.89	2.43	1.84	2.34	1.58	1.89	1.36	1.54	1.26	1.38	1.13	1.19

Values of df_2 (Degrees of Freedom of Denominator)

[Reprinted by permission from *Statistical Methods* by George W. Snedecor and William G. Cochran, 7th ed. © 1980 by The Iowa State Univ. Press, Ames, Iowa 50010.]

TABLE 7.5
Analysis of Variance Table for Data From Two Groups of Table 7.1

Source of Variation	Degrees of Freedom (df)	Sum of Squares (SS)	Mean Square (MS)
Between Groups	1	7.79	7.79
Within Groups	61	3,999.99	65.57
Total	62	4,007.78	

Two Independent Groups

If there were just two independent groups to begin with, say Group 1 and Group 4, and the problem consisted of comparing the mean fasting blood glucose values of these two groups, the above analysis could still proceed. Thus,

$$\text{Between Groups SS} = CT_1 + CT_4 - CT_0 = \frac{(2,886.1)^2}{33} + \frac{(2,062.6)^2}{30}$$

$$- \frac{(2,886.1 + 2,602.6)^2}{33 + 30} = 7.79.$$

And

$$SS_1 + SS_4 = \text{Within Groups SS} = 1,606.92 + 2,393.07 = 3,999.99,$$

$$\text{Total SS} = (254,018.23 + 228,177.30) - \frac{(2,886.1 + 2,602.6)^2}{33 + 30}$$

$$= 4,007.78.$$

As shown in Table 7.5 the analysis of variance would then be:

$$F = \frac{\text{Between Groups MS}}{\text{Within Groups MS}} = \frac{7.79}{65.57} = 0.12, df_1 = 1 \text{ and } df_2 = 61,$$

so that the means of these two groups do not differ significantly from each other.

The identity of the analysis of variance procedure for the two PI groups just described with the analysis of the AAPL data for the Antarctica workers presented in Chapter 5, should be apparent. The test of significance of the difference in means of the two independent samples can also be performed in terms of the t-test. Thus,

$$t = \frac{(87.46 - 86.75) - 0}{\sqrt{65.5736\left(\dfrac{1}{33} + \dfrac{1}{30}\right)}} = \frac{0.71}{\sqrt{4.2478}} = \frac{0.71}{2.06} = 0.34, \text{ with df}$$

$$= N_1 + N_2 - 2 = 61,$$

where

$$s^2 = \frac{SS_1 + SS_4}{(N_1 - 1) + (N_2 - 1)} = \frac{1{,}606.92 + 2{,}393.07}{32 + 29} = \frac{3{,}999.99}{61}$$

$$= 65.5736.$$

The square of t is 0.12, which is the value found for F.

This relationship, $t^2 = F$, holds true whenever there is only one degree of freedom in the numerator of the F ratio which occurs in the case of the contrast between two groups. In the table of the F-distribution, when $df_1 = 1$, the critical value of F is the square of critical value of t. It should be noted that the use of the F-test automatically results in a two-tailed test in the one degree of freedom problem. If a one-tailed test at, say, the 5% level for the comparison of two samples is desired, either the t-test is used or the value of F corresponding to 10% in the upper tail must be used. In any event, for establishing confidence intervals, $\sqrt{F}$, rather than F itself, would be used as the multiplying factor for the estimated standard error.

As noted in Chapter 5, the use of the t-test for comparing the means of two independent groups is robust against moderate departures from normality. It is also robust for heteroscedasticity, particularly if the samples sizes are equal. The extension of the t-test for comparing two or more means, namely the F-test, through the ANOVA procedure is also robust in the same way. In the event of considerable non-normality or heteroscedasticity, one may seek alternative procedures such as mentioned in Chapter 5, e.g., non-parametric procedures and transformations.

Multiple Comparisons Among Groups

Even when there are more than two groups present in the study, one may wish to compare the means of just two of the groups. Since the assumption was made that the variance σ^2 of the various populations is the same, one may use an estimate of σ^2 based on all the groups, i.e., the Within Groups MS with $N - k$ degrees of freedom. Thus to compare Groups 1 and 4, selected from the four groups, the Within

Groups MS (from Table 7.3) of 47.40 with df = 132, would be used, giving

$$t = \frac{(x_1 - x_2) - 0}{\sqrt{s^2\left(\dfrac{1}{N_1} + \dfrac{1}{N_2}\right)}} = \frac{87.46 - 86.75}{\sqrt{47.40\left(\dfrac{1}{33} + \dfrac{1}{30}\right)}} = \frac{0.71}{1.74} = 0.41, df = 132.$$

Equivalently, $t^2 = F = 0.17$, $df_1 = 1$, and $df_2 = 132$. Note that when the MS for only the two groups was used, t was 0.34.

This test is correct if the comparison made was suggested by prior considerations in the planning phase of the study, or at least before viewing the data.

Comparisons Decided à Priori. If *prior considerations* suggest several comparisons among the k groups, it is often desirable to adjust the level of significance of each t-test so as to maintain a desired overall level α for the whole set of comparisons comprising the original null hypothesis. An approximate adjustment would be to make each test at the level of $\alpha \div c$, where α is the level desired for the overall null hypothesis (either 5% or 1%), and c is the number of comparisons to be made.[4]

The suitability of this adjustment is based on the so-called *Bonferroni inequality.*[5] Thus, for example, if 5 comparisons among means are to be made at an overall α of 5%, one would make each comparison at the 5% ÷ 5 or 1% level, i.e., one would use a critical t with 132 df of 2.61 (corresponding to 1%) instead of the value 1.98 corresponding to 5%. This procedure would be conservative since 5, in general, c, comparisons among the k groups are not, in general, independent of each other. For any number, c, of comparisons among means, the critical value of t corresponding to α/c may be obtained by interpolation into tables of the t-distribution or from tables of the Bonferroni t-statistic (Table 7.6).

In certain types of comparisons, more appropriate adjustments of the significance levels were developed by Nair[6] and Dunnett.[7] These usually require equal sample sizes. The critical values for these procedures are usually well approximated by the Bonferroni t-statistic.

Comparisons Indicated by the Data

If the comparisons had been *suggested later,* i.e., "result-guided," then the significance test in terms of the usual t-test is no longer valid. Unfortunately, such t-tests are frequently performed. In a re-

TABLE 7.6
Percentage Points of the Bonferroni t Statistic

$\alpha = .05$

df/c	2	3	4	5	6	7	8	9	10	15	20	25	30	35	40	45	50
5	3.17	3.54	3.81	4.04	4.22	4.38	4.53	4.66	4.78	5.25	5.60	5.89	6.15	6.36	6.56	6.70	6.86
7	2.84	3.13	3.34	3.50	3.64	3.76	3.86	3.95	4.03	4.36	4.59	4.78	4.95	5.09	5.21	5.31	5.40
10	2.64	2.87	3.04	3.17	3.28	3.37	3.45	3.52	3.58	3.83	4.01	4.15	4.27	4.37	4.45	4.53	4.59
12	2.56	2.78	2.94	3.06	3.15	3.24	3.31	3.37	3.43	3.65	3.80	3.93	4.04	4.13	4.20	4.26	4.32
15	2.49	2.69	2.84	2.95	3.04	3.11	3.18	3.24	3.29	3.48	3.62	3.74	3.82	3.90	3.97	4.02	4.07
20	2.42	2.61	2.75	2.85	2.93	3.00	3.06	3.11	3.16	3.33	3.46	3.55	3.63	3.70	3.76	3.80	3.85
24	2.39	2.58	2.70	2.80	2.88	2.94	3.00	3.05	3.09	3.26	3.38	3.47	3.54	3.61	3.66	3.70	3.74
30	2.36	2.54	2.66	2.75	2.83	2.89	2.94	2.99	3.03	3.19	3.30	3.39	3.46	3.52	3.57	3.61	3.65
40	2.33	2.50	2.62	2.71	2.78	2.84	2.89	2.93	2.97	3.12	3.23	3.31	3.38	3.43	3.48	3.51	3.55
60	2.30	2.47	2.58	2.66	2.73	2.79	2.84	2.88	2.92	3.06	3.16	3.24	3.30	3.34	3.39	3.42	3.46
120	2.27	2.43	2.54	2.62	2.68	2.74	2.79	2.83	2.86	2.99	3.09	3.16	3.22	3.27	3.31	3.34	3.37
∞	2.24	2.39	2.50	2.58	2.64	2.69	2.74	2.77	2.81	2.94	3.02	3.09	3.15	3.19	3.23	3.26	3.29

$\alpha = .01$

df/c	2	3	4	5	6	7	8	9	10	15	20	25	30	35	40	45	50
5	4.78	5.25	5.60	5.89	6.15	6.36	6.56	6.70	6.86	7.51	8.00	8.37	8.68	8.95	9.19	9.41	9.68
7	4.03	4.36	4.59	4.78	4.95	5.09	5.21	5.31	5.40	4.79	6.08	6.30	6.49	6.67	6.83	6.93	7.06
10	3.58	3.83	4.01	4.15	4.27	4.37	4.45	4.53	4.59	4.86	5.06	5.20	5.33	5.44	5.52	5.60	5.70
12	3.43	3.65	3.80	3.93	4.04	4.13	4.20	4.26	4.32	4.56	4.73	4.86	4.95	5.04	5.12	5.20	5.27
15	3.29	3.48	3.62	3.74	3.82	3.90	3.97	4.02	4.07	4.29	4.42	4.53	4.61	4.71	4.78	4.84	4.90
20	3.16	3.33	3.46	3.55	3.63	3.70	3.76	3.80	3.85	4.03	4.15	4.25	4.33	4.39	4.46	4.52	4.56
24	3.09	3.26	3.38	3.47	3.54	3.61	3.66	3.70	3.74	3.91	4.04	4.1[a]	4.2[a]	4.3[a]	4.3[a]	4.3[a]	4.4[a]
30	3.03	3.19	3.30	3.39	3.46	3.52	3.57	3.61	3.65	3.80	3.90	3.98	4.13	4.26	4.1[a]	4.2[a]	4.2[a]
40	2.97	3.12	3.23	3.31	3.38	3.43	3.48	3.51	3.55	3.70	3.79	3.88	3.93	3.97	4.01	4.1[a]	4.1[a]
60	2.92	3.06	3.16	3.24	3.30	3.34	3.39	3.42	3.46	3.59	3.69	3.76	3.81	3.84	3.89	3.93	3.97
120	2.86	2.99	3.09	3.16	3.22	3.27	3.31	3.34	3.37	3.50	3.58	3.64	3.69	3.73	3.77	3.80	3.83
∞	2.81	2.94	3.02	3.09	3.15	3.19	3.23	3.26	3.29	3.40	3.48	3.54	3.59	3.63	3.66	3.69	3.72

[a]Obtained by graphical interpolation.

[After Miller; reprinted by permission.[5]]

search situation, a scientist is apt to consider such findings as leads to be pursued, rather than as established facts. There are, however, special tests to cover such situations where the null hypotheses are formulated on the data observed. The simplest of these is the Scheffé procedure since the groups do not have to be equal in size.[8] The critical value that the difference in two means ($\bar{x}_i - \bar{x}_j$) must attain to be significant at the 5% level is $\left[\sqrt{(df_1)F} \right] \left[\sqrt{s^2 \left(\dfrac{1}{N_i} + \dfrac{1}{N_j} \right)} \right]$ where F is the critical value at the 5% level with $df_1 = (k - 1)$ and $df_2 = (N - k)$ needed to adjudge significance in the original ANOVA test and s^2 is the MS Within Groups.

The factor $\left[\sqrt{(df_1)F} \right]$ multiplying the est. SE of the difference is usually quite a bit larger than the usual critical value of t, or than the Bonferroni t-statistic (which *can not* be used for result-guided comparisons). In other words, the difference in means divided by its estimated SE must exceed the factor $\left[\sqrt{(k - 1)F} \right]$ to be significant at the 5% level. In the case of Groups 1 and 4, the difference in means divided by the est. SE is 0.41, and this would have to exceed $\sqrt{(3)(2.68)} = 2.84$ to be significant at the 5% level. We note that when the simple t-test was performed, the critical value of t with 132 df was 1.98. The Bonferroni t-statistic based on $c = 5$ comparisons was 2.61. An interesting feature of the Scheffé procedure is that no differences between means can be significant if the original F does not exceed the critical value. Certainly, in our example the original F was less than the critical value of 2.68 (in fact, less than one), so none of the differences for pairs of groups can be significant. In fact, more complicated contrasts, e.g., the mean of Groups 1 and 2 vs. the mean of Groups 3 and 4 can not be significant either. Of course, if the original F is significant, the simple contrasts looked at need not necessarily be significant.

Another procedure that is widely used for comparisons suggested by the data is the Tukey procedure[9,10] which is based upon the distribution of the Studentized range (Table 7.7). This method requires that all the sample sizes be equal, so that apparently it cannot be used in the present example. For illustrative purposes, however, since the four groups do not differ greatly (33, 38, 35, and 30), it is reasonable to use an average N, in this case, 34. For $k = 4$ means of samples of size 34, the critical difference between two means has to exceed $Q(s/\sqrt{N})$, where $Q = 3.68$ is the upper 5% point (the value exceeded 5% of the time for $k = 4$ and 132 df for the Within Groups MS, and $s/\sqrt{N}$ is the est. SE of a mean based on N readings. Note that the est. SE of a difference is $\sqrt{2}$ times as large as that of a single

TABLE 7.7

Upper 5% Percentage Points, Q, in the Studentized Range

Degrees of Freedom df	Number of Treatments, k																		
	2	3	4	5	6	7	8	9	10	11	12	13	14	15	16	17	18	19	20
1	18.0	27.0	32.3	37.2	40.5	43.1	45.4	47.3	49.1	50.6	51.9	53.2	54.3	55.4	56.3	57.2	58.0	58.8	59.6
2	6.09	8.33	9.30	10.89	11.73	12.43	13.03	13.54	13.99	14.39	14.75	15.08	15.38	15.65	15.91	16.14	16.36	16.57	16.77
3	4.50	5.91	6.33	7.51	8.04	8.47	8.85	9.18	9.46	9.72	9.95	10.16	10.35	10.52	10.69	10.84	10.98	11.12	11.24
4	3.93	5.04	5.76	6.29	6.71	7.06	7.35	7.60	7.83	8.03	8.21	8.37	8.52	8.67	8.80	8.92	9.03	9.14	9.24
5	3.64	4.60	5.22	5.67	6.03	6.33	6.58	6.80	6.99	7.17	7.32	7.47	7.60	7.72	7.83	7.93	8.03	8.12	8.21
6	3.46	4.34	4.90	5.31	5.63	5.89	6.12	6.32	6.49	6.65	6.79	6.92	7.04	7.14	7.24	7.34	7.43	7.51	7.59
7	3.34	4.16	4.58	5.06	5.35	5.59	5.80	5.99	6.15	6.29	6.42	6.54	6.65	6.75	6.84	6.93	7.01	7.08	7.16
8	3.26	4.04	4.53	4.89	5.17	5.40	5.60	5.77	5.92	6.05	6.18	6.29	6.39	6.48	6.57	6.65	6.73	6.80	6.87
9	3.20	3.95	4.42	4.76	5.02	5.24	5.43	5.60	5.74	5.87	5.98	6.09	6.19	6.28	6.36	6.44	6.51	6.58	6.65
10	3.15	3.88	4.33	4.66	4.91	5.12	5.30	5.46	5.60	5.72	5.83	5.93	6.03	6.12	6.20	6.27	6.34	6.41	6.47
11	3.11	3.82	4.26	4.58	4.82	5.03	5.20	5.35	5.49	5.61	5.71	5.81	5.90	5.98	6.06	6.14	6.20	6.27	6.33
12	3.08	3.77	4.20	4.51	4.75	4.95	5.12	5.27	5.40	5.51	5.61	5.71	5.80	5.88	5.95	6.02	6.09	6.15	6.21
13	3.06	3.73	4.15	4.46	4.69	4.88	5.05	5.19	5.32	5.43	5.53	5.63	5.71	5.79	5.86	5.93	6.00	6.06	6.11
14	3.03	3.70	4.11	4.41	4.64	4.83	4.99	5.13	5.25	5.36	5.46	5.56	5.64	5.72	5.79	5.86	5.92	5.98	6.03
15	3.01	3.67	4.08	4.37	4.59	4.78	4.94	5.08	5.20	5.31	5.40	5.49	5.57	5.65	5.72	5.79	5.85	5.91	5.96
16	3.00	3.65	4.05	4.34	4.56	4.74	4.90	5.03	5.15	5.26	5.35	5.44	5.52	5.59	5.66	5.73	5.79	5.84	5.90
17	2.98	3.62	4.02	4.31	4.52	4.70	4.86	4.99	5.11	5.21	5.31	5.39	5.47	5.55	5.61	5.68	5.74	5.79	5.84
18	2.97	3.61	4.00	4.28	4.49	4.67	4.83	4.96	5.07	5.17	5.27	5.35	5.43	5.50	5.57	5.63	5.69	5.74	5.79
19	2.96	3.59	3.98	4.26	4.47	4.64	4.79	4.92	5.04	5.14	5.23	5.32	5.39	5.46	5.53	5.59	5.65	5.70	5.75
20	2.95	3.58	3.96	4.24	4.45	4.62	4.77	4.90	5.01	5.11	5.20	5.28	5.36	5.43	5.50	5.56	5.61	5.66	5.71
24	2.92	3.53	3.90	4.17	4.37	4.54	4.68	4.81	4.92	5.01	5.10	5.18	5.25	5.32	5.38	5.44	5.50	5.55	5.59
30	2.89	3.48	3.84	4.11	4.30	4.46	4.60	4.72	4.83	4.92	5.00	5.08	5.15	5.21	5.27	5.33	5.38	5.43	5.48
40	2.86	3.44	3.79	4.04	4.23	4.39	4.52	4.63	4.74	4.82	4.90	4.98	5.05	5.11	5.17	5.22	5.27	5.32	5.36
60	2.83	3.40	3.74	3.98	4.16	4.31	4.44	4.55	4.65	4.73	4.81	4.88	4.94	5.00	5.06	5.11	5.15	5.20	5.24
120	2.80	3.36	3.69	3.92	4.10	4.24	4.36	4.47	4.56	4.64	4.71	4.78	4.84	4.90	4.95	5.00	5.04	5.09	5.13
∞	2.77	3.32	3.63	3.86	4.03	4.17	4.29	4.39	4.47	4.55	4.62	4.68	4.74	4.80	4.84	4.89	4.93	4.97	5.01

[After Miller; reprinted by permission.[5]]

mean. In our case, the critical difference is $3.68\sqrt{47.40/34} = 4.35$. Obviously, none of the differences between the four means exceeds this value. The critical difference for the two means each based upon $N = 34$ by the Scheffé procedure is $2.84\sqrt{47.40(2/34)} = 4.74$. We note that the Tukey method requires a smaller critical difference for statistical significance than does the Scheffé procedure. This is indeed the case for simple contrasts among means, so that the Tukey method should be used for equal or reasonably equal sample sizes. For more complicated contrasts among means, the Scheffé method is generally more sensitive. It should be pointed out that the overall F might not be significant and yet some of the individual differences might occasionally be significant by the Tukey procedure.

There is a slightly modified version of the Tukey method, the Neuman-Keuls, or sometimes called the Student–Neuman-Keuls procedure, which also uses the Studentized range.[5] If, for example, one mean is dropped as being different from the rest, then the remaining means are compared by using a critical Q based on a smaller number, $k - 1$, of groups. When no further means can be eliminated, the remaining values may be estimates of the same true mean. The Neuman-Keuls method does not lend itself to simultaneous confidence intervals.

Just as we often want to control α at the overall level for significance tests, we want to control the overall confidence for the whole set of confidence intervals at $(1 - \alpha)$. In other words, we are going to give a whole series of confidence intervals, one for each contrast, where the contrasts are often merely the differences between two means. If the individual confidence intervals are set up using the usual critical value of t, the overall confidence is not $(1 - \alpha)$. In the case of result-guided contrasts, the factor multiplying the estimated SE of the difference should be either Q/2 or the Scheffé factor in order to give an overall confidence of at least $(1 - \alpha)$. Again, the Q factor should be used only for equal or approximately equal sample sizes. In the case of contrasts specified à priori, if one wants all of the c intervals to cover the appropriate parameters with a confidence of at least $(1 - \alpha)$, then one should use the Bonferroni t-statistic. The use of the ordinary t-statistic would give an overall confidence of at least $(1 - c\alpha)$.

Random Effects Model

The example of the one-way layout as given by the PI groups would be referred to as the *fixed model* since the inferences are confined to these four groups. It is only in this type of example that one would want to make detailed or multiple comparisons among the groups. If there were a universe of PI groups from which four were selected at random for the study, then the one-way layout would be referred to as the *random effects model*, or more succinctly, as the *random model*. In this case, one would want to make inferences about the whole universe of PI groups. The ANOVA and the associated F-test are used to make this inference. There would be no point, however, in making detailed comparisons among the four groups which happen to be included in the study.

As an example, we have the data from a study in which 20 individuals were selected from a dental and dental hygiene student population and had supragingival plaque scored by the Turesky modification of the Quigley-Hein Index.[11] The data presented in Table 7.8 are from a larger study and show the total plaque score for 12

TABLE 7.8
Total Plaque Scores for Twelve Teeth

Patient Number	Readings		Σx	$\bar{x}$	$\lvert d \rvert$
1	7	10	17	8.5	3
2	21	19	40	20.0	2
3	10	13	23	11.5	3
4	17	18	35	17.5	1
5	22	21	43	21.5	1
6	27	29	56	28.0	2
7	6	12	18	9.0	6
8	21	22	43	21.5	1
9	23	19	42	21.0	4
10	16	18	34	17.0	2
11	15	14	29	14.5	1
12	7	10	17	8.5	3
13	21	19	40	20.0	2
14	50	32	82	41.0	18
15	11	15	26	13.0	4
16	11	15	26	13.0	4
17	34	35	69	34.5	1
18	17	23	40	20.0	6
19	26	30	56	28.0	4
20	25	28	53	26.5	3

$$\overset{40}{\Sigma}x = 789. \qquad \bar{x}_0 = 19.725$$

$$\overset{40}{\Sigma}x^2 = 18,675. \qquad CT_0 = (789)^2/40 = 15,563.0250.$$

$$\overset{20}{\Sigma}CT_i = \frac{(17)^2 + (40)^2 + \ldots + (53)^2}{2} = 36,833/2 = 18,416.5.$$

TABLE 7.9
Analysis of Variance Table of Data from Table 7.8

Source of Variation	df	Sums of Squares	Mean Square
Between individuals	20 - 1 = 19	$\overset{20}{\Sigma}CT_i - CT_0$ = 18,416.5–15,563.0250 = 2,853.475	150.183
Within individuals	40 - 20 = 20	$\overset{40}{\Sigma}x^2 - \overset{20}{\Sigma}CT_i$ = 18,675.0–18,416.5 = 258.500[a]	12.925
Total	40 - 1 = 39	$\overset{40}{\Sigma}x^2 - CT_0$ = 18,675.0–15,563.0250 = 3,119.975	

[a]When there are only two measurements per individual, a simple way of obtaining the Within Individuals SS is: $\Sigma|d|^2/2 = 517/2 = 258.5$.

anterior teeth, with two replications per patient. The subjects did not eat, drink, smoke, or rinse between the readings which were taken about one and a half hours apart. The readings should then be the same for each subject except for any individual variation within that time and any measurement error, i.e., random replications. The universe from which it is visualized that these individuals are drawn is composed of an infinite number of individuals each with his own mean μ_1 and with his own normal distribution of readings having a variance of σ_i^2. We shall assume that we have homoscedasticity so that all individuals have the same σ^2. There is a distribution of μ_1's centered at $\bar{\mu}$ and with a variance of σ^2_μ. The null hypothesis is that $\sigma^2_\mu = 0$, and the alternative is that the variance, σ^2_μ, of the individual means is not equal to 0. The arithmetic of the ANOVA is the same as for the fixed model. (See Table 7.9.)

If the null hypothesis that $\sigma^2_\mu = 0$, is true, then the Between Individuals MS would be estimating the same σ^2 as the Within Individuals MS. On the other hand, if the null hypothesis is false, then the Between Individuals MS tends to be inflated by a factor representing the variance of the μ's, σ^2_μ. In our case,

$$F_{df_1, df_2} = F_{19,20} = 150.1829/12.9250 = 11.62.$$

The critical value of F with 19 degrees of freedom in the numerator and 20 degrees of freedom in the denominator, exceeded 5% of the time, is 2.13. Since our value of F is larger than this critical value, we conclude that σ^2_μ is different from 0. F is also statistically significant at the 1% level and beyond, i.e., $P < .01$.

The fact that the individuals are different from each other means that the whole batch of 40 readings are not independent of each other, but come in clusters (two per individual). That shows that the readings on the same individual tend to be correlated with each other (*intraindividual* or *intraclass correlation*). Parenthetically, we might say that we are only interested in such measurements that distinguish between individuals, i.e., $\sigma^2_\mu \neq 0$.

This random effects model is often called a *Components of Variance* model, since several variances are being estimated. The Within Individuals MS of 12.925 is an estimate of σ^2, the Within Individuals variance. The Between Individuals MS of 150.1829 is an estimate of $\sigma^2 + 2\sigma^2_\mu$. Consequently, σ^2_μ is estimated as est. σ^2_μ = (Between Individuals MS – Within Individuals MS)/2 = 68.629. No comparisons between the individuals are necessary in this model, because the individuals have no identity and would vary from data set to data set. Multiple comparisons are not indicated.

We frequently want the variance of the overall mean $\bar{x}_0$ of 19.725. This was not particularly relevant in the fixed model. The estimated variance of the overall mean $\bar{x}_0$ in this random model is est. $SE_{\bar{x}_0} = \sqrt{\text{Between Individuals MS/Total number of readings}} = \sqrt{150.1829/40} = 1.94$. This value can be used to calculate the confidence interval on the mean of the universe of patients, $\bar{\mu}$. The confidence interval would be $\bar{x}_0 \pm t$ (est. $SE_{\bar{x}_0}$) = 19.72 ± 2.09(1.94) = 15.67 to 23.78, where t is the critical value based on 19 df. This est. $SE_{\bar{x}_0}$ would also be necessary to compare the mean of these individuals with the mean of some other group taken under somewhat different circumstances.

The $SE_{\bar{x}_0}$ can also be estimated from the means of the two readings per individual regarded as a sample of size 20 (= k). From Table 7.8,

$$\overset{20}{\Sigma}\bar{x} = 394.50; \quad \overset{20}{\Sigma}\bar{x}^2 = 9{,}208.25; \quad (\overset{20}{\Sigma}\bar{x})^2/20 = 7{,}781.5125,$$

$$s^2_{\bar{x}} = \frac{\overset{20}{\Sigma}\bar{x}^2 - (\overset{20}{\Sigma}\bar{x})^2/20}{19} = \frac{9{,}208.25 - 7{,}781.51}{19} = \frac{1{,}426.74}{19} = 75.092.$$

The MS or $s^2_{\bar{x}}$ for this sample is exactly half of the Between Individuals MS of 150.1839. For a single sample (see Chapter 4),

$$\text{est. } SE_{\bar{x}_0} = s_{\bar{x}}/\sqrt{20} = 1.94,$$

exactly the same SE as before. If all that is wanted with the data set like this one is to determine the accuracy of the overall mean, we do not need the ANOVA. All that is necessary is to take the mean for each individual, and then fall back on the single sample case.

While no problems arise in the test of the null hypothesis, $\sigma^2_\mu = 0$, when the number of readings per individual is not constant, problems do arise in arriving at a proper estimate of $\bar{\mu}$ and the SE of that estimate. If the number of readings is essentially constant, the method of taking a mean for each individual, and regarding these means as a single sample with its mean, standard deviation and est. $SE_{\bar{x}}$ is appropriate.

TWO-WAY ANALYSIS OF VARIANCE (TWO-WAY LAYOUT)

Another useful type of experimental design in oral biological research is one in which the experimental units (patients, animals, etc.) can be grouped into blocks or strata on the basis of various similarities, such as weight, age, litters, etc. In the simplest case, each block has the same number of units which is equal to a multiple of the number of treatments to be investigated, in fact, often equal to the number of treatments themselves. The treatments are assigned at random to the units within each block, so that each treatment is represented once within each block. This is the so-called *randomized block design*. The block or grouping of experimental units often represents the same patient at different times, or under different treatments, that is, cases in which the individual serves as his own control, as in the case of the paired t-test.

In the one-way analysis of variance of the data in Table 7.1, a source of variation due to differences Between Treatment Groups was separated from the Total Sum of Squares. When a series of treatments or methods are allocated at random to the experimental units within a block, or to the individual on different occasions, a component of variation due to differences Between Blocks (or Individuals) can be separated from the Total SS, as well as that due to differences Between Treatments.

Mixed Model

In order to compare various methods of obtaining total protein values of human parotid saliva, Wolf and Taylor[12] obtained bilateral (pooled) stimulated parotid saliva samples from 21 healthy men and women. Six different methods for determining total protein values were assigned at random to these saliva samples (Method 1 = Micro-Kjeldahl; 2 = Biuret; 3 = Greenburg; 4 = Lowry; 5 = Warburg and Christian; and 6 = Waddell). Duplicate determinations were made for each method. The averages of the two readings for each method for the 21 individuals appear in Table 7.10.

There are now two sets of totals, one set for cases (or individuals) in which each total is based on 6 observations, and one set for methods (or treatments) in which each total is based on 21 observations. The case totals are sums over the methods, and the method totals are sums over the cases. The calculations start like those in the previously illustrated one-way analysis of variance. The correction for the mean (CT) is calculated as the (Grand Total)^2 ÷ number of observations = $(43,529.5)^2/126 = 15,038,233.11$.

$$\text{Total SS} = [(236.0)^2 + (626.0)^2 + \ldots + (291.0)^2] - \text{CT}$$
$$= 18,539,271.14.$$

$$\text{Between Methods SS} = [(5,254.5)^2 + (3,255.0)^2$$
$$+ \ldots + (6,215.0)^2]/21 - \text{CT} = 15,200,889.25.$$

The squared method totals can be summed and then divided by 21, rather than making individual calculations for each method as was done for unequal sample sizes in the one-way analysis of variance, since the number of individuals utilized is the same for each method in the two-way analysis of variance described here. Similarly for cases (or individuals)

$$\text{Between Individuals SS} = [(1,605.5)^2 + (2,896.0)^2$$
$$+ \ldots + (1,381.5)^2]/6 - \text{CT} = 1,220,492.34.$$

The analysis of variance table can then be set up as Table 7.11. The Residual SS is obtained by subtracting the Between Methods SS and Between Individuals SS from the Total SS.

Additive Model, No Interaction

In the simplest case, the individual and method effects are considered additive. This means that there is no interaction between individual and method. In other words, each individual portrays the same pattern of differences between methods so that a "parallelism" is present. In this additive or no interaction model, the Residual MS is an estimate of the variance (σ^2) Within Individuals Within Methods. If it were possible to make repeat determinations on each individual

TABLE 7.10
Average Salivary Protein Determinations (mg%) by Six Different Methods

Case Number	Method 1	2	3	4	5	6	Case Total	Means
1	236.0	117.0	115.5	198.0	625.5	313.5	1,605.5	267.58
2	626.0	371.0	272.5	249.5	1,326.5	50.5	2,896.0	482.67
3	131.0	80.0	57.0	71.0	688.5	254.5	1,282.0	213.67
4	250.5	128.0	102.0	135.0	1,162.5	334.5	2,112.5	352.08
5	371.5	255.0	220.0	199.5	1,102.5	495.0	2,643.5	440.58
6	161.5	103.0	100.5	99.0	954.0	259.5	1,677.5	279.58
7	223.0	148.5	133.5	108.0	1,074.0	247.5	1,934.5	322.42
8	208.5	147.0	130.0	121.5	1,312.5	360.0	2,279.5	379.92
9	245.0	170.0	175.5	133.5	1,345.5	227.0	2,296.5	328.75
10	829.0	379.0	350.0	247.0	979.5	681.0	3,465.0	577.58
11	201.0	140.0	159.0	119.5	783.0	208.0	1,610.5	268.42
12	123.0	83.0	85.5	90.0	1,080.0	208.0	1,669.5	278.25
13	105.5	106.5	79.0	70.5	1,386.0	228.5	1,976.0	329.33
14	248.0	178.0	140.5	164.0	1,980.0	307.5	3,018.0	503.00
15	20.0	36.0	33.0	34.0	732.0	91.5	946.5	157.75
16	214.5	172.0	118.5	124.5	1,370.0	398.0	2,397.5	399.58
17	270.5	152.5	143.0	118.0	1,316.5	353.5	2,354.0	392.33
18	152.5	106.0	99.0	97.0	1,345.5	269.0	2,069.0	344.83
19	179.0	129.0	112.0	100.5	1,044.0	275.0	1,839.5	306.58
20	305.5	160.5	99.0	148.5	999.0	362.0	2,074.5	345.75
21	153.0	93.0	71.5	76.5	696.5	291.0	1,381.5	230.25
Method total	5,254.5	3,255.0	2,796.5	2,705.0	23,303.5	6,215.0	43,529.5	
Means	250.214	155.000	133.167	128.810	1,109.690	295.952		

TABLE 7.11
Analysis of Variance Table for Data of Table 7.10

Source of Variation	df	Sum of Squares	Mean Square	F
Between methods	5	15,200,889.25	3,040,177.85	143.55
Between individuals	20	1,220,492.34	610,246.17	28.81
Residual	100	2,117,889.55	21,178.90	
Total	125	18,539,271.14		

with each method on independent samples of saliva, then these determinations would exhibit a variance σ^2 that is assumed to be the same for all method-individual combinations (cells). It is this σ^2 that the Residual MS is estimating in the additive model.

The Between Methods MS is an estimate of this same σ^2 under the null hypothesis that the methods have the same true or universe means (μ's). If the null hypothesis is false, the Between Methods MS tends to be inflated by the differences among the μ's. The test of the null hypothesis, that there is no difference between the methods, thus requires that the ratio of the mean squares be formed as:

$$F = \frac{\text{Between Methods MS}}{\text{Residual MS}} = \frac{3,040,177.85}{21,178.90}$$

$$= 143.55; df_1 = 5, df_2 = 100.$$

This F is much larger than the critical value (5% point) of F = 2.30 with df = 5,100. The null hypothesis is thus most emphatically rejected, i.e., the means for the various methods differ from each other. P is much less than .01.

The Between Individuals MS similarly is an estimate of σ^2 plus the variance of the true individual means (μ's) in the universe of individuals. The null hypothesis that this variance is zero is thus tested by the ratio of the mean squares:

$$F = \frac{\text{Between Individuals MS}}{\text{Residual MS}} = \frac{610,246.17}{21,178.90}$$

$$= 28.81; df_1 = 20, df_2 = 100.$$

This F is also much larger than the critical value (5% point) of F = 1.68 with df = 20,100. The null hypothesis is again rejected, i.e., the means for individuals in the universe of which the 21 patients comprise a sample differ from each other in their average salivary protein content. This finding of individual differences in salivary protein is not surprising. This was known beforehand and is precisely the reason why the experiment was designed this way — to allow each individual to serve as his own control. In fact, the test just made is usually not necessary.

The fact that the six methods differ significantly from each other in their averages, does not necessarily mean that every method differs from every other method. As in the case with the one-way layout, techniques are available for performing multiple comparisons specified beforehand, and also for "result-guided" comparisons (suggested by the data). In this case, the Residual MS would serve in place of the Within Groups MS in the discussion of the one-way layout.

Nonadditive Model, Interaction

It is frequently the case that the individual and method effects are not additive, so that there is a Method $\times$ Individual Interaction. This means that the pattern of method differences varies among the individuals so that the Residual MS is estimating not merely σ^2 but rather σ^2 *plus* a measure of the interaction. That is, the Residual MS tends to be inflated.

In the two-way layout discussed here, the number of methods is "fixed" at the six chemical techniques included in this study. However, the individuals are thought of as being a random sample from a universe of individuals. The main purpose of the study is to make inferences about the method differences in the universe of individuals from which only a sample of 21 was available. This type of arrangement of the criteria of classification (methods and individuals) is often called a *mixed* model, because one criterion (method) is fixed, i.e., pertains to fixed effects, and the other one (individuals) is random.

Fortunately, in the mixed model the inflation in the Residual MS, because of the presence of an interaction, also enters into the Between Methods MS, so that the appropriate test of the null hypothesis of no method differences is still the ratio Between Methods MS $\div$ Residual MS. If there is an interaction, the resulting inflation in the Residual MS is not present in the Between Individuals MS, so that the ratio Between Individuals $\div$ Residual MS is not the appropriate test that individuals have the same salivary protein content. Because the denominator of this ratio is too large, it would provide, at any rate, a conservative test. A proper test would require that a separate estimate of σ^2 be available to form the ratio Between Individuals MS $\div$ Estimate of σ^2. Such a separate estimate is sometimes obtained by taking repeated measurements appropriately in each individual-method combination, i.e., by having replication in the cell. As pointed out previously, this question of individual differences was not germane to the experiment, since it was known beforehand that individuals differ from each other in their salivary protein content.

Fixed Model

Studies occur in which both the columns (treatments) and the rows (blocks) may be considered as fixed criteria. Such models would be called *fixed*. If there were an interaction present in such data sets, the Residual MS would not be the proper denominator for either Between Columns MS or Between Rows MS. Such data sets where there is only one reading per cell are not frequently encountered in dental and oral research. They are much more common with a number of readings per cell. In such cases, there will be an extra Within Cells MS which will serve as an appropriate denominator for the F-tests. Obviously, when the rows represent individuals, this criterion will hardly ever be considered as fixed.

Missing Values

It is evident that, in the two-way layout with a single value in each cell, there must be the same number of readings in each column (treatment) and the same number of readings in each row (individual) to perform the analysis as described. Occasionally, through some midadventure, a particular cell corresponding to some row-column (individual-treatment) combination will be blank. The cell will be lacking a measurement. This is a simple example of a design with *nonorthogonality*, so that the simple additive properties previously used for the ANOVA do not apply. Methods are available for estimating one (or more) missing value(s) in certain circumstances, and then proceeding with an appropriately modified analysis of variance.[13]

TWO-WAY ANALYSIS OF VARIANCE WITH REPLICATION IN THE CELL (MIXED MODEL)

Bruun, Giskov, and Stoltze performed a study on 20 dental students with a mean age of 20 years.[14] Each subject provided four enamel biopsies taken from either the mesial or distal aspects of the buccal surface of one set of bilateral premolars. At the first visit, a 3 mm^2 enamel biopsy was taken randomly, from one of the four selected untreated sites. Three sample biopsies were taken. These were designated as the Control biopsies (C). Following this, a topical fluoride preparation was applied to both teeth. One week later, three biopsies were taken from a randomly selected one of the three remaining sites (T_1). Immediately afterwards, a second fluoride treatment was applied to the two premolars. One week later, three enamel biopsies were taken from one of the remaining unbiopsied areas on these teeth (T_2). Finally, six months after the beginning of the study, the remaining site was biopsied (T_3). In a few cases where the acid was not quantitatively aspirated, the particular biopsy was discarded and the biopsies of the series were eliminated from the study. The data for only those 14 subjects who provided information on all four "treatments" are presented in Table 7.12 for illustrative purposes.

The first step in the analysis of variance is to obtain the Total SS in the usual way:

$$\text{Correction Term} = (583.7)^2/168 = 2{,}028.0101$$

$$\text{Total SS} = [(2.3)^2 + (3.6)^2 + \ldots + (3.8)^2] - \text{CT}$$
$$= 2{,}523.61 - \text{CT} = 495.5999.$$

The next step is to add the triplicate readings obtained from the biopsies for the 56 individual-treatment cells (Table 7.12). Thus, for individual 1 with Control $(2.3 + 1.6 + 1.3) = 5.2$; for individual 2 with Treatment T_1, $(3.6 + 2.8 + 2.7) = 9.1$, etc. From this Table 7.13, the other SS are obtained. The Between Cells SS is computed as if it were a total SS of this table of sums, keeping in mind that each cell entry is the sum of three readings.

$$\text{Between Cells SS} = \frac{\text{Sum of (cell sum)}^2}{\text{No. readings per cell}} - \text{CT}$$

$$= [(5.2)^2 + (8.1)^2 + \ldots + (14.5)^2]/3 - \text{CT}$$

$$= 7{,}103.4900 - \text{CT} = 339.8199.$$

$$\text{Within Cells SS} = \text{Total SS} - \text{Between Cells SS}$$

$$= 495.5999 - 339.8199 = 155.7800.$$

The Between Cells SS is then subdivided into Between Treatments, Between Individuals, and Residual SS:

TABLE 7.12
Fluoride Levels[a] of Enamel Biopsies of Fourteen Individuals at Four Different Treatment Levels

Individual Number	Control			T_1			T_2			T_3			Individual Total
	1	2	3	1	2	3	1	2	3	1	2	3	
1	2.3	1.6	1.3	3.3	2.9	2.7	4.8	3.0	2.8	4.8	3.0	2.8	35.3
2	3.6	1.9	2.6	3.6	2.8	2.7	5.7	3.5	3.1	4.3	2.7	2.9	39.4
3	3.4	2.8	2.5	9.0	5.6	4.8	13.2	7.5	6.4	4.9	4.2	2.9	67.2
4	2.8	2.7	1.7	3.6	2.6	2.6	5.3	4.5	3.4	3.8	2.8	2.5	38.3
5	1.8	1.0	1.0	3.2	2.3	2.0	5.0	3.8	3.3	4.4	2.5	2.3	32.6
6	2.5	1.2	1.2	5.4	3.0	2.6	4.7	2.9	2.9	3.1	2.1	2.1	33.7
7	3.4	1.9	2.0	5.0	3.4	3.3	5.3	4.9	3.1	3.0	2.7	2.3	40.3
8	2.1	1.0	0.8	3.2	2.5	2.3	4.8	3.3	3.3	3.7	3.3	2.7	33.0
9	1.8	1.2	1.1	4.2	3.2	2.6	5.7	3.8	2.9	3.8	2.7	2.5	35.5
10	3.6	2.0	1.5	5.0	2.9	2.6	6.3	4.7	3.4	3.9	4.3	2.4	42.6
11	2.5	1.7	1.2	3.0	2.1	2.1	6.4	4.0	3.9	4.6	3.5	2.9	37.9
12	3.0	1.9	1.6	4.8	2.9	2.9	9.0	5.0	4.5	5.7	4.0	4.0	49.3
13	1.5	1.1	1.1	4.5	3.0	2.3	5.9	3.8	3.2	3.0	2.2	2.1	33.6
14	6.4	5.3	3.7	8.9	4.3	4.1	7.4	5.8	4.6	6.2	4.5	3.8	65.0
Treatment Total	40.7	27.3	23.3	66.7	43.5	39.6	89.5	60.5	50.7	59.2	44.5	38.2	583.7

[a] pp 1000.

TABLE 7.13
Cell Totals of Table 7.12

Individual Number	Cont.	T_1	T_2	T_3	Individual Totals	Means
1	5.2	8.9	10.6	10.6	35.3	2.94
2	8.1	9.1	12.3	9.9	39.4	3.28
3	8.7	19.4	27.1	12.0	67.2	5.60
4	7.2	8.8	13.2	9.1	38.3	3.19
5	3.8	7.5	12.1	9.2	32.6	2.72
6	4.9	11.0	10.5	7.3	33.7	2.81
7	7.3	11.7	13.3	8.0	40.3	3.36
8	3.9	8.0	11.4	9.7	33.0	2.75
9	4.1	10.0	12.4	9.0	35.5	2.96
10	7.1	10.5	14.4	10.6	42.6	3.55
11	5.4	7.2	14.3	11.0	37.9	3.16
12	6.5	10.6	18.5	13.7	49.3	4.11
13	3.7	9.8	12.8	7.3	33.6	2.80
14	15.4	17.3	17.8	14.5	65.0	5.42
Treatment total	91.3	149.8	200.7	141.9	583.7	
Means	2.17	3.57	4.78	3.38		

$$\text{Between Treatments SS} = \frac{\text{Sum of (treatment sum)}^2}{\text{No. readings per treatment}} - CT$$

$$= [(91.3)^2 + (149.8)^2 + \ldots + (141.9)^2]/42$$

$$- CT = 143.2239;$$

$$\text{Between Individuals SS} = \frac{\text{Sum of (individual sum)}^2}{\text{No. readings per individual}} - CT$$

$$= [(35.3)^2 + \ldots + (65.0)^2]/12 - CT$$

$$= 137.7057;$$

$$\text{Residual SS} = \text{Between Cells SS} - (\text{Between Treatments SS}$$
$$+ \text{Between Individuals SS}) = 58.2211.$$

The analysis of variance table would then be as shown in Table 7.14.

There are a total of 168 readings in the original Table 7.12 so that there are $(168 - 1) = 167$ degrees of freedom assigned to the Total SS. There are 56 readings in the table of sums (Table 7.13), so that there are $(56 - 1) = 55$ degrees of freedom associated with the Between Cells SS derived from this table. Of these, 3 df are associated

TABLE 7.14
Analysis of Variance Table of Data in Table 7.12

Source of Variation	df	SS	MS
Between Treatments	3	143.2239	47.7413
Between Individuals	13	137.7057	10.5927
Residual	39	58.8903	1.5100
(Between Cells)	(55)	(339.8199)	
Within Cells	112	155.7800	1.3909
Total	167	495.5999	

with Treatments, and 13 are associated with Individuals, leaving 39 df for the Residual. The number of df for the Residual SS may also be obtained by multiplying the degrees of freedom for Between Treatments and Between Individuals. Thus, $3 \times 13 = 39$.

Tests of Significance (Mixed Model)

The Within Cells MS is an estimate of σ^2, the variation within an individual when subjected repeatedly to the same treatment. The Residual MS is an estimate of the same σ^2 if there is no Interaction Between Individuals and Treatments. If there is an Interaction, the Residual MS is inflated by the presence of a term involving the Interaction. The significance of an inflation can be tested by forming an F based on the Residual MS and the Within Cells MS, — namely,

$$F_{39,\,112} = \frac{\text{Residual MS}}{\text{Within Cells MS}} = \frac{1.5100}{1.3909} = 1.09.$$

This is statistically not significant since the critical value of $F_{39,\,112}$ is 1.51 at the 5% level. The fact that the Interaction is not statistically significant means that the treatment differences may be the same for each individual, although the F ratio is larger than 1. It is a frequent experience that while the test for Interaction may not be statistically significant, the ratio is greater than 1, indicating that there may well be some Interaction present.

When the Interaction is found not to be statistically significant, some workers like to combine the Residual MS with the Within Cells MS to obtain a pooled denominator or *Error* term for testing Between Treatments with many more degrees of freedom. This may be a serious mistake, because the Residual MS is often larger than the Within Cells MS, even though it is statistically not significant. The fact that the pooled MS has more degrees of freedom is no argument for pooling, especially since, in this example, there are ample degrees of freedom (39) for the Error MS for Between Treatments in this mixed model. In fact, the critical values of F decrease very little as the degrees of freedom in the denominator increase. In general, the most robust procedure should be used to test Between Treatments. In this case of the mixed model this would use the Residual MS (i.e., Treatment $\times$ Individual Interaction MS) even though perhaps one was entitled to use the Within Cells MS or, indeed, a pooling of the Residual MS with the Within Cells MS. Comparing the Between Treatments MS with the Residual MS,

$$F_{3,39} = \frac{\text{Between Treatments MS}}{\text{Residual MS}} = \frac{47.7413}{1.5100} = 31.62,$$

which is statistically significant, since it exceeds the 5% level of $F_{3,39}$ of 2.85. In fact, it is statistically significant beyond the 1% level. It is possible to make comparisons among the four treatments using the Residual MS and the methods discussed in the section on Multiple Comparisons Among Groups.

There is no particular merit in testing the statistical significance of the Between Individuals MS since it was known à priori that individuals differ with respect to enamel fluoride levels. It was precisely for this reason that the investigators elected to use the individual as a block. Nevertheless, it is possible to make this test since the Between Individuals MS is estimating σ^2 plus a function of the variance among individual means and the Within Cells MS is estimating σ^2. Consequently, the test consists of

$$F_{13,112} = \frac{\text{Between Individuals MS}}{\text{Within Cells MS}} = \frac{10.5927}{1.3909} = 7.62,$$

which exceeds the critical value of $F_{13,112}$ of 1.81 at the 5% level, in fact, $P < .01$.

Advantages of Replication in the Cell

The most important advantage of having replicate measurements of fluoride concentration in enamel sample readings is that one can test for the presence of a Treatment $\times$ Individual Interaction. While this interaction may often be expected to be present, it could not easily be demonstrated with a single reading per cell. A second advantage is that each treatment-individual combination or cell is represented by a mean of three readings, so that in the case of the mixed model, the test that compares the Between Treatments MS with the Residual MS is slightly more sensitive than if there were a single reading in the cell. Third, and least important, at least in the mixed model, one could test the differences among individuals for enamel fluoride levels in spite of the presence of interaction.[15]

The calculation of the ANOVA for the two-way layout with replication in the cells is often illustrated somewhat differently. The repeat readings in the cell are replaced by their average; the data set then corresponds to the two-way layout with one value per cell. The data are then analyzed as illustrated previously for this type of model. The resulting Between Treatments, Between Individuals, and Residual SS are exactly one-third of the values appearing in Table 7.14, and may be multiplied by the constant number of readings per cell, in this case, 3, to give the original sums of squares illustrated in this table. The Within Cells SS is computed separately. The various F-tests may then be performed. This method has the advantage, in the case of the mixed model, that, if all that is wanted is a test of significance between treatments, this can be obtained by comparing with the Residual MS. Of course, if one wants to test the significance of the Interaction, then one has to complete the analysis as indicated.

TWO-WAY ANALYSIS OF VARIANCE WITH REPLICATION IN THE CELL (FIXED MODEL)

Skier and Mandel recorded the Löe-Silness Gingival Index (GI) scores of 24 male and 15 female patients, age 22–68 years, who were classified as caries-resistant, and another group of 24 male and 15 female patients classified as caries-susceptible.[16] The data are presented in Table 7.15.

The two criteria of classification are sex and caries resistance or susceptibility. These are fixed criteria in the sense that only two modalities of sex and caries status are recognized. This is a 2 × 2 layout of Rows and Columns. The individuals are *nested* within the other two factors so that the Within Cells SS might, in fact, be called *Between Individuals Within Sex* and *Within Caries Status*. We note that the number of readings per cell is not constant as it was in the preceding problem. The number of readings however, is proportional.* This makes the calculations just a little more tedious, but

---

*Number of readings in cell

$$= \frac{(\text{total no. of readings in row})(\text{total no. of readings in column})}{\text{total number of readings}}.$$

TABLE 7.15
GI Scores of Male and Female Patients Classified According to Caries Resistance and Caries Susceptibility[a]

	Male GI Scores				Female GI Scores		
Patient Number	Caries-Resistant	Patient Number	Caries-Susceptible	Patient Number	Caries-Resistant	Patient Number	Caries-Susceptible
1	1.50	25	0.58	49	0.47	64	1.27
2	0.52	26	0.75	50	1.00	65	0.78
3	0.22	27	0.92	51	0.61	66	1.44
4	0.11	28	2.11	52	0.11	67	0.50
5	0.61	29	0.86	53	0.44	68	1.44
6	0.66	30	0.33	54	0.80	69	1.38
7	0.19	31	0.86	55	0.03	70	0.17
8	0.53	32	0.94	56	0.55	71	0.80
9	0.58	33	1.80	57	0.05	72	1.02
10	0.10	34	0.78	58	1.11	73	1.05
11	1.00	35	0.83	59	0.36	74	0.92
12	0.58	36	0.89	60	0.81	75	0.52
13	0.83	37	1.00	61	1.11	76	1.75
14	1.00	38	0.72	62	0.30	77	0.58
15	1.08	39	0.28	63	0.81	78	0.64
16	2.00	40	1.05				
17	1.69	41	0.50				
18	0.30	42	1.11				
19	2.50	43	0.61				
20	2.08	44	1.05				
21	0.97	45	0.69				
22	0.47	46	0.86				
23	1.75	47	1.44				
24	0.38	48	0.42				

[a] [Skier and Mandel.[16]]

does not vitiate the additivity properties of the sums of squares in the ANOVA. In the arithmetic, all that it means is that, in the calculation of the various correction terms, the squared sums cannot just be added and then divided by a constant number of readings as was done in the previous example. Rather, each correction term must be computed step-by-step.

Table 7.16 presents various summary values for the cells of Table 7.15. Then, the first step in the analysis is to obtain the Total SS in the usual way, and the ANOVA appears in Table 7.17.

In the case of the fixed model, all of the MS's referring to the two factors, the main effects, as well as the Interaction MS, are referred to the Within Cells MS. If the null hypothesis were false, the expected value of the MS's would be σ^2 plus a factor reflecting the falseness of the null hypothesis. In the case of the fixed model, the interaction does not enter into the expected value for either of the fixed effect MS's. We see that none of the values of F having df = 1, 74 exceed the critical value of 3.96. Consequently, none of the effects is statistically significant.

If there were significant interaction, it would mean that the sex difference in GI scores varies significantly from one caries status to another, or, equivalently, that the difference in caries statuses in GI scores varies significantly from one sex to another. In that case, the main effects, namely, the status and sex, would lose a lot of their meaning.

The fact that each of the F values has 1 df in the numerator, implies that all of these tests could have been made by some appropriate form of a t-test — not the simple one discussed in Chapter 5. For example, to see whether the sex averages are significantly different from each other, it would not be permissible just to take all the males as one sample and all the females as the other sample and run a two sample t-test. The fact that the males and females, respectively, are divided according to the strata, i.e., caries status, would have to be taken into consideration.

Inequality of Number of Readings Per Cell

The analysis of data of this kind becomes complicated if the frequencies in the cells are neither equal nor proportional. With such *nonorthogonal* ANOVA, the SS do not have the usual additivity property. In the case of the fixed model, there are what appear to be the exact solutions.

Before the availability of computer programs, constants were

TABLE 7.16
Summary Values for the Four Cells of Table 7.15

Male	Female	Total
	Caries *Resistant*	
N $= 24$	15	39
$\Sigma x = 21.74$	8.56	30.30
$\bar{x}$ $=$ 0.9058	0.5707	
s^2 $=$ 0.4551	0.1325	
	Caries *Susceptible*	
N $= 24$	15	39
$\Sigma x = 21.38$	14.26	35.64
$\bar{x}$ $=$ 0.8908	0.9507	
s^2 $=$ 0.1771	0.1931	
	Total	
N $= 48$	30	78
$\Sigma x = 43.12$	22.82	65.94

Summary Calculations

Correction Term $= (\overset{78}{\Sigma} x)^2/N = (65.94)^2/78 = 55.7447$.

Total SS $= \overset{78}{\Sigma} x^2 - CT = 76.2818 - 55.7447 = 20.5370$.

Between Cells SS $= \dfrac{(21.74)^2}{24} + \dfrac{(8.56)^2}{15} + \dfrac{(21.38)^2}{24} + \dfrac{(14.26)^2}{15} - CT$

$$= 1.4356.$$

Within Cells SS = Total SS − Between Cells SS = 19.1014.

Between Status SS $= \dfrac{(30.30)^2 + (35.64)^2}{39} - CT = 0.3655$.

Between Sexes SS $= \dfrac{(43.12)^2}{48} + \dfrac{(22.82)^2}{30} - CT = 0.3498$.

Status $\times$ Sex Interaction SS = Between Cells SS

− (Between Status SS + Between Sexes SS)

$$= 0.7203.$$

TABLE 7.17
Analysis of Variance Table of Data in Table 7.16

Source of Variation	df	SS	MS
Within Cells	74	19.1014	0.2581
(Between Cells)	(3)	1.4356	0.4785
Between Status	1	0.3655	0.3655
Between Sexes	1	0.3498	0.3498
Status × Sex Interaction	1	0.7203	0.7203
Total	77	20.5370	

$$F_{1,74} = \frac{\text{Status} \times \text{Sex Interaction MS}}{\text{Within Cells MS}} = \frac{0.7203}{0.2581} = 2.7908.$$

$$F_{1,74} = \frac{\text{Between Status MS}}{\text{Within Cells MS}} = \frac{0.3655}{0.2581} = 1.4161.$$

$$F_{1,74} = \frac{\text{Between Sexes MS}}{\text{Within Cells MS}} = \frac{0.3498}{0.2581} = 1.3553.$$

fitted by the Method of Least Squares to measure the main effects in the absence of interaction, as well as to obtain a measure of interaction. Main effects in the presence of interaction were usually computed by Yates' procedure for unweighted cell means.[17] Computer programs are now available to accomplish these purposes. In the Appendix are presented edited printouts of the SAS General Linear Models Procedure, which is actually a regression procedure with dummy variables.

A convenient and frequently used approximate solution, especially if the number of readings per cell does not vary widely, is to replace each cell by its mean. Then one is confronted by a two-way layout with one reading per cell, even though these means are based on varying numbers of readings. The SS in this two-way layout are multiplied by an average of the number of readings per cell. The preferable average is the harmonic mean, $\overline{N}_H$, where

$$\overline{N}_H = \frac{\text{Number of Cells}}{\text{Sum of Reciprocals of Cell Frequencies}}.$$

The Within Cells SS can, of course, be computed separately by the ordinary formula as Within Cells SS = Total SS − Between Cells SS. Within Cells MS is still estimating σ^2. Now, the MS computed from the SS inflated by the harmonic mean are compared with the Within Cells MS by the usual F-test.

If the number of readings per cell were constant, the ANOVA calculated as described would correspond exactly to the ANOVA in which the original cell readings were not used. While the method using the harmonic mean is not exact, the approximation is remarkably good if the frequencies do not vary too widely. Also, interestingly in the special case of the 2 × 2 example just discussed, the method yields the correct ANOVA.

As an example of this method which utilizes the harmonic mean, the following data on the duration of local anesthesia are presented in Table 7.18. One of four local anesthetic solutions was employed on 79 patients who came to a private office for endodontic therapy

TABLE 7.18
Duration[a] of Anesthesia for Four Solutions[b] Employed for Endodontic and Periodontic Procedures Using Inferior Alveolar Nerve Block

Anesthetic Solution			
Sol. 1	Sol. 2	Sol. 3	Sol. 4
Endodontic			
20	20	9	19
17	18	25	18
17	22	24	24
15	19	20	23
19	16	18	13
20	11	18	8
18	7	17	24
	22	19	9
Periodontic			
30	21	24	20
23	24	38	28
16	27	26	25
18	26	17	20
23	23	20	15
16	21	20	32
12	21	17	23
20	19	26	22
21	13	23	15
24	16	21	
	24	20	
	21	20	
	29	17	
	7	26	
	23		

[a] Duration given in 10-minute units.

[b] Solutions = 1.8 ml. each.

or periodontal surgery. The data for the 31 who had inferior alveolar nerve block for endodontics and the 48 who had nerve block for periodontal surgery are presented.[17]

Table 7.19 (see page 136) summarizes the data in Table 7.18 in terms of cell means, etc; the ANOVA is given in Table 7.20. (See page 137.)

We compute the Correction Term and the Total SS in the usual way. The Between Cells SS takes into account the unequal frequency in each cell. Thus, for x,

$$CT = (\overset{79}{\Sigma}x)^2/79 = (1{,}582)^2/79 = 31{,}680.0506.$$

$$\text{Total SS} = \overset{79}{\Sigma}x^2 - CT = 34{,}018.0000 - CT = 2{,}337.9494.$$

$$\begin{aligned}
\text{Between Cells SS} &= \Sigma(\text{cell sum})^2/N - CT \\
&= [(126)^2/7 + \ldots + (200)^2/9] - CT \\
&= 32{,}006.9694 - CT = 326.9188.
\end{aligned}$$

$$\begin{aligned}
\text{Within Cells SS} &= \text{Total SS} - \text{Between Cells SS} \\
&= 2{,}337.9494 - 326.9188 = 2{,}011.0306.
\end{aligned}$$

Next, we compute the various sums of squares on the cell means and perform an ANOVA as if it were a two-way layout without replication in the cells. Thus, for $\bar{x}$,

$$CT = (\Sigma\bar{x})^2/8 = (156.897)^2/8 = 3{,}077.0836.$$

$$\text{Total SS} = \Sigma\bar{x}^2 - CT = 33.9643.$$

$$\begin{aligned}
\text{Between Procedures SS} &= (70.875)^2/4 + (86.022)^2/4 - CT \\
&= 3{,}105.7625 - CT = 28.6789.
\end{aligned}$$

$$\begin{aligned}
\text{Between Solutions SS} &= (38.300)^2/2 + \ldots + (39.472)^2/2 - CT \\
&= (3{,}080.5035 - CT = 3.4198.
\end{aligned}$$

$$\begin{aligned}
\text{Interaction SS} &= \text{Total SS} - (\text{Procedures SS} + \text{Solutions SS}) \\
&= 1.8656.
\end{aligned}$$

It is not surprising that the patients alloted one procedure or the other — namely, endodontic or periodontic — differ in their average duration of anesthesia. This was not an experimental factor, but the treatments were.

With unequal cell frequencies in the mixed model there appears to be no exact solution as there was in the case of the fixed model.[18] If the numbers were equal, one could use cell means and then inflate

TABLE 7.19
Summary Table of Data of Table 7.17

| | Anesthetic Solution | | | | |
	Sol. 1	Sol. 2	Sol. 3	Sol. 4	Total
Endodontic					
Number of measurements	7	8	8	8	31
Sum of measurements	126	135	150	138	549
Cell mean	18.000	16.875	18.750	17.250	$70.875 = \overset{4}{\Sigma}\overline{x}$
Periodontic					
Number of measurements	10	15	14	9	48
Sum of measurements	203	315	315	200	1,003
Cell means	20.300	21.000	22.500	22.222	$86.022 = \overset{4}{\Sigma}\overline{x}$
Total					
Number of measurements	17	23	22	17	79
Sum of measurements	329	450	465	338	1,582
$\overset{2}{\Sigma}\overline{x} =$	38.300	37.875	41.250	39.472	$165.897 = \overset{8}{\Sigma}\overline{x}$

$\overset{8}{\Sigma}\overline{x}^2 = 3,111.0479.$

$\overset{79}{\Sigma}x^2 = 34,018.000.$

$\overline{N}_H = 8/(1/7 + 1/8 + \ldots + 1/9) = 8/8.6706 = 9.2265.$

TABLE 7.20
Analysis of Variance on Cell Means Using Harmonic Mean

Source of Variation	df	SS	$(SS) \times \overline{N}_H$	MS
Between Procedures	1	28.6789	264.6070	264.6070
Between Solutions	3	3.4198	31.5529	10.5176
Procedure $\times$ Solution				
Interaction	3	1.8656	17.2130	5.7377
Total	7	33.9643	313.3729	
Within Cells	71		2,011.0306	28.3244

$$F_{3,71} = \frac{\text{Procedure} \times \text{Solution Interaction MS}}{\text{Within Cells MS}}$$

$$= 5.7377/28.3244 = 0.2026; P > .05.$$

$$F_{3,71} = \frac{\text{Between Solutions MS}}{\text{Within Cells MS}}$$

$$= 10.5176/28.3244 = 0.3593; P > .05.$$

$$F_{1,71} = \frac{\text{Between Procedures MS}}{\text{Within Cells MS}}$$

$$= 264.6070/28.3244 = 9.3420; P < .01.$$

the Between Rows and Columns and Residual SS by the constant number, which is also $\overline{N}_H$. This would give the same analysis as using the original readings. This suggests that an approximate solution is to perform an ANOVA on the cell means and compare the Between Procedures MS (fixed effect) directly with the Residual (actually, Interaction) MS without inflating by $\overline{N}_H$ because $\overline{N}_H$ would appear in both the numerator and denominator of F. In addition, we can take the Residual MS, inflate it by $\overline{N}_H$ and compare it with the usual Within Cells MS to have an approximate test of the Interaction of the fixed factor (Procedures) with the random factor (Individual). Also, the MS for the random factor can be inflated by $\overline{N}_H$ and compared with the Within Cells MS to have an approximate test of that factor. Often, when one has data of this type, one is interested only in the fixed factor and in that case, we merely perform a two-way ANOVA on the means and then compare Between Procedures with the Residual. Of course, if there are only two modalities of the fixed factor, the latter suggestion amount to just a paried t-test on the differences between the two means. The approximate method suggested becomes better and better as the cell frequencies approach constancy.

Two Related Samples (Paired Samples)

In the development of a new adhesive vehicle for obtaining long contact with oral mucous membranes, different formulations or preparations were studied.[19] After preliminary screening, two preparations (A and B) were each applied four times, according to a prearranged random scheme, to specific areas of the oral cavity of nine dental students. The repeated applications were made to the same sites and the duration of contact of the preparation with the tissue in that area was determined to the nearest five minutes. It was not disclosed to the subject which preparation was being applied. The average of the four observations for the alveolar mucosa on the labial of the upper right canine appear in Table 7.21. The completed analysis of variance table appears in Table 7.22.

TABLE 7.21
Average Duration of Contact of Two Preparations With Oral Mucous Membrane of Nine Individuals

Individual	Duration in Minutes Prep A	Prep B	Difference (d) (B − A)	Total (B + A)	Mean
SS	156.25	232.50	+ 76.25	388.75	194.375
PT	71.25	70.00	− 1.25	141.25	70.625
SR	101.25	115.00	+ 13.75	216.25	108.125
TS	121.25	128.75	+ 7.50	250.00	125.000
KS	87.50	86.25	− 1.25	173.75	86.875
DS	70.00	143.75	+ 73.75	213.75	106.875
SC	60.00	112.50	+ 52.50	172.50	86.250
HB	227.50	181.25	− 46.25	408.75	204.375
RS	215.00	233.75	+ 18.75	448.75	224.375
Total	1,110.00	1,303.75	+193.75	2,413.75	
Mean	123.333	143.861	+ 21.528		

The two-analysis of variance of the data in Table 7.21 proceeds as follows:

Correction Term = $(2,413.75)^2/18 = 323,677.1710$.

Between Preparations SS = $[(1,110.00)^2 - (1,303.75)^2]/9 - CT = 2,085.5035$.

Between Individuals SS = $[(388.75)^2 + (141.25)^2 + \ldots + (448.75)^2]/2 - CT$
$$= 53,537.6736.$$

Total SS = $[(156.25)^2 + (71.25)^2 + \ldots + (233.75)^2] - CT = 61,911.8924$.

Residual SS = Total SS − (Between Preparations SS + Between Individuals SS)
$$= 6,288.7153.$$

TABLE 7.22
Analysis of Variance Table of Data in Table 7.20

Source of Variation	df	SS	MS
Between preparations	1	2,085.5035	2,085.5035
Between individuals	8	53,537.6736	6,692.2092
Residual	8	6,288.7153	786.0894
Total	17	61,911.8924	

$$F = \frac{\text{Between Preparations MS}}{\text{Residual MS}} = \frac{2,085.5035}{786.0894} = 2.65; df_1 = 1, df_2 =$$

8, so that F is not statistically significant at the 5% level. The preparation means do not differ significantly from each other.

t-Test

The means of the two treatments (preparations) can also be compared by the t-test, working directly with the preparation differences for each individual as illustrated on pages 5.12ff. The estimate of the variance of the difference (d) between the mean values of preparation A and preparation B is obtained as

$$s_d^2 = \frac{\Sigma d^2 - (\Sigma d)^2 / N}{N - 1} = 1,572.1788$$

The average of the differences between the means ($\bar{d}$) is compared with the est. $SE_{\bar{d}}$, to obtain Student's t ratio as $t = \bar{d}/\text{est. } SE_{\bar{d}}$ where

$$\text{Est. } SE_{\bar{d}} = \sqrt{s_d^2/N} = \sqrt{1,572.1788/9} = 13.22, \text{ so that}$$

$$t = \frac{21.53}{13.22} = 1.63, df = 8.$$

The difference in means is not statistically significant at the 5% level. Again, it should be noted that in this special case with just two treatments, $t^2 = (1.63)^2 = 2.65 = F$ (except for rounding off differences).

INCOMPLETE TWO-WAY ANALYSIS OF VARIANCE

In a frequent type of design, there are two criteria of classification, but the data are incompletely cross-classified. One of the criteria is nested within another criterion. An illustration of this type of problem is the following: As part of a larger study, Chilton and Maher[20] studied the gingival crevicular fluid (GCF) volume from the buccal aspect of the maxillary right first molar of 19 young adults with mild chronic marginal gingivitis. Two readings were taken with a standardized technique, one half hour apart. The subjects refrained from all eating, drinking, rinsing, and all oral hygiene procedures during this period. The two readings should be the same for each patient, except for individual variation within that time and any measurement error, i.e., random replications.

After the readings had been obtained, the subjects were randomly assigned, using a predetermined random scheme, to one of two groups (A and B) which would later be subjected to different oral hygiene regimens. The GCF data generated before institution of the oral hygiene regimens for 9 patients in Group A and 10 patients in Group B appear in Table 7.23. The purpose of the statistical analysis of these data is to check on the comparability of the two groups at the beginning of the study. Indeed, they should be comparable if we have confidence in the randomization scheme.

The data for each of the two groups conform to a one-way random effects model. When the data are viewed as a whole, we see that there are two criteria, namely, group and individual. The individuals, however, are nested within the groups and are not cross-classified between groups, which is why this model has been labelled an incomplete two-way layout. The individuals are said to be hierarchical

TABLE 7.23

GCF for Tooth Number 3, for Two Groups of Nine and Ten Individuals, Respectively

Group A					Group B			
Individual Number	Readings		Σx	$\bar{x}$	Individual Number	Readings		Σx	$\bar{x}$
1	32	10	42	21.0	10	78	73	151	75.5
2	69	49	118	59.0	11	10	13	23	11.5
3	14	28	42	21.0	12	65	76	141	70.5
4	36	51	87	43.5	13	87	84	171	85.5
5	33	25	58	29.0	14	52	62	114	57.0
6	16	24	40	20.0	15	38	37	75	37.5
7	22	20	42	21.0	16	49	39	88	44.0
8	16	4	20	10.0	17	40	62	102	51.0
9	23	22	45	22.5	18	27	16	43	21.5
					19	9	1	10	5.0
$\overset{18}{\Sigma}x$			494		$\overset{20}{\Sigma}x$			918	
$\bar{x}$			27.444		$\bar{x}$			45.9000	
$\overset{18}{\Sigma}x^2$			17,878.		$\overset{20}{\Sigma}x^2$			56,102.	

within groups. In spite of the hierarchy, the model would be said to be mixed since one criterion, group, is fixed, while the other criterion, individual, is random.

While there are many ways of computing the ANOVA on the data presented in Table 7.23, a convenient method would be to perform an ANOVA for each of the two groups of subjects. The necessary calculations to obtain the appropriate sums of squares are given below. The ANOVA for each group appears in Table 7.24.

Summary Calculations of GCF Data of Table 7.23

Group A (N = 9)	Group B (N = 10)
$(494)^2/18 = 13,557.5556 \qquad = CT =$	$(918)^2/20 = 42,136.2000$
$[(42)^2 + (118)^2 + \ldots + (45)^2]/2 - CT = $ Between Indiv $SS = [(151)^2 + (23)^2 + \ldots + (10)^2]/2 - CT$	
$= 34,174.0000/2 - CT = 17,082.0000 - CT$	$= 111,170.0000 - CT = 55,585.0000 - CT$
$= 3,529.4444$	$= 13,448.8000$
$\overset{18}{\Sigma}x^2 - CT = [(32)^2 + (69)^2 + \ldots + (22)^2] - CT = $ Total $SS = \overset{18}{\Sigma}x^2 - CT = [(78)^2 + (10)^2 + \ldots + (1)^2] - CT$	
$= 17,878.0000 - CT = 4,320.4444$	$= 56,102.0000 - CT = 13,965.8000$

It is worthwhile to make certain comparisons between the make up of these two groups. It is noted, for example, that the Within Individuals MS is approximately the same for the two groups, 87.89, and 51.70, respectively. An F-test (two-tailed; see footnote, page 105) can be performed.

$$F_{9, 10} = 87.89/57.10 = 1.70.$$

The critical value of $F_{9, 10}$ corresponding to 2.5% in one tail (5% in two tails) is given as 3.78 (see Snedecor and Cochran[2]), so that the value of F is statistically not significant. Hence, the intraindividual variation may be the same in the two groups, as indeed it should be. We are still assuming, of course, that all the individuals in either group have the same intraindividual variability. We may also compare the two interindividual MS (441.18 and 1,494.31) which measure the heterogeneity of the two groups with respect to differences among individual levels.

TABLE 7.24
ANOVA Table for Group A and for Group B From Table 7.23

Source of Variation	Group A			Group B		
	df	SS	MS	df	SS	MS
Between Individuals	8	3,529.4444	441.18	9	13,448.8000	1,494.31
Within Individuals	9	791.0000	87.89	10	517.0000	51.70
Total	17	4,320.4444		19	13,965.8000	

$$F_{9,8} = 1,494.31/441.18 = 3.39.$$

The critical value of $F_{9,8}$ for 2.5% in one tail (5% in two tails) is 4.36. Thus, the mean squares do not differ significantly, nor should they, because the two groups were a random subdivision of a larger group.

In view of the demonstrated similarity, the two ANOVAS can be pooled into one analysis. There is an extra term to be calculated, namely, the Between Groups SS, in this case with one degree of freedom. This is calculated as:

Between Groups SS = (CT Group A + CT Group B – Overall CT
   = [(494)^2/18 + (918)^2/20] – (494 + 918)/38 = 3,226.8082.

The final table which presents the ANOVA of all these data is Table 7.25.

The major purpose of these data was to compare Groups A and B with respect to the mean levels of GCF. To do this, the Between Groups MS is compared with the Between Individuals (Within Groups) MS:

$$F_{1,17} = \frac{\text{Between Groups MS}}{\text{Between Individuals (Within Groups) MS}} = \frac{3,226.81}{998.72} = 3.23.$$

This is appropriate for the particular model we have, where individuals are nested within groups and individuals represent a random criterion. In the rare case where individuals are fixed and the inference is made solely for these individuals, the F would be formed differently.

It should be noted that the F, although not large, is close to being statistically significant at the 5% point. At any rate, we would evidently have to attribute it to the flukes of randomization. When the

TABLE 7.25
Two-Way Analysis of Variance for GCF Values of Groups A and B of Table 7.21

Source of Variation	df	SS	MS
Between Groups	1	3,226.8082	3,226.81
Between Individuals (Within Groups)	17	16,978.2444	998.72
Within Individuals	19	1,308.0000	68.84
Total	37	21,513.0526	

study proceeds to the next phase — namely, the different oral hygiene regimens — it is possible to make some adjustment for the initial differences in level.

Since there are only two groups involved, it would be entirely possible to perform a two-sample t-test. The nine individual means of Group A and the ten of Group B represent two samples whose means are 27.44 and 45.90, respectively. The pooled s^2 is computed in the usual way from the two samples of individual means with df = 17. The standard error of the difference in means is $s\sqrt{1/9 + 1/10}$. The resulting t_{17} should be exactly equal to the square root of the $F_{1,17}$ just calculated.

INCOMPLETE THREE-WAY ANALYSIS OF VARIANCE

In another frequent type of design, there are three criteria of classification, but the data are incompletely cross-classified. One of the criteria is nested within another criterion. An illustration of this type of problem, which the dental research worker may often meet, occurs when he compares the results of a treated and control group over a period of time. If there are only two time intervals, say before and after, the analysis can be performed by comparing the two groups with respect to the average difference between the before and after values by the t-test (see pages 73–77). When there are more than two time periods, however, an ANOVA can be performed. This type of ANOVA is more involved than those discussed previously. In Table 7.26, data are presented on the *L. acidophilus* counts in logarithms of seven vaccinated patients, before and at two and five months after vaccination with this organism.[21] Data are also given for six unvaccinated patients over the same time intervals. Patients are nested within vaccination status. The bacterial counts are highly variable and more closely approximate normal distributions if converted to logarithms.

From the data presented, we are primarily interested in determining: (1) whether the two groups differ significantly in their average level of *L. acidophilus* counts over this period of time; (2) whether the trends (variation between periods) differ significantly between the two groups; and (3) whether there is a significant overall trend (variation over time). While there are various ways of computing the ANOVA on the data in Table 7.26, a convenient method would be as follows: Compute a two-way ANOVA for both groups of patients.

TABLE 7.26
Logarithms of Salivary Lactobacilli Counts in Thousands

Patient Number	Vaccinated Patients				Patient Number	Control Patients			
	Before	2 Mo.	5 Mo.	Patient Total		Before	2 Mo.	5 Mo.	Patient Total
1	2.07	2.03	1.46	5.56	1	1.15	1.00	0.60	2.75
2	2.75	2.52	2.63	7.90	2	1.30	1.20	1.00	3.50
3	2.86	1.94	1.41	6.21	3	1.78	1.57	1.18	4.53
4	2.38	1.65	1.75	5.78	4	1.74	1.58	1.41	4.73
5	2.23	2.17	1.84	6.24	5	2.12	2.17	2.18	6.47
6	2.02	2.21	1.58	5.81	6	2.47	2.37	1.46	6.30
7	1.84	1.90	1.75	5.49					
Period Total	16.15	14.42	12.42	42.99	Period Total	10.56	9.89	7.83	28.28

Summary Calculations of Lactobacilli Data of Table 7.24

Vaccinated Group	Control Group

$(42.99)^2/21 = 88.0067 =$ *Correction Term* $= (28.28)^2/18 = 44.4310$

$[(16.15)^2 + \ldots + (12.42)^2]/7 - CT =$ $= [(10.56)^2 + \ldots + (7.83)^2]/6 - CT =$

$89.0022 - CT = 0.9955 =$ *Periods SS* $= 45.1058 - CT = 0.6748$

$[(5.56)^2 + \ldots + (5.49)^2]/3 - CT =$ $[(2.75)^2 + \ldots + (6.30)^2]/3 - CT$

$268.1299/3 - CT = 1.3699 =$ *Individuals SS* $= 144.2572/3 - CT = 3.6547$

$[(2.07)^2 + \ldots + (1.79)^2] - CT =$ $[(1.15)^2 + \ldots + (1.46)^2] - CT =$

$91.3343 - CT = 3.3276 =$ *Total SS* $= 49.1554 - CT = 4.7244$

Individual $\times$ Period Interaction SS* =
$0.9622 =$ Total SS $-$ (Periods SS + Individuals SS) $= 0.3943$

Next, the two two-way ANOVAS calculated for the two vaccination groups are added together, giving Table 7.27.

Because Periods are crossed with Groups, the Between Periods (Within Groups) SS can be divided into two parts: Between Periods and Period $\times$ Group Interaction, each with two degrees of freedom.

$$\text{Correction Term} = \frac{(42.99 + 28.28)^2}{39} = 130.2414.$$

$$\text{Between Periods SS} = \frac{(16.15 + 10.56)^2 + \ldots + (12.42 + 7.83)^2}{7 + 6} - CT$$

$$= 131.8817 - CT = 1.6403.$$

Period $\times$ Group Interaction SS = Between Periods (Within Groups)
$$- \text{Between Periods}$$
$$= 1.6703 - 1.6403 = 0.0300.$$

TABLE 7.27

Two-Way Analysis of Variance for Both Vaccination Groups of Table 7.24

Source of Variation	df	SS
Between Periods (Within Groups)	4	1.6703
Between Individuals (Within Groups)	11	5.0246
Individual $\times$ Period Interaction		
(Within Groups)[a]	22	1.3571
Total (Within Groups)	37	8.0520

[a]We are not calling this term *Residual* in view of its probable inflation by an interaction.

When the two groups are compared, there is still one other source of variation, Between Groups SS, with df = 1. The calculation of the SS for this new source of variation follows:

$$\text{Between Groups SS} = \frac{(42.99)^2}{21} + \frac{(28.28)^2}{18} - CT = 132.4377 - CT$$

$$= 2.1963.$$

The final ANOVA appears in Table 7.28.

The answer to the first question as to whether the two groups differ in their average level of *L. acidophilus* counts, is given by determining whether they differ more from each other than do the individuals of the same group differ among themselves. We calculate:

$$F_{1,11} = \frac{\text{Between Groups MS}}{\text{Between Individuals (Within Groups) MS}} = \frac{2.1963}{0.4568} = 4.81.$$

This F value is almost statistically significant at the 5% point. We note that since we are comparing the means of the logarithms we are also comparing the geometric means (antilogs of the means of the logs).

The answer to the second question as to whether the two groups exhibit different period to period trends, can be found by comparing the group differences in trend with the differences in trend for individuals of the same group. We calculate:

$$F_{2,22} = \frac{\text{Period} \times \text{Group Interaction MS}}{\text{Individual} \times \text{Period Interaction (Within Groups) MS}}$$

$$= \frac{0.0150}{0.0617} = 0.2431, P > 5\%.$$

We can, therefore, state that the two groups do not exhibit significantly different period to period trends. In other words, the trends may be parallel.

The answer to the third question as to whether there is an overall trend (variation over time) is answered by

$$F_{2,22} = \frac{\text{Between Periods MS}}{\text{Individual} \times \text{Period Interaction (Within Groups) MS}}$$

$$= \frac{0.8202}{0.0617} = 13.29.$$

TABLE 7.28
Analysis of Variance of Data of Table 7.25

Source of Variation	df	SS	MS
Between Individuals (Within Groups)	11	5.0246	0.4568
Between Groups	1	2.1963	2.1963
Between Periods	2	1.6403	0.8202
Period $\times$ Group Interaction	2	0.0300	0.0150
Individual $\times$ Period Interaction			
(Within Groups)	22	1.3571	0.0617
Total	38	10.2483	

This is highly significant. For both the vaccinated and control patients, the mean bacterial count (or rather, the geometric mean) decreases consistently over time.*

The example of the incomplete three-way layout presented here is a special type of mixed model in which the two criteria, Period and Group, are fixed, whereas the other, Individual, is random. This type of problem is frequently encountered in dental and oral research. The selection of the *Error* mean squares for the denominators of the suggested F-tests apply to this particular type of mixed model.

Repeat Measurements Over Time

In the above example, for each of the groups the block is the individual who is measured at various times so that time is considered as a fixed factor. No randomization of the modalities of this factor is possible, however, since one time period naturally precedes the next. In such cases, there are frequently defects in the ANOVA model in the sense that the intercorrelations of the measurements at the various times are not constant as demanded in the usual model. Data of this type are said to represent repeat readings over time. In fact, when another factor such as in this case, Group, is involved, the whole design is often called a *split plot* design, the term originating in agricultural studies. If there are only two times involved, e.g., with a single group, no problem would arise, since, by virtue of taking dif-

---

*The data in Table 7.26 were selected for illustrative purposes from a larger study, so that the conclusions drawn from the preceding analyses may not apply to the study as a whole. It is obvious that an actual design would require more than 13 individuals.

ferences only one variance would have to be estimated (see discussion of the paired t-test in Chapter 5). If two groups are involved, as in the present case, again there is no problem if there are only two time periods, since then the average difference for one group may be compared with the average difference for the other group (see, for example, the discussion in Chapter 5). For more than two time periods, however, either with a single group or with two or more groups, the ANOVA model and the corresponding F-tests involving time, may be incorrect. Alternatives have been suggested in the sense of using multivariate methods which are beyond the scope of this book.[22,23]

THREE-WAY ANALYSIS OF VARIANCE

A study was made of plasma salicylate levels obtained at four time periods (10, 15, 20, and 30 minutes) on 28 individuals after taking standard tablets of Code Drug A or Code Drug B.[24] After an overnight fasting period, and following withdrawal of a blood sample, each subject received two tablets of one of the drugs, which were swallowed without chewing and followed by 100 ml of water. One-half of the group was chosen at random to receive Drug A, while the other half received Drug B. After an interval of at least three days (to eliminate residual effects of prior medication) those individuals who had received Drug A first were then given Drug B, and those who had received Drug B first were given Drug A after three days. Whether an individual received A first was determined by randomization. Approximately half of the individuals received the sequence AB, the remainder BA.* (The data are presented in Table 7.29 on page 150.)

In this experiment, the plasma salicyclic levels were completely cross-classified with respect to three criteria: individuals, drugs, and periods (or time intervals). In this type of experimental model, the investigators regarded two of the criteria or factors as "fixed": the two specific drugs and the four specific time periods after the subjects took the drug preparations. The 28 individuals on whom the data were drawn, however, constituted a "random" sample of all

---

*The original study, analyzed in the previous edition, included a second run of the experiment that made statistical analysis conform to a four-way analysis of variance, using Runs as an additional criterion. To simplify the discussion, this has been eliminated from this edition.

individuals who could have been studied. The type of experimental model that we have may, therefore, be regarded as a *mixed model*. As previously mentioned, the mixed model is used frequently in clinical experimentation, although there are certainly not always three criteria. The methods of statistical analysis to be employed and the interpretations to be made from them are dictated by the model.

Two-Way Analysis of Variance

There are seven sources of variation, as follows: Between Individuals, Between Periods, Between Drugs, Individual × Period Interaction, Individual × Drug Interaction, Period × Drug Interaction, and Individual × Period × Drug Interaction (or Triple Interaction). A convenient method for calculating the various terms of the analysis of variance with three criteria would be (a) to analyze the data for each drug as a two-way analysis of variance; (b) to perform a two-way analysis of variance on the sum of the measurements of Drug A and B to obtain the terms of the three-way analysis of variance not involving drugs; and (c) to subtract the terms under (b) from the sums of the corresponding terms in (a), to obtain the interaction terms of the three-way analysis of variance involving drug, d. to compute the Between Drugs SS separately.

The method to be used for the separate two-way analyses of variance on Drug B and Drug A using the data from Table 7.29, has been illustrated previously (page 141). We also need a summary table showing the values for each individual when Drug B and Drug A are added at each of the four time periods. Thus, for the first individual, 0.75 + 0.15 = 0.90; 1.05 + 0.25 = 1.30; 1.70 + 1.35 – 3.05; 3.10 + 2.35 = 5.45, and similarly for the 27 other individuals. This summary table appears as Table 7.30 on page 151.

From Table 7.30 the correction term (CT) is obtained as follows:

$$CT = \frac{(\text{Grand total of 224 readings})^2}{224} = \frac{(409.53)^2}{224} = 748.7269.$$

$$\text{Between Individuals SS} = \frac{\text{Sum of 28 (individual total)}^2}{(2)(4)} - CT$$

$$= \frac{(10.70)^2 + (12.45)^2 + \ldots + (8.25)^2 + (13.40)^2}{8} - CT$$

$$= 106.9602.$$

TABLE 7.29
Plasma Salicylate Levels (mg%) for Drug B and Drug A

Individual Number	Drug B/Minutes					Drug A/Minutes				
	10	15	20	30	Individual Total	10	15	20	30	Individual Total
1	0.15	0.25	1.35	2.35	4.10	0.75	1.05	1.70	3.10	6.60
2	1.20	2.20	3.30	4.25	10.95	0.10	0.15	0.50	0.75	1.50
3	0.30	1.50	1.85	2.70	6.35	0.30	0.80	1.30	2.20	4.60
4	0.50	1.60	3.15	3.70	8.95	0.65	1.35	1.75	2.35	6.10
5	1.20	1.40	1.70	3.35	7.65	0.30	0.55	1.10	1.30	3.25
6	0.65	2.50	5.00	5.60	13.75	0.80	1.70	1.80	2.80	7.10
7	0.40	1.15	1.40	1.60	4.55	0.40	0.60	0.75	1.55	3.30
8	0.90	2.40	3.75	5.00	12.05	1.25	2.50	2.90	4.15	10.80
9	1.00	2.00	3.75	4.80	11.55	0.70	1.05	2.00	3.70	7.45
10	1.40	3.30	3.50	5.85	14.05	0.10	0.18	0.85	1.10	2.23
11	0.45	1.15	2.35	4.05	8.00	0.40	0.60	0.83	1.30	3.13
12	1.15	4.15	6.05	6.95	18.30	0.50	0.75	0.95	2.50	4.70
13	1.08	1.10	2.15	2.34	6.67	0.25	0.55	0.80	1.15	2.75
14	1.60	2.75	3.56	5.10	13.01	0.45	0.55	0.95	1.35	3.30
15	0.20	0.40	0.95	1.15	2.70	0.35	0.65	1.55	2.05	4.60
16	0.40	0.42	1.95	2.40	5.17	0.70	0.80	1.45	2.80	5.75
17	0.60	0.65	1.50	3.70	6.45	0.10	0.25	0.30	0.80	1.45
18	2.40	4.10	4.45	6.15	17.10	0.45	0.55	0.85	1.00	2.85
19	0.90	3.00	3.10	4.00	11.00	0.00	0.35	0.70	1.15	2.20
20	2.00	3.45	4.35	6.05	15.85	0.25	1.90	2.18	3.70	8.03
21	0.65	0.80	1.15	2.40	5.00	0.55	0.75	0.95	1.45	3.70
22	1.45	2.95	3.95	4.85	13.20	0.70	1.20	1.62	1.95	5.47
23	1.70	2.35	2.65	5.05	11.75	0.65	1.10	1.65	2.35	5.75
24	2.35	3.20	4.15	4.45	14.15	1.10	3.25	3.60	4.77	12.72
25	1.65	3.40	3.50	3.60	12.15	0.60	1.10	1.30	2.25	5.25
26	0.20	0.55	1.70	3.45	5.90	0.20	0.25	0.80	1.70	2.95
27	0.00	0.45	1.50	2.70	4.65	0.10	1.00	1.20	1.30	3.60
28	1.70	1.85	2.10	3.35	9.00	0.60	0.65	1.40	1.75	4.40
Period total	28.18	55.02	79.86	110.94	274.00	13.30	26.18	37.73	58.32	135.53
Period mean	1.01	1.97	2.85	3.96		0.48	0.94	1.35	2.08	

TABLE 7.30
Plasma Salicylate Levels[a] for Drug B Plus Drug A

Individual Number	Periods/Minutes				Individual Total
	10	15	20	30	
1	0.90	1.30	3.05	5.45	10.70
2	1.30	2.35	3.80	5.00	12.45
3	0.60	2.30	3.15	4.90	10.95
4	1.15	2.95	4.90	6.05	15.05
5	1.50	1.95	2.80	4.65	10.90
6	1.45	4.20	6.80	8.40	20.85
7	0.80	1.75	2.15	3.15	7.85
8	2.15	4.90	6.65	9.15	22.85
9	1.70	3.05	5.75	8.50	19.00
10	1.50	3.48	4.35	6.95	16.28
11	0.85	1.75	3.18	5.35	11.13
12	1.65	4.90	7.00	9.45	23.00
13	1.33	1.65	2.95	3.49	9.42
14	2.05	3.30	4.51	6.45	16.31
15	0.55	1.05	2.50	3.20	7.30
16	1.10	1.22	3.40	5.20	10.92
17	0.70	0.90	1.80	4.50	7.90
18	2.85	4.65	5.30	7.15	19.95
19	0.90	3.35	3.80	5.15	13.20
20	2.25	5.35	6.53	9.75	23.88
21	1.20	1.55	2.10	3.85	8.70
22	2.15	4.15	5.57	6.80	18.67
23	2.35	3.45	4.30	7.40	17.50
24	3.45	6.45	7.75	9.22	26.87
25	2.25	4.50	4.80	5.85	17.40
26	0.40	0.80	2.50	5.15	8.85
27	0.10	1.45	2.70	4.00	8.25
28	2.30	2.50	3.50	5.10	13.40
Period total	41.48	81.20	117.59	169.26	409.53

[a] Levels given in mg%.

$$\text{Between Periods SS} = \frac{\text{Sum of 4 (period total)}^2}{(2)(28)} - CT$$

$$= \frac{(41.48)^2 + (81.20)^2 + (117.59)^2 + (169.26)^2}{56} - CT$$

$$= 158.2443.$$

$$\text{Between Cells SS} = \frac{\text{Sum of 112 (cell reading)}^2}{2} - CT$$

$$= \frac{(0.90)^2 + (1.30)^2 + \ldots + (3.50)^2 + (5.10)^2}{2} - CT$$

$$= 288.4853.$$

Each individual-period cell reading represents the sum of a reading for Drug B and for Drug A.

Individual × Period Interaction SS = Between Cells SS
                 − (Between Individuals SS + Between Periods SS) = 23.2808.

From the individual totals specific for drug in Table 7.16, we compute the following:

$$\text{Between Drugs SS} = \frac{\text{Sum of 2 (drug total)}^2}{(28)(4)} - CT$$

$$= \frac{(274.00)^2 + (135.53)^2}{112} - CT = 85.5979.$$

The sums of the terms for the separate two-way analyses performed on Drug A and Drug B, as well as the terms of the two-way analysis performed on the data of Table 7.30 and Between Drugs SS, are given in Table 7.31.

It may be noted here that the data correspond to repeat readings over time, but the assumption has been made that time may be used as a fixed criterion in the ANOVA. Reference to this type of problem has been made on page 147 in connection with the incomplete three-way ANOVA. A more elegant way, which would avoid some of the assumptions inherent in the ANOVA, would be to regard the readings at the four time periods as readings on four different variables and resort to some type of multivariate analysis. This type of analysis for a three-way layout has been illustrated by Fertig, Chilton, and Varma.[25]

Check on SS Involving Drugs

The four SS involving drugs can be checked very easily by an independent procedure, since there are only two drugs involved. For this purpose, a table of differences of the values of Drug B minus the values of Drug A for each patient at each time period is constructed. Thus, for the first patient, the difference between B and A at 10

TABLE 7.31
Sums of Squares for Two-Way and Three-Way Analysis of Variance

Source of Variation	df	Sum of Squares For Drug A and Drug B	df	SS For (Drug A + Drug B)	Difference (Interaction with Drug)
Between Individuals (I)	$2(28 - 1) = 54$	170.9822	27	106.9602	64.0220
Between Periods (P)	$2(4 - 1) = 6$	172.5922	3	158.2443	14.3479
Individual × Period Interaction (IP)	$2(28 - 1)$ $\times (4 - 1) = 162$	42.6313	81	23.2808	19.3505
Individual × Drug Interaction (ID)			$(28 - 1)(2 - 1) = 27$	64.0220	
Period × Drug Interaction (PD)			$(4 - 1)(2 - 1) = 3$	14.3479	
Individual × Period × Drug Interaction (IPD)			$(28 - 1)(4 - 1)$ $\times (2 - 1) = 81$	19.3505	
Between drugs (D)			$(2 - 1) = 1$	85.5979	
Total			223	471.8036	

minutes is 0.15 - 0.75 = -0.60; at 15 minutes, 0.25 - 1.05 = -0.80; at 20 minutes, 1.35 - 1.70 = -0.35; and at 30 minutes, 2.35 - 3.10 = -0.75; and so on for the other 27 patients. This summary table appears as Table 7.31.

From this table, we calculate

$$CT = \frac{(\text{Grand total of 112 readings})^2}{(112)(2)} = \frac{(+138.47)^2}{224}$$

$$= 85.5979 = \text{Between Drugs SS.*}$$

$$\text{Between Individuals SS} = \frac{\text{Sum of 28 (individual total)}^2}{(4)(2)} - CT$$

$$= \frac{(-2.50)^2 + (+9.45)^2 + \ldots + (+1.05)^2 + (+4.60)^2}{8} - CT$$

$$= 64.0219 = \text{Individual} \times \text{Drug Interaction SS.}$$

$$\text{Between Periods SS} = \frac{\text{Sum of 4 (period total)}^2}{(28)(2)} - CT$$

$$= \frac{(+14.88)^2 + (+28.84)^2 + (+42.13)^2 + (+52.62)^2}{56} - CT$$

$$= 14.3478 = \text{Period} \times \text{Drug Interaction SS.}$$

$$\text{Between Cells SS} = \frac{\text{Sum of 112 (cell reading)}^2}{2} - CT$$

$$= \frac{(-0.60)^2 + (-0.80)^2 + \ldots + (+0.70)^2 + (+1.60)^2}{2}$$

$$- CT = 97.7203.$$

---

*Since the *main effects* Between Drugs involve only one degree of freedom, it is evident that the test of significance of this effect could have been performed by an appropriate t-test. The correction term in the table of differences is the Between Drug SS and this will be tested for significance by Between Individuals MS from the table of differences (actually, the Individual $\times$ Drug Interaction MS). Alternatively, from scratch, the average difference for every individual can be calculated by averaging the four differences for each individual thus obtaining a single sample of 28 differences, from which a value of t is readily calculated.

TABLE 7.32
Difference in Plasma Salicylate Levels (mg%) Drug B – Drug A

Individual Number	Periods/Minutes				Individual Number
	10	15	20	30	
1	− 0.60	− 0.80	− 0.35	− 0.75	− 2.50
2	+ 1.10	+ 2.05	+ 2.80	+ 3.50	+ 9.45
3	0.00	+ 0.70	+ 0.55	+ 0.50	+ 1.75
4	− 0.15	+ 0.25	+ 1.40	+ 1.35	+ 2.85
5	+ 0.90	+ 0.85	+ 0.60	+ 2.05	+ 4.40
6	− 0.15	+ 0.80	+ 3.20	+ 2.80	+ 6.65
7	0.00	+ 0.55	+ 0.65	+ 0.05	+ 1.25
8	− 0.35	− 0.10	+ 0.85	+ 0.85	+ 1.25
9	+ 0.30	+ 0.95	+ 1.75	+ 1.10	+ 4.10
10	+ 1.30	+ 3.12	+ 2.65	+ 4.75	+ 11.82
11	+ 0.05	+ 0.55	+ 1.52	+ 2.75	+ 4.87
12	+ 0.65	+ 3.40	+ 5.10	+ 4.45	+ 13.60
13	+ 0.83	+ 0.55	+ 1.35	+ 1.19	+ 3.92
14	+ 1.15	+ 2.20	+ 2.61	+ 3.75	+ 9.71
15	− 0.15	− 0.25	− 0.60	− 0.90	− 1.90
16	− 0.30	− 0.38	+ 0.50	− 0.40	− 0.58
17	+ 0.50	+ 0.40	+ 1.20	+ 2.90	+ 5.00
18	+ 1.95	+ 3.55	+ 3.60	+ 5.15	+ 14.25
19	+ 0.90	+ 2.65	+ 2.40	+ 2.85	+ 8.80
20	+ 1.75	+ 1.55	+ 2.17	+ 2.35	+ 7.82
21	+ 0.10	+ 0.05	+ 0.20	+ 0.95	+ 1.30
22	+ 0.75	+ 1.75	+ 2.33	+ 2.90	+ 7.73
23	+ 1.05	+ 1.25	+ 1.00	+ 2.70	+ 6.00
24	+ 1.25	+ 0.05	+ 0.55	− 0.32	+ 1.43
25	+ 1.05	+ 2.30	+ 2.20	+ 1.35	+ 6.90
26	0.00	+ 0.30	+ 0.90	+ 1.75	+ 2.95
27	− 0.10	− 0.55	+ 0.30	+ 1.40	+ 1.05
28	+ 1.10	+ 1.20	+ 0.70	+ 1.60	+ 4.60
Period Total	+14.88	+28.84	+42.13	+52.62	+138.47

Each individual-period cell involves a difference between two drugs; consequently, there are two readings:

Individual × Period Interaction SS = Between Cells SS
− (Between Periods SS + Between Individuals SS)
= 19.3506 = Individual × Period × Drug Interaction SS.

Interpretations

While the calculations of the seven components in the three-way analysis of variance can be performed readily, considerable difficulty may be encountered in the selection of the appropriate numerator and denominator for the F-ratios which are used for testing the statistical significance of the various effects or interactions. The numerator is the particular effect or interaction that the investigator is interested in testing, with its degrees of freedom, df_1. The difficulty usually lies in the selection of the appropriate denominator, i.e., the error MS, with its degrees of freedom, df_2. For example, do the two drugs differ with respect to the level of plasma salicylate obtained? In this case the numerator for the F-ratio is obviously Between Drugs MS, $df_1 = 1$. In this experiment, where the only random criterion is individual, the appropriate denominator for testing the difference between drugs is that term which measures how the drug difference fluctuates from individual to individual, namely, Individual $\times$ Drug Interaction MS (ID), $df_2 = 27$.

Selection of the appropriate error term, i.e., the denominator of the F-ratio, will depend on the type of model to which the experiment conforms. In our example, on which the three-way analysis of variance is based, there are three criteria: drugs (D), periods (P), and individuals (I). The investigators were interested in two specific drugs and the plasma levels of salicylate at four specific time periods. They selected 28 individuals at random from some universe of all individuals who could have been selected. Thus, we shall consider the criteria drug and period, as "fixed," and the criterion individuals as "random."

In this type of model, with two criteria fixed and one random, the error MS (the denominator of the F-ratio) for any fixed effect or interaction involving only fixed effect is the interaction of that same effect (or interaction) with individual (I), the random criterion. There are simple rules of thumb for determining the expected values of the mean squares and also for selecting the appropriate numerators and denominators for the F-tests under the various models. If the effect (or interaction) includes I, then there is no proper denominator unless certain higher-order interactions can be assumed to be truly zero. The investigators, however, were not usually interested in testing the sources of variation involving I, because it was recognized at the outset that there would be individual differences. It was precisely for this reason that this "nuisance" variable, I, was controlled in the design by cross-classifying the other criteria with individual, i.e., by using the same individuals over again.

In the plasma salicylate experiment, used as an example, the investigators were primarily interested in answering three questions:

1. Does the plasma salicylate level change with time, regardless of drug? In other words, is the absorption curve depicted in Figure 7.1 (B + A curve) different from a horizontal line?

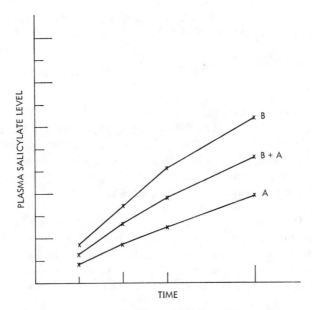

FIG. 7.1 D/ID Significant; PD/IPD Significant.

2. Is there a difference between the two drugs in the plasma salicylate level obtained, regardless of time? This question calls for a
comparison of the average readings over the four time periods for
Drug B with those of Drug A (Fig. 7.1).

3. Is the change in plasma salicylate level with time different for
the two drugs? This question refers to the parallelism of the two absorption curves as well as to the constancy of the drug differences
for the various periods (Figure 7.1).

In answering the first question, the numerator of the F-ratio is
obviously Between Periods MS (P). The denominator is the interaction of period with individual, i.e., Individual × Period Interaction
MS (IP). Thus,

$$F = \frac{P}{IP} = \frac{102.8433}{0.3945} = 260.69; \, df_1 = 3, df_2 = 81 \text{ (significant)}.$$

The absorption curve (B + A) in Figure 7.1 differs from a horizontal
line. Similarly, the numerator of the F-ratio for answering Question 2
is Between Drugs MS (D), and the denominator is the interaction of
drug with individual, i.e., Individual × Drug Interaction MS (ID):

$$F = \frac{D}{ID} = \frac{143.4199}{2.8593} = 50.16; \, df_1 = 1, df_2 = 27 \text{ (significant)}.$$

The B and the A curves in Figure 7.1 are at different vertical levels. The third question is answered by

$$F = \frac{PD}{IPD} = \frac{9.9321}{0.2609} = 38.17; df_1 = 3, df_2 = 81 \text{ (significant)}.$$

The B and A curves in Figure 7.1 are not parallel.

Actually, Questions 2 and 3 are more important for the investigators than Question 1, since they know from prior experience that there is some sort of plasma salicylate absorption curve. In general, there are four possible combinations of significance and nonsignificance of the ratios referring to Questions 2 and 3.

A. D/ID significant and PD/IPD significant. There is an average drug difference over the time periods, but the average difference is not constant, i.e., the absorption curves are not parallel. This is the actual situation in the plasma salicylate example, as shown in Figure 7.1. Drug B gives higher plasma salicylate levels and has a faster absorption curve than Drug A.

B. D/ID significant and PD/IPD not significant. There is a drug difference which is constant, within chance error, from period to period, i.e., the absorption curves may be parallel, without consideration of their shapes (see Fig. 7.2 for hypothetical examples).

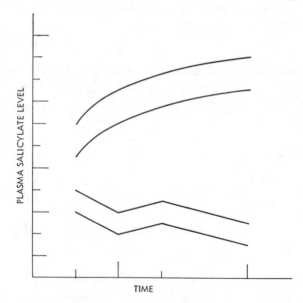

FIG. 7.2 D/ID Significant; PD/IPD Not Significant.

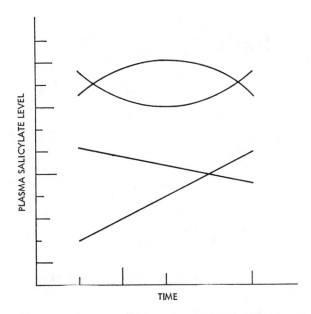

FIG. 7.3 D/IP Not Significant; PD/IPD Significant.

C. D/ID not significant and PD/IPD significant. The two absorption curves are different, but there is some sort of comparison (or crossing over), so that, over the periods studied, there is no significant difference between the average drug readings (see Figure 7.3 for hypothetical examples).

D. D/ID not significant and PD/IPD not significant. There is no average drug difference for the periods, and the curves may be parallel, i.e., the curves essentially coincide except for chance variation (see Figure 7.4 for hypothetical examples).

When there is a significant interaction (Case A,D) the statement with respect to the effect of the Drug, i.e., the main effect, lacks some clarity because the difference (the effect) is not uniform, but depends on the time at which it is measured.

It is evident that each cell should have a reading. If any of the cells are empty, we run into the same problem as in the two-way layout, except that it is a little more complicated. Occasionally, we have three-way layouts in which the number of readings per cell is more than one. If the number of readings per cell is constant, there is no difficulty; nor is there any difficulty with certain types of proportionality of the numbers. If the numbers in the cells are neither equal nor proportional, however, then the same sort of difficulties exist as

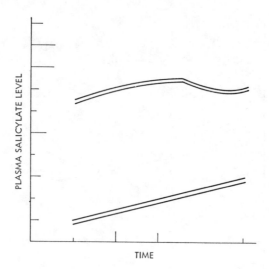

FIG. 7.4 D/ID Not Significant; PD/IPD Not Significant.

in the two-way layout with replications in the cell except it is much worse.

A three-way model has been illustrated in which only two criteria were fixed and the other was random. Obviously, there are many other possibilities, such as two of the criteria might be random and only one fixed, or all three might be random. While the arithmetic of these models is exactly the same as for the three-way layout just illustrated, the selection of the proper Error terms is not the same.[26]

The method of assigning the patients to an AB sequence or a BA sequence was purely random. There was no restriction on the numbers falling into the two sequences. If, however, a restriction were made such that half should follow the AB sequence and half the BA sequence, then there is an extra restriction corresponding to a crossover design (see Chapter 17). If there were a three-way layout with the extra restriction of a crossover, then, if the extra restriction were considered important, a somewhat different ANOVA is called for in which an extra main effect and extra interactions are isolated.

REFERENCES

1. Shannon, I. L., and Gibson, W. A.: Oral glucose tolerance responses in healthy young adult males classified as to caries experience and periodontal status, Periodontics 2:293, 1964.

2. Snedecor, G. W., and Cochran, W. G.: Statistical Methods, 7th ed., Ames, Iowa, Iowa State College Press, 1980.

3. Dixon, W. J., and Massey, F. J., Jr.: Introduction to Statistical Analysis, 3rd ed. New York, McGraw-Hill, 1969.

4. Dunn, O. J.: Multiple comparisons among means, J Amer Stat Assn 56:52, 1961.

5. Miller, R. G.: Simultaneous Statistical Inference, 2nd ed., New York, Springer-Verlag, 1981.

6. Nair, K. R.: The studentized form of the extreme mean square test in the analysis of variance, Biometrika 35:16, 1948.

7. Dunnett, C. W.: New tables for multiple comparisons with a control, Biometrics 20:482, 1965.

8. Scheffé, H.: A method of judging all contrasts in the analysis of variance, Biometrika 40:87, 1953.

9. Tukey, J. W.: Some selected quick and easy methods of statistical analysis, Trans NY Acad Sci 16:88, 1953.

10. Kurtz, T. E., Link, R. F., Tukey, J. W., and Wallace, D. C.: Shortcut multiple comparisons for balanced single and double classifications. Part I, Results. Technometrics 7:95, 1965.

11. Mann, J., Greene, J. J., Stoller, N. H., Byrne, J., and Chilton, N. W.: Inter- and intra-examiner variability in scoring supragingival plaque. I. The clinical study. Pharm & Thera in Dent 5:1, 1980.

12. Wolf, R. O., and Taylor, L. L.: A comparative study of saliva protein analysis, Arch Oral Biol 9:135, 1964.

13. Steel, R. G. D., and Torre, J. H., Principles and Procedures of Statistics, 2nd ed., New York, McGraw-Hill, 1980.

14. Bruun, C., Giskov, H., and Stoltze, K.: *In vivo* uptake and retention of fluoride in human surface enamel after application of a fluoride-containing lacquer (Fluor-Protector), Caries Res, 14:103, 1980.

15. Anderson, R. L., and Bancroft, T. A.: Statistical Theory in Research, New York, McGraw-Hill, 1952.

16. Skier, J., and Mandel, I. D.: Comparative periodontal status of caries resistant versus susceptible adults, J Periodont 5:614, 1980.

17. Fertig, J. W., and Chilton, N. W.: A dental local anesthetic study, fixed model, two-way layout design, Arch Oral Biol 13:1477, 1968.

18. Chilton, N. W., and Fertig, J. W.: Studies in the design and analysis of dental experiments. I. The importance of equal sample sizes in experiments, J Dent Res 39:53, 1960.

19. Kutscher, A. H., Zegarelli, E. V., Roland, N., Chilton, N. W., and Mercadente, J. L.: A new, long-acting vehicle for the application of drugs to the oral mucous membranes, J Amer Dent Assn 62:666, 1961.

20. Chilton, N. W., and Maher, T.: The variability of gingival crevicular fluid determinations. School of Dental Medicine, University of Pennsylvania, 1981 (unpublished).

21. Williams, N. B.: Immunization of human beings with oral lactobacilli, J Dent Res 23:403, 1944.

22. Morrison, D. A.: Multivariate Statistical Analysis, 2nd ed., New York, McGraw-Hill, 1976.

23. Fertig, J. W., Varma, A. O., and Senning, R.: Techniques for the analysis of repeat measurements over time. In Chilton, N. W., ed.: Proceedings of an international conference on clinical trials of agents used in the prevention/treatment of periodontal diseases, J Perio Res (Supplement 14), 1974.

24. Truitt, E. B., and Morgan, A. M.: A comparison of the gastrointestinal absorption of plain and buffered acetylsalicylic acid, Fed Proc Abstract: March 1959.

25. Fertig, J. W., Chilton, N. W., and Varma, A. O.: A multivariate analysis of pulpal responses of bilateral intact teeth, Arch Oral Biol 17:1255, 1972.

26. Schultze, E. F., Jr.: Rules of thumb for determining expectations of mean squares in the analysis of variance, Biometrics 11:123, 1955.

8

Regression and Correlation

This chapter deals primarily with some of the simpler aspects of regression and correlation involving two variables as illustrated in the literature on dental research.

REGRESSION

The enzymatic hydrolysis of procaine was studied by incubating human plasma samples containing 3.7×10^{-4} moles of procaine per liter. At various time intervals samples were withdrawn and the quantity hydrolyzed determined.[1] The results for one plasma, given below, will illustrate linear regression technique.

The times at which the samples of plasma were measured for quantity hydrolyzed were fixed by the investigator. The determinations of quantity hydrolyzed are independent random values, subject

TABLE 8.1
Quantity of Hydrolyzed Procaine [(moles/liter) $\times$ 10^5]
by Incubation Time (minutes) of Human Plasma

Time (min)	Quantity Hydrolyzed [(moles/liter) $\times$ 10^5]
2	3.5
3	5.7
5	9.9
8	16.3
10	19.3
12	25.7
14	28.2
15	32.6

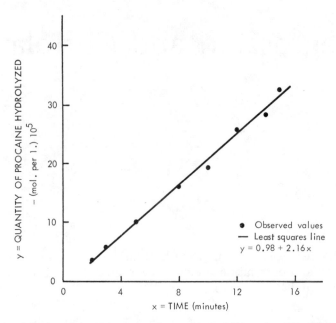

FIG. 8.1 Relationship Between Quantity of Procaine Hydrolyzed in Plasma 1 and Time.

to measurement error. In graphing the material on arithmetic paper, the fixed variable, Time, is usually represented on the x-axis and the random variable, Quantity Hydrolyzed, along the y-axis (Figure 8.1). From theoretical chemical considerations the relationship should be linear and, indeed, this is shown. The points follow a straight line closely so that it would not be difficult to find a freehand straight line that would adequately describe the relationship of enzymatic hydrolysis of procaine to time. However, the straight line that "best" represents the relationship of Quantity Hydrolyzed to Time can be constructed by the *Method of Least Squares.** In this method a straight line is so fitted that the sum of the squares of the vertical deviations of the *graphed points* from the corresponding y values on the fitted line is minimized. The method of least squares can also be used to fit other curves, such as parabolas, hyperbolas, etc., to data. The fitting of only the simplest type of curve, the straight line, will be illustrated here.

The formula for a straight line fitted to the data may be given as

---

*The line depicted in Figure 8.1 has been constructed by the method of least squares.

Y = a – bx. This means that the values (Y) on the vertical or ordinate scale are equal to a constant (a) plus the product of the values (x) on the horizontal or abscissa scale multiplied by another constant (b). The value of b is the slope of the line, i.e., change in y per unit change in x. b is often called the *regression coefficient* of y on x. The value of a is the intercept of the line, i.e., the value of y when x = 0.*

The method of least squares which minimizes $\Sigma(y - Y)^2$, results in two simultaneous equations (the so-called *normal equations*) from which we can determine the appropriate values of the constants "a" and "b":

$$(1) \quad Na + b\Sigma x = \Sigma y$$

$$(2) \quad a\Sigma x + b\Sigma x^2 = \Sigma xy.$$

The only unknowns in these two equations are a and b, since we can calculate everything else from the data available. Thus:

N = the number of (x, y) points = 8

$\Sigma x = 2 + 3 + 5 + 8 + 10 + 12 + 14 + 15 = 69$

$\Sigma y = 3.5 + 5.7 + 9.9 + 16.3 + 19.3 + 25.7 + 28.2 + 32.6 = 141.2$

$\Sigma x^2 = (2)^2 + (3)^2 + (5)^2 + (8)^2 + (10)^2 + (12)^2 + (14)^2 + (15)^2 = 767$

$\Sigma xy = 2(3.5) + 3(5.7) + 5(9.9) + 8(16.3) + 10(19.3)$
$\qquad\qquad\qquad + 12(25.7) + 14(28.2) + 15(32.6) = 1,589.2.$

Substituting these values in the two equations, we obtain:

$$(1) \quad 8a + 69b = 141.2$$

$$(2) \quad 69a + 767b = 1,589.2.$$

One convenient way of solving these simultaneous equations is by first dividing each one by the respective coefficient of "a", obtaining:

$$(1)' \quad a + 8.6250b = 17.6500$$

$$(2)' \quad a + 11.1159b = 23.0319$$

Subtracting $(2)'$ from $(1)'$ we obtain:

---

*y is often called the *dependent variable* and x is the *independent* or *predictor variable*.

$-2.4909b = -5.3819$

$b = +2.1606$ $+2.16 \times 10^{-5}$ moles per liter per min.

Substituting this value of "b" in Equation (1) above:

(1) $8a + 69(2.16) = 141.2$

$8a + 149.04 = 141.2$

$8a = 141.2 - 149.04 = -7.84$

$a = -0.98 \times 10^{-5}$ moles.

As an alternative, a and b may be calculated quickly by using formulae

$$b = \frac{\Sigma xy - \dfrac{\Sigma x \Sigma y}{N}}{\Sigma x^2 - \dfrac{(\Sigma x)^2}{N}} = \frac{1{,}589.2 - \dfrac{69(141.2)}{8}}{767 - \dfrac{(69)^2}{8}} = \frac{371.35}{171.875} = 2.16.$$

The numerator of b is usually called the *Sum of Products* (SP_{xy})*
and represents an algebraic rearrangement of $\Sigma(x - \bar{x})(y - \bar{y})$. (Σx)
$(\Sigma y)/N$ is usually called the *Correction Term* (CT) for products.
$SP_{xy}/(N - 1)$ is called the covariance of x and y. The denominator is,
of course, SS_x, the Sum of Squares of the x's.

From the first normal equation, dividing by N, it is seen that
$a + b\bar{x} = \bar{y}$, showing that the line passes through the point of means
$\bar{x}, \bar{y}$, where $\bar{x} = 8.6205$; $\bar{y} = 17.6500$. Thus,

$$a = \bar{y} - b\bar{x} = [(141.2)/8) - (2.16)(69/8)]$$
$$= 17.6500 - 18.6300 = -0.98.$$

Substituting these values of a and b in the formula for a straight line,
we obtain the formula of the fitted line†:

$$Y = -0.98 + 2.16x.$$

---

*While the numerial value of SS must always be positive, SP values may
well be negative. In regression, a negative SP denotes a negative r, or a negative b.

†The points on the fitted line are designated as Y to distinguish them from
the observed y values. The values given by the line are also frequently designated
as y or Y.

While only one point is necessary in addition to $(\bar{x}, \bar{y})$ to graph a straight line, a third point will serve as a check. Thus,

$$\text{when } x = 2, \; Y = -0.98 + 2.16(2) = +3.34$$
$$x = 15, \; Y = -0.98 + 2.16(15) = +31.42.$$

Drawing a straight line through these points will enable one to compare the observed readings with the fitted trend line, as seen in Figure 8.1.

Variation of Observed Points Around the Fitted Line

It is important to know how much the eight points (N) differ from the fitted trend. Even if we had the true straight line $Y' = \alpha + \beta x$ (based on a universe of hydrolyzed procaine values at each x), we would certainly expect that the observed procaine values at a given x value would deviate from Y' or $\mu_{y.x}$, the universe mean value at that x. In fact, at each x we would find a distribution of y values, hopefully with a constant standard deviation $\sigma_{y.x}$ (homoscedasticity). The sample estimate of $\mu_{y.x}$ is Y.

The sample estimate of $\sigma_{y.x}$ is $s_{y.x} = \sqrt{\dfrac{\Sigma(y - Y)^2}{N - 2}}$ with (N - 2)

degrees of freedom,* where Y is the value on the line estimated from the sample and (y - Y) is the deviation of an observed point from the corresponding value on the line. $s_{y.x}$, the standard deviation of y specific for x, corresponds to the usual standard deviation except that the mean upon which it is based is not constant but changes with different values of x. The calculations of $s_{y.x}$ are illustrated in Table 8.2 on page 168.

$$s_{y.x} = \sqrt{\frac{\Sigma(y - Y)^2}{N - 2}}$$

$$= \sqrt{\frac{(.2)^2 + (.2)^2 + \ldots + (-1.1)^2 + (1.2)^2}{6}}$$

$$= \sqrt{\frac{5.07}{6}} = 0.92 \times 10^{-5} \text{ moles.}$$

---

*The N values of (y - Y) are subject to two restrictions: $\Sigma(y - Y) = 0$ and $\Sigma[x(y - Y)] = 0$. $\sigma_{y.x}$ is often called the *standard error of estimate*.

TABLE 8.2

Deviation of Observed Values From Calculated Values of Data in Table 8.1

x	Observed y	$Y = -0.98 + 2.16x$	$(y - Y)$	$(y - Y)^2$
2	3.5	3.3	+0.2	0.04
3	5.7	5.5	+0.2	0.04
5	9.9	9.8	+0.1	0.01
8	16.3	16.3	0.0	0.00
10	19.3	20.6	-1.3	1.69
12	25.7	24.9	+0.8	0.64
14	28.2	29.3	-1.1	1.21
15	32.6	31.4	+1.2	1.44
			+0.1	5.07

Note: $\Sigma(y - Y) = +0.1$. If it were not for rounding off errors, $\Sigma(y - Y)$ would equal zero. For the same reason, $\Sigma(y - Y)^2$ is subject to rounding errors.

It is worth noting that a and b, calculated by the method of least squares, are subject to less sampling variation than any other a and b calculated by any other method. If the conditions of homoscedasticity in the universe at the various x's are not met, then, although it is still true that the line fits the observed points with a minimum $\Sigma(y - Y)^2$, a and b do not have this same optimum property.

The Significance of a Linear Trend

Even if the true relationship is linear, one must recognize that the fitted line is merely an estimate of the true line. Because of the limited number of procaine measurements made in the study, the fitted constants a and b will be subject to chance variation. It is of particular interest to evaluate the chance variation of the slope, b, since this is usually the more important characteristic of the fitted line. If repeated data of the kind represented in Table 8.1 were taken, the estimated slope would vary around the true slope, β. In fact, it can be shown that if the distributions of y at the various x's are normal, then the distribution of the sample slope is a normal curve centered at the true slope, β, and with a standard error: $SE_b = \dfrac{\sigma_{y.x}}{\sqrt{\Sigma(x - \bar{x})^2}}$. The denominator in the formula was obtained in calculating the slope previously as SS of the x's = 171.875.

To test the significance of the slope of the fitted line from zero, we then compare it with the slope of a horizontal line (which is zero), since the null hypothesis in this case ($\beta = 0$) is that in the universe of procaine values, the average quantity of procaine hydrolyzed does not vary with time, for the range of times under study. In accordance with this null hypothesis, we calculate

$$z = \frac{b - 0}{SE_b} \text{ when } SE_b = \frac{\sigma_{y.x}}{\sqrt{\Sigma (x - \bar{x})^2}}.$$

Since $\sigma_{y.x}$ is unknown, as indeed it usually is, the SE_b is estimated as

$$\text{est. } SE_b = \frac{s_{y.x}}{\sqrt{\Sigma (x - \bar{x})^2}} \text{ with } (N - 2) \text{ degrees of freedom.}$$

Therefore,

$$\text{est. } SE_b = \frac{0.92 \times 10^{-5}}{\sqrt{171.875}} = 0.07 \times 10^{-5} \text{ moles per liter per minute.}$$

We then calculate

$$t = \frac{b - 0}{\text{est. } SE_b} = \frac{(2.16 \times 10^{-5}) - 0}{0.07 \times 10^{-5}} = 30.8,$$

with $(N - 2) = 6$ degrees of freedom since $s_{y.x}$ has been used in the estimate of SE_b.

Since this t exceeds the critical value of 2.45 (5% point), we can conclude that the slope of the fitted line is significantly different from zero, i.e., β is not equal to zero. In fact, P is exceedingly small. This is not surprising in view of the theoretical chemical considerations.

The confidence range for the true slope, β, can be calculated very simply by the use of the t-distribution. The 95% confidence range for β extends from

$$b - 2.45 \text{ est. } SE_b \text{ to } b + 2.45 \text{ est. } SE_b =$$

$$2.16 - (2.45)(0.07) \text{ to } 2.16 + (2.45)(0.07) = 1.99 \text{ to } 2.33.$$

Occasionally problems arise in which there is more than one measurement of y at each x. The calculation of the regression line and of $s_{y.x}$ and of the test of significance of the slope proceed in exactly the same way as when there is only one y at each x. However, in this type of problem, it is possible to subdivide the sum of squares of the deviations about the line into two parts, namely, the SS for the deviations of the means of the y's about the line and the SS of the y's about their respective means at the various x's. In this case, a separate test may be made for the significance of the departures from linearity.

If the distributions of the y's at the various x's are not normal, the sampling distribution of b around β will still be a normal curve generally with the standard error as given, except perhaps for gross departures from normality (Central Limit Theorem). Similarly, the use of the t-test with such data is robust as it was in the case of problems involving means (see Chapter 5). Obviously, if the distribution of the y's at the various x's is very far from normal, we may not want to deal with the means of such distributions or the lines fitted to such means.

Test of Significance of Slope by ANOVA

The total variation of the y's about their overall mean (y), i.e., the total SS_y with N - 1 df, can be broken down into two parts: one part is the SS of the points around the line, namely, the sum of the $\Sigma(y - Y)^2$ with N - 2 df; the other part is the Regression SS with 1 df which may be calculated as (Total SS - SS about the line).

The Regression SS is a function of the slope and is 0 if the slope is 0. The Regression SS can be more easily calculated as b^2SS_x, or bSP_{xy}, or $(SP_{xy})^2/SS_x$. All of these expressions are equal. Obviously, a rapid way of computing the SS about the line, $\Sigma(y - Y)^2$, would be to subtract the Regression SS from the Total SS.

For example,

$$SS_y = \Sigma y^2 - CT = [(3.9)^2 + (10.7)^2 + \ldots + (36.6)^2] - (141.2)^2/8 =$$
$$3,299.4200 - 2,492.1800 = 807.2400.$$

$$b = SP_{xy}/SS_x = 371.3500/171.8750 = 2.1606.$$

$$\text{Regression SS} = b^2SS_x = (2.1606)^2(171.8750) = 802.3456$$
$$= bSP_{xy} = (2.1606)(371.3500) = 802.3388$$
$$= (SP_{xy})^2/SS_x = 802.3321.$$

The slight inequalities in values of Regression SS are due to rounding b. Probably the most frequently used expression for Regression SS is b^2SS_x.* Note that $SS_y - b^2SS_x = 4.8944$ which differs from the

---

*The expression involving the least rounding error is $(SP_{xy})^2/SS_x$.

TABLE 8.3
Analysis of Variance Table for Line Fitted to Data of Table 8.2

Source of Variation	df	SS	MS
Regression of y on x	1	$b^2\Sigma(x - \bar{x})^2 = 802.3456$[a]	802.3456
Deviation from Line	$(N - 2) = 6\Sigma(y - Y)^2 = 4.8944$		0.8159
Total	$(N - 1) = 7\Sigma(y - \bar{y})^2 = 807.2400$		

$$F_{1,6} = \frac{802.3456}{0.8159} = 983.39;$$

$$t_6 = \sqrt{F_{1,6}} = 31.4.$$

This value differs from the previous t on page 169 of 30.8 which was subject to various rounding errors.

[a] Regression SS/Total SS = 802.3456/807.2400 = 0.9939, is frequently called the *Coefficient of Determination*. It measures the closeness of the points to the fitted line. As will be seen in the section on correlation (p. 178), the coefficient of determination is equal to the square of the correlation coefficient, r^2. $(1 - r^2)$ is frequently called the *Coefficient of Alienation*. Thus, even though r has no intrinsic meaning in a pure regression problem, it is still a convenient index.

previously computed $\Sigma(y - Y)^2 = 5.07$ because of rounding errors previously mentioned. The ANOVA table appears as Table 8.3.

Comparison of Two Linear Trends

The slope of the line just fitted to procaine values refers to procaine in the plasma of one specific individual. It would be of interest to compare this trend with the trend for a second individual. The data for Plasma 2 are given in Table 8.3.

The data, together with those of Plasma 1, have been graphed in Figure 8.2, and straight lines, fitted by the method of least squares, have been drawn. The fitted points, the residuals, and the residuals squared appear in the last three columns of Table 8.4.

$$s_{y.x} = \sqrt{\frac{\Sigma(y - Y)^2}{N - 2}} = \sqrt{\frac{5.86}{4}} = \sqrt{1.4650} = 1.2$$

$$\text{est. } SE_b = \frac{s_{y.x}}{\sqrt{\Sigma(x - \bar{x})^2}} = \frac{1.21}{\sqrt{106}} = \frac{1.21}{10.3} = 0.117.$$

The slope of the line fitted to these data, b = 2.70, is also significant at the .05 level, since

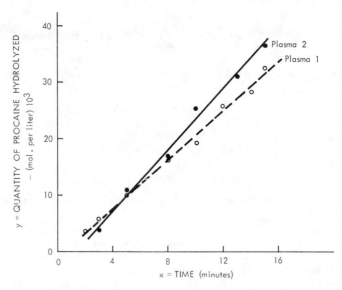

FIG. 8.2 Relationship Between Quantity of Procaine Hydrolyzed in Plasma 1 and Plasma 2 and Time.

$$t = \frac{2.70 - 0}{0.12} = 22.5 \text{ with 4 degrees of freedom.}$$

For each plasma, then, there is a positive relation of amount of procaine hydrolyzed to incubation time, under the conditions of the experiment.

The next question that may be asked about the data is whether the two trends are significantly different from each other. The difference in the two slopes must then be compared. To make the comparison, we calculate the standard error of the difference between two slopes from the formula:

$$SE_{b_1 - b_2} = \sqrt{SE_{b_1}{}^2 + SE_{b_2}{}^2},$$

where a common estimate of $\sigma_{y.x}$ is used in the calculations on the assumption that $\sigma_{y.x}$ is the same for both lines. This common estimate is

$$s_{y.x} = \sqrt{\frac{(N_1 - 2)s_{y1.x}^2 + (N_2 - 2)s_{y2.x}^2}{N_1 + N_2 - 4}} = \sqrt{\frac{5.07 + 5.86}{10}}$$

$$= \sqrt{1.095}$$

TABLE 8.4
Quantity of Hydrolyzed Procaine [(moles/liter) $\times$ 10^5] by Incubation Time (minutes) of Human Plasma 2[1]

x	Observed y	$Y = -3.60 + 2.70x$	$(y - Y)$	$(y - Y)^2$
3	3.9	4.5	-0.6	0.36
5	10.7	9.9	+0.8	0.64
8	16.8	18.0	-1.2	1.44
10	25.2	23.4	+1.8	3.24
13	31.2	31.5	-0.3	0.09
15	36.6	36.9	-0.3	0.09

$N = 6$; $\Sigma x = 54$; $\Sigma x^2 = 592$; $\Sigma y = 124.4$; $\Sigma y^2 = 3,359.98$; $\Sigma xy = 1,406.2$.

$$\text{est. } SE_{b_1} = \sqrt{\frac{1.095}{171.875}} = \sqrt{0.0064}$$

$$\text{est. } SE_{b_2} = \sqrt{\frac{1.095}{106.000}} = \sqrt{0.0103}$$

$$\text{est. } SE_{b_1 - b_2} = \sqrt{0.0064 + 0.0103} = 0.13 \times 10^{-5} \text{ with}$$

$$(N_1 + N_2 - 4) = 10 \text{ degrees of freedom.}$$

Comparing the difference between the two slopes $(b_1 - b_2)$ with zero,

$$t = \frac{(b_1 - b_2) - 0}{SE_{b_1 - b_2}} = \frac{(2.16 - 2.70) - 0}{0.13} = 4.15 \text{ with}$$

$$(N_1 + N_2 - 4) = 10 \text{ degrees of freedom.}$$

The difference between the two slopes is statistically significant at the .05 level.

ANOVA Test of Parallelism

The testing of the significance of the difference between two slopes is actually an ANOVA problem. Separate lines are fitted to the data of Table 8.1 and 8.4, and the respective SS_y subdivided into Regression SS and SS around line.

Line 1		Line 2
$N_1 = 8$, $SS_{x_1} = 171.8750$		$N_2 = 6$, $SS_{x_2} = 106.0000$
$SS_{y_1} = 807.2400$		$SS_{y_2} = 780.7533$
$SP_{x_1 y_1} = 371.3500$		$SP_{x_2 y_2} = 286.6000$
$b_1 = 2.1606$		$b_2 = 2.7038$

	df	Source of Variation		df
$b_1{}^2 SS_{x_1} = 802.3456$	1	Regression	$b_2{}^2 SS_{x_2} = 774.9167$	1
$\Sigma(y - Y_1)^2 = 4.8944$	6	Deviations from Line	$\Sigma(y - Y_2)^2 = 5.8366$	4
$SS_{y_1} = 807.2400$	7	Within Sample	$SS_{y_2} = 780.7533$	5

We now fit two parallel lines to see how much variation there is about these lines and what the regression SS is. The slope of the two parallel lines is the weighted average of b_1 and b_2.

$$b = \frac{SP_{x_1 y_1} + SP_{x_2 y_2}}{SS_{x_1} + SS_{x_2}} = \frac{SP_{xy} \text{ Within Samples}}{SS_x \text{ Within Samples}}$$

$$= \frac{371.3500 + 286.6000}{171.8750 + 106.0000} = 2.3678.$$

The Regression SS for the two parallel lines is

$$b^2 (SS_{x_1} + SS_{x_2}) = 1{,}557.8998 \text{ with 1 df.}$$

The SS for deviations about two parallel lines is Within Samples SS_y – Regression SS =

$$SS_{y_1} + SS_{y_2} - b^2(SS_{x_1} + SS_{x_2}) =$$
$$807.2400 + 780.7533 - 1{,}557.8998 = 30.0935.$$

with $N_1 + N_2 - 3 = 11$ df. The difference between this and the pooled SS for deviations about two separate lines is

$$30.0935 - (4.8944 + 5.8366) =$$
$$30.0935 - 10.7310 = 19.3625 \text{ with 1 df.}$$

We note that this is the same quantity as the difference between the Regression SS for two separate lines with 2 df and the Regression SS for two parallel lines with 1 df.

$$b_1{}^2 SS_{x_1} + b_2{}^2 SS_{x_2} - b^2 (SS_{x_1} + SS_{x_2}) = 802.3456 + 774.9167 -$$

$$1{,}557.8998 = 1{,}577.2623 - 1{,}557.8998 = 19.3625 \text{ with 1 df.}$$

The difference of 19.3625 is a function of the differences in slopes. The ANOVA is presented in Table 8.5. (See page 176.)

To test the departure from parallelism, i.e., difference in slopes,

$$F_{1,10} = \frac{19.3625}{s_{y.x}^2} = 18.0435; \ \sqrt{F_{1,10}} = t_{10} = 4.2478,$$

which agrees with the previous solution by the t-test except for rounding, particularly in $\Sigma (y - Y)^2$.

To test the significance of the average slope,

$$F_{1,10} = b^2 SS_x / s_{y.x}^2 = 1{,}451.$$

The advantage of the ANOVA method over t is that more than two slopes can be compared.

Nonlinear Trends

Although the linear trend is the simplest type and lends itself to many comparatively simple analyses, not all relationships can be described by straight line trends.

There are a number of curvilinear trends involving only two parameters, which can be linearized by using a new independent variable. For example, in drug studies the response y is often considered as a function of the logarithm of the dose, e.g., $y = a + b(\log x)$. Obviously, if log x is replaced by a new variable, say z, a straight line problem results, and the formulas for least squares already given can be used.

Another curvilinear relationship with two parameters is the exponential which is expressed in various forms, a frequent one being $y = AB^x$. While this curve cannot readily be fitted by least squares, if we are content to fit a line to the logarithms of y, then,

$$\log y = \log A + (\log B)x,$$

so that now a straight line problem results, where

$$a = \log A \text{ and } b = \log B.$$

TABLE 8.5
Analysis of Variance of Data in Tables 8.1 and 8.4

Source of Variation	df	SS	MS
Regression for 2 separate lines	2	$b^2SS_{x1} + b^2SS_{x2} = 1,577.2623$	
{ Regress. for 2 parallel lines	1	$b^2SS_x = 1,557.8998$	1,557.8998
{ Difference in slopes	1	Difference = 19.3625	19.3625
Deviations about 2 separate lines	10	Difference = 10.7310	$1.0731 = s_{y \cdot x}^2$
Within Samples	12	$SS_{y1} + SS_{y2} = 1,587.9933$	

There are many such two parameter curves which can be linearized either by using a function of the independent variable, x, or of y, or sometimes of both.

Many curvilinear trends involve more than two parameters. Many of these can be fitted by the method of least squares but the techniques are generally beyond the scope of this book.

For example, a second order parabolic trend has been fitted to the caries experience of children of 21 communities and the fluoride concentration of their public water supply (Table 8.6, Figure 8.3). While the parabola fits the observed points rather well, in this case it is certainly not a good curve for extrapolation purposes as the fluoride concentration increases, since the curve will inevitably rise to higher values of caries experience again. In fact, other curves, such as some type of an exponential, might be more appropriate for these data.

Growth curves are frequently of a nonlinear type, as illustrated in Figure 8.4. (See page 179.) Ten normal male rats of the Holtzman strain, averaging 44 grams in weight, were selected at weaning and followed for 37 weeks before being sacrificed. The average weight of these animals, which constituted the control group for a histochemical study of the effect of estrogen on bone, was graphed against time.[3] It is difficult to decide what type of curve best fits these data. Some modified form of an exponential may be suitable.

TABLE 8.6
Dental Caries Experience of 7257 Children 12–14 Years of Age of 21 Communities, According to the Fluoride Concentration of the Public Water Supply[2]

Community	DMF Teeth Per 100 Children	Fluoride Concentration in ppm	Community	DMF Teeth Per 100 Children	Fluoride Concentration in ppm
1	236	1.9	12	652	0.3
2	246	2.6	13	673	0.0
3	252	1.8	14	703	0.2
4	258	1.2	15	706	0.1
5	281	1.2	16	722	0.0
6	303	1.2	17	733	0.2
7	323	1.3	18	772	0.1
8	343	0.9	19	810	0.0
9	412	0.6	20	823	0.1
10	444	0.5	21	1,037	0.1
11	556	0.4			

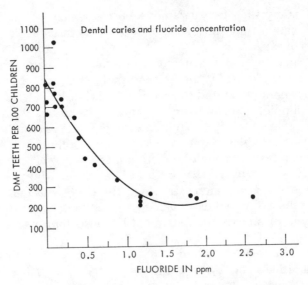

FIG. 8.3 Dental Caries Experience of Children Residing in 22 Different Communities, According to the Concentration of Fluoride in the Public Water Supply.

CORRELATION

Simultaneous Readings on a Selected Group of Individuals

In the procaine hydrolysis problems just discussed, desired times to be studied were selected and then readings were taken at these times. In other types of problems, the data may be obtained for two quantitative characteristics (often simultaneously), for each of a group of individuals *without* selection on the basis of either of the two characteristics. It is with such data that we can examine the relation of each variable to the other, in contradistinction to the previous problem where we could examine only the trend of procaine hydrolysis (y) with time (x).

The series of measurements of the amount of calcium dissolved in saliva (mg/100 cc)* and the amylolytic (ptyalin) index for 34 individuals,[4] will serve to illustrate the type of data in which simul-

---

*In this study, the amount of calcium dissolved in saliva is an index of acid formation in the saliva.

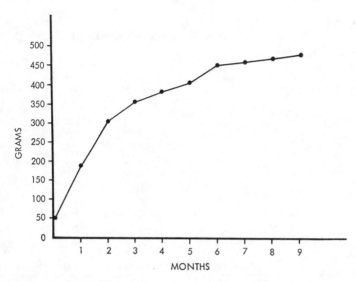

FIG. 8.4 Average Weight of 10 Normal Male Rats Over a Period of 37 Weeks After Weaning.[3]

taneous measurements are made (Table 8.7). In this study, the calcium solubility and enzyme activity were determined for each of the 34 individuals studied. When such quantitative data of two characteristics are available for a group of individuals, it is always of interest to see whether any relationship exists between these two measurements, and if so, just how strong this relationship may be.

Graphical Representation of the Relationship Between Two Variables

One variable (calcium dissolved) is plotted on the ordinate scale and the other variable (amylolytic index) on the abscissa scale. The scales need not start at zero, but it is important to lay out the units so that the ranges of both variables cover about the same distance on the graph paper. Thus, the range of amylolytic index is from 1–5 and should occupy about the same space on the abscissa scale as the range from 0–30 for calcium dissolved occupied on the ordinate scale. The measurements of all 34 subjects are graphed as points corresponding to the respective calcium and index values so that the resulting picture is that of a scatter of spots on the graph paper, hence the name *Spot Graph* or *Scatter Diagram* (*Scattergram*).

TABLE 8.7

Simultaneous Determination of Calcium Solubility in Saliva (mg/100 cc) and Amylolytic Index[4]

Patient Number	Amylolytic Index (x)	Calcium Dissolved (y)	Patient Number	Amylolytic Index (x)	Calcium Dissolved (y)
1	1.0	4.5	18	2.8	18.0
2	2.6	18.0	19	1.3	5.0
3	4.2	29.0	20	3.6	15.0
4	1.5	10.0	21	3.4	21.0
5	1.1	8.0	22	2.0	8.5
6	2.6	24.0	23	4.2	15.5
7	2.6	17.0	24	4.7	24.5
8	4.0	26.5	25	1.4	8.5
9	1.1	10.0	26	2.2	23.0
10	2.4	21.5	27	3.4	10.0
11	3.0	8.0	28	3.3	24.5
12	3.0	10.5	29	4.0	24.5
13	3.2	26.0	30	3.6	13.0
14	3.2	6.5	31	2.6	12.0
15	2.1	13.0	32	2.2	11.0
16	1.4	19.0	33	1.2	15.0
17	1.2	11.5	34	1.5	10.0

When we examine the swarm of spots in the scatter diagram illustrating these data (Figure 8.5), we see that most of these points can be included within the outline of an ellipse whose greater diameter extends from the lower left to the upper right corner of the paper. When we see such an elliptical clustering (with a definite upward slope), it is indicative of a positive relationship — i.e., if an individual has a high amylolytic index, he also tends to have a higher amount of calcium capable of being dissolved in his saliva. Similarly, those individuals with a low index tend to have a low calcium solubility in saliva.

When no relationship exists between the two variables, the swarm of points will have no slope and will be arranged like grains of salt shaken from a saltcellar, hit or miss. If the scale divisions are chosen as described, the cluster of points will tend to be circular in outline when there is no relationship between the two variables. Even though a few outlying spots might give an appearance of an ellipse, our impression of no relationship, based on the fact that most of the spots are clumped in a circle, should not be changed by a few outlying points.

The simplest type of perfect relationship is represented by a straight line. Some perfect relationships, however, may be repre-

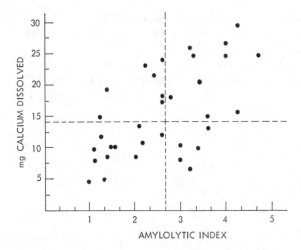

FIG. 8.5 Scatter Diagram of 34 Individuals According to the Amount of Calcium Dissolved in Their Saliva and the Amylotytic Index of Their Saliva.

sented by other simple curves. Perfect relationships rarely occur with biological data, though in physics and chemistry we find many such relationships, as in Boyle's and Charles' laws of the behavior of the volume of a gas according to pressure and temperature. Even here, negligible measurement errors detract from a perfect relationship.

Not all relationships between two variables are positive, i.e., a low x associated with low y and high x associated with high y. In other cases, the slope may be from upper left to lower right, a negative direction. In these instances, an inverse relationship exists, so that when one variable is high the other tends to be low, and vice versa. In the data we are studying, there appears to be an upward slope to the graphed points. We, therefore, have some reason to believe that there is a positive relationship between these two variables.

Examination of the Relationship by Dividing
Data into Two Groups

One simple way of examining the relationship is to divide the data into two broad groups with respect to one of the variables, say y. The two groups should be approximately equal in numbers. If we were to draw a horizontal line at y = 14 mg of calcium dissolved, the swarm of points in Figure 8.5 would be divided into two broad groups — a low calcium group (below 14 mg) and a high calcium group (above 14 mg). We can then refer to the original raw data and tabulate the amylolytic index values according to the low calcium and high calcium groups (Table 8.8).

We can test the significance of the relationship by performing a comparison of means test between the mean values of amylolytic indices for the low calcium and the high calcium groups (independent samples). Thus,

$$s = \text{pooled } s = 0.95$$

$$\text{est. SE}_{\bar{x}_1} = \frac{s}{\sqrt{N}} = \frac{0.95}{\sqrt{17}} = 0.230$$

$$\text{est. SE}_{\bar{x}_2} = \frac{s}{\sqrt{N}} = \frac{0.95}{\sqrt{17}} = 0.230.$$

TABLE 8.8
Amylolytic Index Values, Grouped According to High and Low Calcium Values

Low Calcium $(y < 14 \text{ mg})$	High Calcium $(y > 14 \text{ mg})$
1.0	1.2
1.3	1.4
1.1	2.6
1.4	2.6
1.1	2.8
2.0	2.4
1.5	2.2
1.5	2.6
1.2	3.6
2.2	3.4
2.1	3.3
2.6	3.2
3.0	4.0
3.2	4.0
3.0	4.2
3.4	4.7
3.6	4.2

$\Sigma x_1 = 35.2$ $\Sigma x_2 = 52.4$
$N_1 = 17$ $N_2 = 17$
$\bar{x}_1 = 2.07$ $\bar{x}_2 = 3.08$
$s_1 = 0.90$ $s_2 = 1.00$

Pooled $s = 0.95$, df $= 32$.

$$\text{est SE}_{\bar{x}_1 - \bar{x}_2} = \sqrt{(\text{SE}_{\bar{x}_1})^2 + (\text{SE}_{\bar{x}_2})^2} = \sqrt{2(0.230)^2} = 0.33$$

$$t = \frac{(\bar{x}_1 - \bar{x}_2) - 0}{\text{est. SE}_{\bar{x}_1 - \bar{x}_2}} = \frac{(2.07 - 3.08)}{0.33} = -3.06 \text{ with df} = 32; P < .01.$$

The average amylolytic index thus differs significantly between the high and low calcium groups, indicating the significance of the relationship.

The Coefficient of Correlation (Ungrouped Data)

There is a more elaborate way of examining the relationship between the amylolytic index and the amount of calcium dissolved in saliva, as in the previous problem. This is by calculating Pearson's product-moment correlation coefficient (r). The limitations and interpretations of the coefficient will be discussed later, but this problem will serve to illustrate the calculation of r for an ungrouped series.

A defining formula for the product-moment coefficient of correlation is

$$r = \frac{\Sigma(x - \bar{x})(y - \bar{y})}{\sqrt{[\Sigma(x - \bar{x})^2][\Sigma(y - \bar{y})^2]}} \, .$$

This formula can be rearranged algebraically in many ways for ease of computation. One convenient rearrangement is

TABLE 8.9
Calculation of r from Ungrouped Data

Individual Number	Amylolytic Index x	Calcium Dissolved y	x^2	y^2	xy
1	1.0	4.5	1.00	20.25	4.50
2	2.6	18.0	6.76	324.00	46.80
3	4.2	29.0	17.64	841.00	121.80
4	1.5	10.0	2.25	100.00	15.00
5	1.1	8.0	1.21	64.00	8.80
6	2.6	24.0	6.76	576.00	62.40
7	2.6	17.0	6.76	289.00	44.20
8	4.0	26.5	16.00	702.25	106.00
9	1.1	10.0	1.21	100.00	11.00
10	2.4	21.5	5.76	462.25	51.60
11	3.0	8.0	9.00	64.00	24.00
12	3.0	10.5	9.00	110.25	31.50
13	3.2	26.0	10.24	676.00	83.20
14	3.2	6.5	10.24	42.25	20.80
15	2.1	13.0	4.41	169.00	27.30
16	1.4	19.0	1.96	361.00	26.60
17	1.2	11.5	1.44	132.25	13.80
18	2.8	18.0	7.84	324.00	50.40
19	1.3	5.0	1.69	25.00	6.50
20	3.6	15.0	12.96	225.00	54.00
21	3.4	21.0	11.56	441.00	71.40
22	2.0	8.5	4.00	72.25	17.00
23	4.2	15.5	17.64	240.25	65.10
24	4.7	24.5	22.09	600.25	115.15
25	1.4	8.5	1.96	72.25	11.90
26	2.2	23.0	4.84	529.00	50.60
27	3.4	10.0	11.56	100.00	34.00
28	3.3	24.5	10.89	600.25	80.85
29	4.0	24.5	16.00	600.25	98.00
30	3.6	13.0	12.96	169.00	46.80
31	2.6	12.0	6.76	144.00	31.20
32	2.2	11.0	4.84	121.00	24.20
33	1.2	15.0	1.44	225.00	18.00
34	1.5	10.0	2.25	100.00	15.00
Total	87.6	522.0	262.92	9,622.00	1,489.40

TABLE 8.10.
Calculation of r From Data in Table 8.9

$\Sigma x = 87.6$	$\Sigma x^2 = 262.92$	$\Sigma xy = 1,489.40$	$\Sigma y = 522.0$	$\Sigma y^2 = 9,622.00$
$\bar{x} = 2.58$			$\bar{y} = 15.35$	

$$SS_x = 262.92 - \frac{(87.6)^2}{34} = 37.2212 \qquad SSy = 9,622.00 - \frac{(522.00)^2}{34} = 1,607.7647$$

$$s_x^2 = 2.1279 \qquad\qquad\qquad s_y^2 = 48.7201$$

$$SP_{xy} = 1,489.40 - \frac{(87.6)(522.0)}{34} = 144.4824$$

$$r = \frac{SP_{xy}}{\sqrt{(SS_x)(SS_y)}} = +.591.$$

$$r = \frac{\Sigma xy - \dfrac{(\Sigma x)(\Sigma y)}{N}}{\sqrt{\left[\Sigma x^2 - \dfrac{(\Sigma x)^2}{N}\right]\left[\Sigma y^2 - \dfrac{(\Sigma y)^2}{N}\right]}} = \frac{SP_{xy}}{\sqrt{(SSx)\,(SSy)}}.$$

It should be noted that the sum of squares (SS) of the x's and of the
y's appears in the denominator. The term in the numerator is often
called the sum of products (SP) of x and y. The only new arithmetical computation is that for Σxy, which is the sum of the products of
each y value and its corresponding x value. This is the same Σxy that
was used earlier in the fitting of a straight line. A summary of the
data and the calculation of r are given in Table 8.10.

A complete exploration of the relationship between the two
variables would require that we determine whether the observed
relationship ($r = +0.591$) differs significantly from no relationship
($r = 0$). A discussion of this significance test comes later. The regression line for predicting y from x (or x from y) should also be part of
the exploration.

The Coefficient of Correlation (Grouped Data)

The method for the calculation of the coefficient of correlation just
illustrated can be used most conveniently for up to about 50 pairs of
measurements. When the number of pairs of observations is much
larger than 50, however, direct calculation from the ungrouped data
becomes quite cumbersome, so that it may be better to construct a
correlation table.

The construction of a correlation table and the calculations that
can be made from it can be illustrated by data (Table 8.11) on the

TABLE 8.11
Vital Capacity (cc of Air) of 200 Patients Before and After Operative Oral Surgery[5]

Patient Number	Preop x	Postop y	Patient Number	Preop x	Postop y
1	97	97	51	95	93
2	92	98	52	97	85
3	96	99	53	99	93
4	101	96	54	74	74
5	82	83	55	69	65
6	78	88	56	82	82
7	89	79	57	61	61
8	62	79	58	71	71
9	77	73	59	71	71
10	92	89	60	110	105
11	65	69	61	91	97
12	79	70	62	96	90
13	85	85	63	86	87
14	95	90	64	112	105
15	80	85	65	77	82
16	88	90	66	94	93
17	97	103	67	89	89
18	81	73	68	78	87
19	89	101	69	97	90
20	96	101	70	116	113
21	64	54	71	108	108
22	69	81	72	90	87
23	90	88	73	67	67
24	48	48	74	80	82
25	102	99	75	76	83
26	80	73	76	101	104
27	80	75	77	79	89
28	89	89	78	74	77
29	78	80	79	77	81
30	96	96	80	94	82
31	75	70	81	69	62
32	62	62	82	87	89
33	89	92	83	87	89
34	93	93	84	94	90
35	89	82	85	109	101
36	113	113	86	87	87
37	89	89	87	84	83
38	84	91	88	75	73
39	95	97	89	50	46
40	62	60	90	70	79
41	75	80	91	101	95
42	91	88	92	104	109
43	66	73	93	91	91
44	92	88	94	84	87
45	109	101	95	89	88
46	89	91	96	76	73
47	85	82	97	58	62
48	69	66	98	108	108
49	111	111	99	94	96
50	92	92	100	99	92

TABLE 8.11 *(continued)*

Patient Number	Preop x	Postop y	Patient Number	Preop x	Postop y
101	87	97	151	72	72
102	84	82	152	91	89
103	87	85	153	75	82
104	87	97	154	73	65
105	83	87	155	82	84
106	100	107	156	92	97
107	101	98	157	80	71
108	77	74	158	62	49
109	68	70	159	97	99
110	87	79	160	93	83
111	90	95	161	76	74
112	71	72	162	44	46
113	82	79	163	91	94
114	83	89	164	81	82
115	90	95	165	62	74
116	94	91	166	80	82
117	96	96	167	56	53
118	87	89	168	92	92
119	87	89	169	68	71
120	92	92	170	75	79
121	97	97	171	92	80
122	85	89	172	75	72
123	80	74	173	87	91
124	89	71	174	83	88
125	95	98	175	77	84
126	93	89	176	82	79
127	84	77	177	92	89
128	109	107	178	101	99
129	100	90	179	76	82
130	110	105	180	90	86
131	91	95	181	65	70
132	58	58	182	92	89
133	90	92	183	111	120
134	80	82	184	84	89
135	66	66	185	66	62
136	72	68	186	99	105
137	84	75	187	65	76
138	64	71	188	96	91
139	67	67	189	102	102
140	75	75	190	102	102
141	83	85	191	71	71
142	83	83	192	66	66
143	79	69	193	83	81
144	53	52	194	59	55
145	40	62	195	82	78
146	85	83	196	96	103
147	66	66	197	55	59
148	130	130	198	107	107
149	69	62	199	69	68
150	100	102	200	107	97

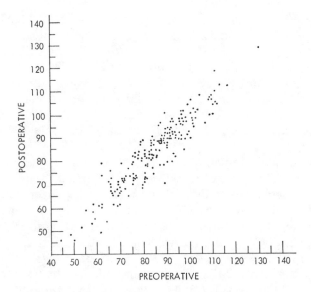

FIG. 8.6 Scatter Diagram of 200 Patients According to Their Vital Capacity Before and After Operative Oral Surgery.

vital capacity of air in cc (to the nearest cc) of 200 patients, measured before and after oral surgery.[5] In order to examine these measurements to determine visually whether there is any relationship between the pre- and postoperative vital capacity for these patients, a scatter diagram may be constructed (Figure 8.6). The swarm of these points can be enclosed in an ellipse whose greater diameter extends from the lower left to the upper right of the graph, denoting a positive relationship. While the relationship can be examined by grouping the points into two broad groups, as previously illustrated, it would be appropriate to use a number of intervals for both variables, thereby constructing a correlation table.

In constructing the correlation table, the number of classes or intervals depends on the number of readings. With 200 pairs of readings, about 10 classes would be appropriate. It is advisable to have approximately the same number of classes for both variables. In this problem dealing with preoperative (x) and postoperative (y) vital capacity, both variables refer to the same physiological measurements and the range of the two variables is about the same.* For these reasons, the 10 class intervals chosen are the same for both

---

*There are many examples when x and y do not represent the same physiological measurements.

variables: 40-49, 50-59, 60-69, 70-79, 80-89, 90-99, 100-109, 110-119, 120-129, and 130-139 cc of air. Each individual is tallied according to the classes of x and y into which he falls. Individual number 1 (97, 97) would therefore be tallied in 90-99 for the pre-operative group and 90-99 in the postoperative group, i.e., a single tally at the intersection of the two intervals. Individual number 21 (64, 54) would be tallied at the intersection of the intervals 60-69 and 50-59, and so on. The final result of the tallies appears in Table 8.12.

This correlation table presents the two overall frequency distributions (preoperative, x; postoperative, y) as marginal totals. Within the body of the table, the individual frequencies have been listed simultaneously for both variables. Thus we find that 8 individuals have an x value from 60-69 and, at the same time, a y value from 70-79; that 18 individuals have an x value from 70-79 and also a y value from 70-79, etc. The overall distribution of y given in the total column at the right of the table can be obtained by adding the frequencies in the various rows. Thus, we find that the number of patients in the first row (y = 40-49 cc of air) is $2 + 1 + 1 = 4$; in the second row (y = 50-59 cc of air), it is $5 + 1 = 6$; in the third row (y = 60-69 cc of air), it is $1 + 1 + 15 + 3 = 20$; and so on. The overall distribution of y does not differ greatly from a normal curve, an important theoretical consideration in the use of the correlation coefficient.

In a similar manner, the overall frequency of the 200 patients according to preoperative vital capacity (x), was obtained (bottom row) by adding the frequencies in the various columns. Thus, the number of patients in the first column (x = 40-49 cc of air) is $2 + 1 = 3$; in the second column (x = 50-59 cc of air), it is $1 + 5 + 1 = 7$; in the third column (x = 60-69 cc of air), it is $1 + 1 + 15 + 8 + 1 = 26$, and so on. The overall frequency distribution of x also resembles a normal curve.

In making any calculations from such a correlation table, the technique of coding the midpoints of the class intervals is of great assistance in easing the burden of arithmetic. We have coded the midpoint of the interval 40-49, which is 44.5, as 0 for both x and for y, and have the class interval of 10 cc as the working unit. Then, in this coding system, $54.5 = 1$, $64.5 = 2$, $74.5 = 3 \ldots 124.5 = 8$, and $134.5 = 9$.

The necessary calculations are facilitated by the construction of a calculation table (Table 8.13). This table is essentially the same as Table 8.12, with the addition of calculations in the margins. The marginal frequencies of y and x have been transcribed from Table

TABLE 8.12
Correlation Table of Pre- and Postoperative Vital Capacity of Lungs, in cc of Air, of 200 Patients[5]

Postoperative Vital Capacity in cc of Air (y)	Preoperative Vital Capacity in cc of Air (x)										Frequency (f)
	40–49	50–59	60–69	70–79	80–89	90–99	100–109	110–119	120–129	130–139	
40–49	2	1	1								4
50–59		5	1								6
60–69	1	1	15	3							20
70–79			8	18	13						39
80–89			1	11	34	14					60
90–99					7	32	7				46
100–109					1	4	12	3			20
110–119								3			3
120–129								1			1
130–139										1	1
Frequency	3	7	26	32	55	50	19	7	0	1	200

TABLE 8.13
Calculation Table for r

Preoperative Vital Capacity (x)
(midpoints of class intervals)

POSTOPERATIVE VITAL CAPACITY (y) (midpoints of class intervals)	44.5	54.5	64.5	74.5	84.5	94.5	104.5	114.5	124.5	134.5	1 f	2 y	3 fy	4 fy^2	5 Σx_y	6 $y\Sigma x_y$
44.5	2	1	1								4	0	0	0	3	0
54.5		5	1								6	1	6	6	7	7
64.5	1	1	15	3							20	2	40	80	40	80
74.5			8	18	13						39	3	117	351	122	366
84.5			1	11	34	14					60	4	240	960	241	964
94.5					7	32	7				46	5	230	1,150	230	1,150
104.5					1	4	12	3			20	6	120	720	117	702
114.5								3			3	7	21	147	21	147
124.5								1			1	8	8	64	7	56
134.5										1	1	9	9	81	9	81
1 f	3	7	26	32	55	50	19	7	0	1	200		791 (Σfy)	3,559 (Σfy^2)	797 (Σfx)	3,553 (Σxy)
2 x	0	1	2	3	4	5	6	7	8	9						
3 fx^2	0	7	52	96	220	250	114	49	0	9	797 = Σfx					
4 fx^2	0	7	104	228	880	1,250	684	343	0	81	3,577 = Σfx^2					
5 Σy_x	2	7	59	104	216	240	107	47	0	9	791 = Σfy					
6 $x\Sigma y_x$	0	7	118	312	864	1,200	642	329	0	81	3,553 = Σxy					

8.12 and appear as column 1 and row 1. The coded midpoint values appear as y (column 2) and x (row 2).

The first step in the calculations is to summarize the overall distributions of y and x. This requires the determination of Σfy, Σfy^2, Σfx, and Σfx^2. Each value of fy is obtained in the usual manner, by multiplying the coded y value by the respective f, and appears in column 3. Each value of fy^2 is obtained by multiplying the value of fy by the respective y, and appears in column 4. The values of fx and fx^2 were calculated similarly, and are given in rows 3 and 4 at the bottom of the table.

Each value of Σx in column 5 is the sum of the x measurements
  y
corresponding to that particular value of y. Thus, at y = 0, we find that 2 cases have an x value of 0, 1 case has a value of x = 1 and 1 case has a value of x = 2, so that:

$$\Sigma x = 2 \times 0 + 1 \times 1 + 1 \times 2 = 3.$$
  y

At y = 1, we find 5 cases at x = 1 and 1 case at x = 2, so that:

$$\Sigma x = 5 \times 1 + 1 \times 2 = 7.$$
  y

At y = 2, we find:

$$\Sigma x = 1 \times 0 + 1 \times 1 + 15 \times 2 + 3 \times 3 = 40,$$
  y

and so on for the rest of the y values. Adding the column of Σx, we
                                                          y
obtain 797, the same total which we have already found for Σfx in row 3.

Similarly, by examining the table in a vertical manner, we can obtain the Σy values (row 5), each of which is the sum of the y
           y
values corresponding to that particular value of x. Thus,

at x = 0, $\Sigma y = 2 \times 0 + 1 \times 2 = 2$
    x

at x = 1, $\Sigma y = 1 \times 0 + 5 \times 1 + 1 \times 2 = 7$
    x

at x = 2, $\Sigma y = 1 \times 0 + 1 \times 1 + 15 \times 2 + 8 \times 3 + 1 \times 4 = 59,$
    x

and so on. The total of the $\sum_x y$ values is found to be 791, which is the same as $\sum fy$, which we have already found in column 3.

In order to calculate the coefficient of correlation, r, we need the value of $\sum xy$. This can be obtained as follows: Each value of $\sum_y x$ (column 5) is multiplied by the appropriate value of y (column 2) to give $y(\sum_y x)$ (column 6). Thus,

$$\text{at } y = 0, y\sum_y x = 3 \times 0 = 0$$

$$\text{at } y = 1, y\sum_y x = 7 \times 1 = 7$$

$$\text{at } y = 2, y\sum_y x = 40 \times 2 = 80, \text{and so on.}$$

The sum of the values in column 6 is 3,553, and is the desired $\sum xy$. The value of $\sum xy$ may also be obtained by computing $x\sum_x y$ (row 6), the product of each $\sum_x y$ (row 5), and the respective x values (row 2). Thus,

$$\text{at } x = 0, x\sum_x y = 0 \times 2 = 0$$

$$\text{at } x = 1, x\sum_x y = 1 \times 7 = 7$$

$$\text{at } x = 2, x\sum_x y = 2 \times 59 = 118, \text{and so on.}$$

The sum of the values in row 6 is 3,553, the same value of $\sum xy$ as obtained previously.

To calculate r, the appropriate values from Table 8.13 are substituted in the formula:

$$r = \frac{\sum xy - \dfrac{(\sum fx)(\sum fy)}{N}}{\sqrt{\left[\sum fx^2 - \dfrac{(\sum fx)^2}{N}\right]\left[\sum fy^2 - \dfrac{(\sum fy)^2}{N}\right]}} = \frac{SP_{xy}}{\sqrt{(SS_x)(SS_y)}}.$$

At this point, it is convenient to summarize the marginal distribution of x and y.

Coded Units

x = Preoperative vital capacity	y = Postoperative vital capacity
$\Sigma fx = 797$	$\Sigma fy = 791$
$\Sigma fx^2 = 3{,}577$	$\Sigma fy^2 = 3{,}559$
$\bar{x} = \dfrac{797}{200} = 3.985$	$\bar{y} = \dfrac{791}{200} = 3.955$
$s_x^2 = \dfrac{1}{199}\left[3{,}577 - \dfrac{(797)^2}{200}\right] = 2.0148$	$s_y^2 = \dfrac{1}{199}\left[3{,}599 - \dfrac{(791)^2}{200}\right] = 2.1638$
$s_x = 1.419$	$s_y = 1.471$
Decoded (original) values:	*Decoded (original) values:*
$\bar{x} = 10(3.985) + 44.5 = 84.35$	$\bar{y} = 10(3.955) + 44.5 = 84.05$
$s_x = 10(1.419) = 14.19$	$s_y = 10(1.471) = 14.71$

$$r = \frac{3{,}553 - \dfrac{(797)(791)}{200}}{\sqrt{\left[3{,}577 - \dfrac{(797)^2}{200}\right]\left[3{,}559 - \dfrac{(791)^2}{200}\right]}} = \frac{3{,}553.000 - 3{,}152.135}{\sqrt{(400.955)(430.595)}}.$$

$$r = +.965.*$$

Although r is found to be close to its maximum value of +1.0, there is still an appreciable scatter of the points in the scatter diagram. The fact that the means of pre- and postop are so similar as well as the standard deviations, is due to the fact that the same physiological variables are used at the different time periods.

The coefficient of correlation serves a twofold purpose: first, it gives a numerical index of the relationship between two variables, and second, it assists greatly in the calculation of trend or regression lines.

Regression Lines

In examining the relationship between two variables, it is important to see how the mean of one variable changes with specific values of the other. Thus, we can readily calculate how the means of the post-

---

*Since r is a pure number, decoding this value is not necessary.

operative vital capacity of individuals vary according to their preoperative vital capacity. This is somewhat comparable to the examination of the linear regression of hydrolyzed procaine on time for Plasma 1 (page 163 ff.). There is a slight distinction in how the x's were obtained, however. In the procaine analysis, there were 8 distinct x values, predetermined and measured without error, while in the present problem, the x values represent a random sampling from a universe of x values. From Table 8.13, the means of postoperative vital capacity $(\bar{y}_x)$ for specific values of preoperative vital capacity (x) can be calculated by dividing each Σy (row 5) by the respective f (row 1).

$$At\ x = 0, \bar{y}_x = 2/3 = 0.67;$$
$$at\ x = 1, \bar{y}_x = 7/7 = 1.00,$$

and so on, obtaining the coded values in Table 8.14. These $\bar{y}_x$ values can be decoded very simply, since 44.5 cc was made equal to zero, and since each working unit was equivalent to 10 cc. A coded $\bar{y}_x$ value of 0.67 thus equals

$$44.5\ cc + (0.67)(10\ cc) = 51.2\ cc.$$

A coded $\bar{y}_x$ value of 1.00 is equivalent to

$$44.5\ cc + (1.00)(10\ cc) = 54.5\ cc,\ etc.$$

TABLE 8.14
Mean Postoperative Vital Capacity Values (y), According to Preoperative Vital Capacity (x)

Original Values Preop Midpoints (x)	Coded Values		Decoded Original Values Postop Means $(\bar{y}_x)$
	Preop Midpoints (x)	Postop Means $(\bar{y}_x)$	
44.5	0	0.67	51.2
54.5	1	1.00	54.5
64.5	2	2.27	67.2
74.5	3	3.25	77.0
84.5	4	3.93	83.8
94.5	5	4.80	92.5
104.5	6	5.63	100.8
114.5	7	6.71	111.6
124.5	8	—	—
134.5	9	9.00	134.5

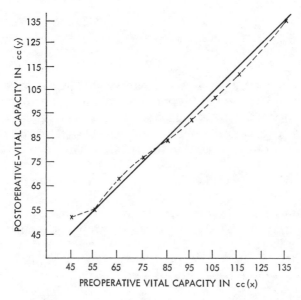

FIG. 8.7 **Mean Values of Postoperative Vital Capacity with Respect to Preoperative Vital Capacity, with Fitted Straight Line Trend.**

Graphing these mean values of y according to the preoperative value (x) shows us that the trend can apparently be described by a straight line (Figure 8.7).* The slope of this line can be estimated in a freehand manner, but we can very readily fit a straight line to this trend and calculate the slope by the method of least squares. In fitting the line, the frequency at each x must, of course, be used as a weight to get the same SS_x and SP_{xy} as were obtained from the original data on page 193.

Since, $b = SP_{xy}/SS_x$ and $r = SP_{xy}/\sqrt{(SS_x)(SS_y)}$, it follows that $b = r\sqrt{SS_y/SS_x} = r(s_y/s_x)$, illustrating that the calculation of b is readily made if r is available.†

r is also useful in calculating the SS for Deviations about the Line. Thus, SS for Deviations about the Line = $SS_y(1 - r^2)$. Evidently, the standard error of estimate,

---

*Since there is more than one y at each x, the goodness of fit of the line can be tested as suggested on page 289 ff.

†Note that r^2 can be expressed as b SP_{xy}/SS_y = Regression SS/Total SS. This ratio was previously referred to as the Coefficient of Determination in the regression problem.

$$s_{y.x} = s_y \sqrt{\frac{(N-1)}{(N-2)} \cdot (1 - r^2)}$$

The calculation of r from the means given in Table 8.14 is not possible since SS_y cannot be obtained. A direct calculation of r, as if each $\bar{y}_x$ pertained to a single observation, would yield a grossly exaggerated correlation coefficient. We have already found the decoded values of s_y = 14.71 and s_x = 14.19. Thus,

b = (+0.965)(14.71/14.19) = +1.000 cc per cc.

The constant a, determining the height of the line, is obtained from the formula, a = $\bar{y}$ – b$\bar{x}$. We have already found decoded $\bar{y}$ = 84.05 and decoded $\bar{x}$ = 84.35:

a = (84.05) – (1.000)(84.35) = –0.30 cc.

The formula for the straight line estimating the trend of the universe mean values of y with respect to x (Y' or $\mu_{y.x}$) i.e., postoperative vital capacity predicted from preoperative vital capacity, is therefore Y = a + bx = –0.30 + 1.000x. The calculated line has been drawn on the graph depicting the mean values of postoperative vital capacity.

The slope, b, of the trend line is commonly referred to as the *regression coefficient* of y on x. It is the average difference in postoperative vital capacity (y) between two groups of individuals whose preoperative vital capacity (x) differs by one unit. That is, if one group of individuals has a preoperative vital capacity 1 cc higher than another group, we expect that the first group will have an average postoperative vital capacity 1.000 cc higher than that of the second group. Similarly, if one group of individuals has a preoperative vital capacity which is 10 cc higher than another group of patients, we expect that its postoperative vital capacity will be higher by 10.00 cc, on the average. Our regression coefficient of 1.000 cc/cc does *not* mean that if an individual increases his preoperative vital capacity by 1 cc, he may be expected to increase his postoperative vital capacity by 1.000 cc. In other words, our data present an *interindividual* rather than an *intraindividual* relation.

It is interesting to note that in this case the intercept of the regression line is practically zero, and the slope is one. In other words, we have a 45° line passing through the origin. Examples of this type occur frequently when the same variable is measured at

different times or when the same variable is measured by two different but equivalent methods.

Up to this point, we have investigated how the average postoperative vital capacity varies with the preoperative vital capacity. The
relationship may also be examined in another way — how does the
preoperative vital capacity vary with postoperative vital capacity? In
this case, we wish to examine the regression of x on y. The formula
for this regression line is $X = A + By$. Once again we can calculate the
slope of the fitted straight line trend (knowing that the values of $\bar{x}_y$
fall essentially on a straight line). The slope of this trend, B, is
calculated as:

$$B = r(s_x/s_y) = +0.933 \text{ cc per cc, and}$$
$$A = \bar{x} - B\bar{y} = 5.931 \text{ cc.}$$

The regression coefficient is then $B = +0.933$ cc/cc. This means that
if a group of individuals is found to have a postoperative vital capacity
higher by 1 cc than another group, then the preoperative vital capacity of the first group is 0.933 cc higher than that of the second, on
the average.

In the particular problem at hand, the regression of preoperative
vital capacity on postoperative vital capacity, while formally correct,
does not seem as pertinent as the regression of postoperative vital
capacity on preoperative vital capacity because of the time sequence.
In other problems, where x and y refer to distinct variables — such
as, for example, serum calcium and serum phosphorus, blood phosphorus and total cholesterol — the examination of either regression
would appear to carry the same import. It is seldom necessary to use
both regression lines. It is worth noting that in the "pure" regression
problem illustrated in Table 8.1, only one regression has any meaning, namely that of y on x.

Correlation Coefficient When There Is
Little Relationship

Before discussing the meaning of the correlation coefficient in detail,
let us examine the correlation table of the amount of phosphate
(mg%) and total cholesterol (mg%) found in the peripheral blood of
136 patients with marked periodontal disease.[6] The scatter diagram
of these data (Figure 8.8) shows no definite elliptical clustering of
the points; in fact, the main swarm of points can be included in a

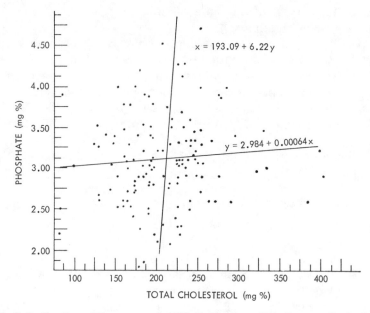

FIG. 8.8 Scatter Diagram of 136 Patients with Severe Periodontal Disease, According to the Phosphate and Total Cholesterol Content of Their Peripheral Blood.

circle centered near 3.00 mg% phosphate and 225 mg% cholesterol. Since practically no slope exists for this swarm, we can conclude, from mere inspection, that little or no relationship exists between phosphate and total cholesterol in these patients.

Examination of the correlation table (Table 8.15) shows that the frequency distribution of each variable simulates a normal curve. In addition, the distributions of y for specific values of x are assumed to be normal curves, and the distribution of x for specific values of y likewise. This calculation table was constructed in a manner similar to that for Table 8.13. From this table, we can readily calculate the coefficient of correlation, r = +.058, and the regression lines. Thus, from the scatter diagram, the correlation coefficient and either of the regression lines, we see that the quantity of total cholesterol in the patients studied bears practically no relation to the amount of phosphate in their blood.

Interpretation of the Coefficient of Correlation

The use of the coefficient of correlation, r, as an index of the relation between two variables is frequently encountered in dental research

TABLE 8.15
Correlation Table of Blood Phosphate and Total Cholesterol of 136 Patients with Periodontal Disease[7]

Phosphate mg% (y)	Total Cholesterol mg% (x)							f	y	fy	fy^2	$\sum_y x$	$y\sum_y x$	$\bar{x}_y$
	100	150	200	250	300	350	400							
1.75			2					2	0	0	0	4	0	2.00
2.25	1	1	7	3				12	1	12	12	24	24	2.00
2.75	1	14	13	10	3	1	2	44	2	88	176	99	198	2.25
3.25		14	12	22	1	2		51	3	153	459	118	354	2.31
3.75	1	3	8	3	2			17	4	68	272	36	144	2.12
4.25		1	2	4	1			8	5	40	200	21	104	2.62
4.75			2					2	6	12	72	4	24	2.00
f	3	33	46	42	7	3	2	136		373	1,191	306	849	
x	0	1	2	3	4	5	6							
fx	0	33	92	126	28	15	12	306						
fx^2	0	33	184	378	112	75	72	854						
$\sum_x y$	7	88	123	121	22	8	4	373						
$x\sum_x y$	0	88	246	363	88	40	24	849						
$\bar{y}_x$	2.33	2.67	2.67	2.88	3.14	2.67	2.00	2.00						

literature. We have already found that $r = +.965$ when a rather strong positive relationship existed between pre- and postoperative vital capacity, and that $r = +.058$ when practically no relationship existed between blood phosphate and total cholesterol. The maximum correlation that can exist would give $r = +1$ or $r = -1$, whereas the minimal relationship would give $r = 0$. Thus, the possible values of the coefficient of correlation, r, vary from -1 through 0 to $+1$, inclusive. The perfect negative relationship ($r = -1$) would appear on a graph as a straight line extending from the upper left to the lower right, whereas a perfect positive relationship ($r = +1$) would appear as a straight line extending from the lower left to the upper right. In either of these perfect relationships, all the graphed points would fall exactly on a straight line. In addition, the two regression lines would coincide. Biological variables do not usually occur in such perfect relationships, so that elliptical configurations of the graphed points, rather than straight lines, indicate relationship. This has already been seen, just as it has been noted that a configuration of graphed points appearing circular denotes little or no relationship.

The nearness of r to 1 is somewhat deceptive in the impression it gives of the completeness of the relation between y and x. For example, if $r = .7$, certainly rather close to 1, it does not mean that a predictability of 70% exists. Nor does it mean that there is a 70% perfect relation. The meaning of r can perhaps be understood a little better if one thinks of the reduction in the variation, i.e., variance or standard deviation, of y when x is specified, as compared to the variation of y when x is not utilized. Thus, if $r = .7$, this would mean that

$$\sigma^2_{y.x} / \sigma^2_y = (1 - r^2) = [1 - (.7)^2)] = .51,$$

i.e., the variance of y given x is 51% of what it was originally when x was not considered, or, in terms of the standard deviation,

$$\text{when } \sigma_{y.x} / \sigma_y = \sqrt{.51} = .71, \text{ or } 71\%.$$

Obviously, then, the correlation coefficient of .7 may not be so strong because a good deal of variation remains. Using an $r = .8$, we find

$$\sigma^2_{y.x} / \sigma^2_y = 1 - (8)^2 = .36 \text{ or } \sigma_{y.x} / \sigma_y = \sqrt{.36} = .6.$$

The standard deviation of the y's, taking account of x, is still 60% of the standard deviation when x is not being considered at all. Thus, a correlation coefficient of .8 may not be so important. In the example of vital capacity before and after oral surgery (Table 8.12), r was .965, certainly close to 1.0 and yet, examining the table it is found that y is still quite variable when the preoperative vital capacity (x) is fixed. Thus, in terms of predictability, one should not be overly optimistic when the value of r is getting close to 1.

Limitations on the Use of the Coefficient of Correlation

Although the correlation coefficient is widely used, it is not always correctly applied nor properly interpreted. Theoretically, the simultaneous measurements should be a sample from a normal bivariate distribution. This implies that the marginal distributions of x and y are normal curves, that both regressions are linear, that the distributions of y specific for x are normal curves with a constant standard deviation, $\sigma_{y.x}$, and that the distributions of x specific for y are normal curves with a constant standard deviation $\sigma_{x.y}$. The best way of checking these features is to examine the spot graph and, further, to plot the mean values of one variable for specific values of the other. If a straight line does not appear to describe the trend of these mean values, r should not be used. Even if all the points fell exactly on some curve — say, a parabola — r could not assume the maximum value of ±1, since these points would always deviate from a straight line.

Curves other than the straight line can be fitted by the method of least squares and appropriate correlation indices obtained, but these are not correlation coefficients and will not be discussed in this text. An illustration of the scatter diagram of two related variables with a curvilinear configuration is the hydrogen ion concentration and rate of flow of saliva,[8] which appears in Figure 8.9.

For r to be used validly, it must be able to vary from 0 to 1, in either a positive or negative direction. This criterion is met only when the distribution of each variable resembles a normal curve and the regression lines are linear. In the correlation table of the amount of milk taken per day and the calcium intake of 135 women (Table 8.16),[9] we see that the frequency distribution of milk intake does not resemble a normal curve. The calcium intake distribution is skewed to a slightly lesser extent. The scatter diagram of these data (Figure 8.10) discloses a markedly elliptical grouping with a definite slope. While the positive relationship here is fairly obvious, it is not appropriate to utilize r. Possibly a mere description of the strong relationship by table and graph may suffice.

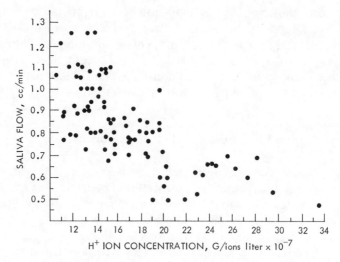

FIG. 8.9 Scatter Diagram of 85 Individuals, According to the Rate of Flow and Acidity of Their Saliva.

We thus see that the coefficient of correlation is merely a numerically convenient device for measuring the relationship between two variables when certain definite conditions are satisfied. It must be remembered, however, that a definite relationship may exist between two variables even though r may not be a very satisfactory index. In interpreting the coefficient of correlation, one must always remem-

TABLE 8.16
Correlation Table of Calcium and Milk Intake of 135 Women[9]

Calcium in Grams	Milk in Tablespoons								Frequency (f)
	0-9	10-19	20-29	30-39	40-49	50-59	60-69	70-	
0.050-0.149	1								1
0.150-0.249	10	2							12
0.250-0.349	17	10							27
0.350-0.449	4	24							28
0.450-0.549		14	6						20
0.550-0.649		4	11						15
0.650-0.749			6	5	1				12
0.750-0.849				8	3				11
0.850-0.949					2	1			3
0.950-1.049					1	1			2
1.050-0.149					1	2			3
1.150-								1	1
Frequency (f)	32	54	23	13	8	4	0	1	135

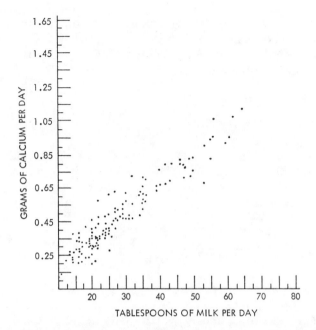

FIG. 8.10 Scatter Diagram of 135 Women, According to Their Daily Calcium Intake and Milk Consumption.

ber that r is a measure of association, and that association is not causation. The occurrence of certain phenomena may be based on the interaction of a multiplicity of causes, so that an association between two variables does not necessarily imply a cause and effect relationship. Attributing a cause and effect relationship where only association exists is a pitfall that we must avoid at all costs.

Testing the Significance of the Coefficient of Correlation

The correlation coefficient is determined from a limited sample of simultaneous measurements, drawn from a universe of such measurements. It therefore is subject to sampling error. When we compare r with 0, we are asking: "Could the value of r we found have arisen by chance in taking a sample of our size (N) from a universe in which there is no relationship between the two variables under consideration (true correlation coefficient = 0)?" When the true correlation coefficient in a bivariate normal surface is 0, then the ratio, $\dfrac{r\sqrt{N-2}}{\sqrt{1-r^2}}$ follows the t-distribution value of (N – 2) degrees of freedom. Consequently, we use the t-test to compare r with 0.

Testing the correlation coefficient, r = .058, found in the phosphate-cholesterol problem for significance, we find:

$$t = \frac{+.058\sqrt{136 - 2}}{\sqrt{1 - (0.058)^2}} = +0.67 \text{ with df} = 134.$$

We can therefore conclude that the coefficient of correlation, r = +.058 is statistically not significant. Testing for significance the correlation coefficient, r = +.967, found in the pre- and postoperative vital capacity problem, we find

$$t = \frac{+.967\sqrt{200 - 2}}{\sqrt{1 - (0.967)^2}} = 535.7 \text{ with df} = 198.$$

r, in this case, is highly significant.

On occasion, we may meet a problem in which the coefficient of correlation is applicable, and in which r is found to be about .3 or .4 in a positive or negative direction. Further, when a significance test is performed, r is found to be statistically significant. For example, a coefficient of correlation of +.32 was found for 60 individuals measured for salivary citrate content and erosion index, and this value was found to be statistically significant. Although such a value of r could not have readily occurred through the action of chance alone, it must be realized that a value of r = +.32 is not important for many purposes. The appropriate scatter diagram would not differ greatly from the circular configuration indicating an r of 0. As in all significance tests, a distinction must be made between statistical significance and practical importance.

Testing the Significance of Regression Coefficients

Another way of testing the significance of the relationship between two simultaneously recorded variables is to compare the regression coefficient of y on x (or x on y) with zero. This is often a more convenient way of assessing the relationship. This test has been illustrated for a simple regression problem, on page 168 ff. We must first calculate $s_{y.x}$ (or $s_{x.y}$) which is the variation of y (or x) values around the regression line of y on x (or x on y), and an estimate of $\sigma_{y.x}$ (or $\sigma_{x.y}$) as discussed previously. r serves as a useful computing tool in this connection.

$$s_{y.x} = \sqrt{\frac{(SS\ of\ y)(1 - r^2)}{N - 2}} \qquad s_{x.y} = \sqrt{\frac{(SS\ of\ x)(1 - r^2)}{N - 2}}$$

$$SE_b = \frac{s_{y.x}}{\sqrt{SS\ of\ x}} \qquad SE_B = \frac{s_{x.y}}{\sqrt{SS\ of\ y}}$$

For the data on blood phosphate and total cholesterol from Table 8.15,

$$SS\ of\ y = 1{,}191 - \frac{(373)^2}{136} \qquad SS\ of\ x = 854 - \frac{(306)^2}{136}$$

$$= 167.993 \qquad\qquad\qquad = 165.500$$

$$s_{y.x} = \sqrt{\frac{\left[1{,}191 - \frac{(373)^2}{136}\right] \times [1 - (.058)^2]}{136 - 2}} \qquad s_{x.y} = \sqrt{\frac{\left[854 - \frac{(306)^2}{136}\right] \times [1 - (.058)^2]}{136 - 2}}$$

$$s_{y.x} = \sqrt{1.2494} = 1.118 \qquad s_{x.y} = \sqrt{1.2308} = 1.109$$

$$SE_b = \frac{1.118}{\sqrt{167.993}} = 0.0862 \qquad SE_B = \frac{1.109}{\sqrt{165.500}} = 0.0862$$

$$t = \frac{(b - 0)}{SE_b} = \frac{0.058}{0.086} = 0.674 \qquad t = \frac{(B - 0)}{SE_B} = \frac{0.058}{0.086} = 0.674$$

It should be noted that the value of t is numerically the same and leads to the same conclusions whether the t-test involves the regression of y on x, x on y, or r.

REFERENCES

1. Aven, M., and Foldes, F. F.: The chemical kinetics of procaine and chloroprocaine hydrolysis, Science 114:206, 1951.

2. Dean, H. T.: Epidemiological studies in the United States. In Moulton, F. R., ed.: Dental Caries and Fluorine, Washington (D.C.), Amer Assn Advancement of Science, 1946, p. 26.

3. Bernick, S., and Ershoff, B. H.: Histochemical study of bone in estrogen-treated rats, J Dent Res 42:981–989, 1963.

4. Fosdick, L. S., and Rapp, G. W.: The effect of amylolytic enzymes on acid production in saliva, J Dent Res 23:85, 1944.

5. Frank, V. H., and Frasher, C. B.: Evaluation of pre-operative risks for anesthetics, Amer J Orthodont 26:473, 1940.

6. Tenenbaum, B., and Karshan, M.: Blood studies in periodontoclasia I, J Amer Dent Ass 32:1272, 1945.

7. Karshan, M., Tenenbaum, B., Karlan, F., and Leonard, H.: Blood studies in periodontoclasia II, J Dent Res 25:257, 1946.

8. Anderson, D. J.: The hydrogen-ion concentration of the saliva, II. The relationship between hydrogen-ion concentration and rate of flow of saliva, J Dent Res 28:305, 1949.

9. Radusch, D. F.: The relationship between periodontal conditions and certain dietary factors, J Dent Res 18:305, 1939.

9

Multiple Regression

In the previous chapter, attention was devoted to the regression of y on a single independent or *predictor* variable, x. In a "real life" situation, however, there may be more than one such predictor variable $(x_1, x_2, \ldots x_k)$. The statistical treatment of this relationship is known as *multiple regression*. Some of the purposes of multiple regression are to formulate an appropriate equation which would yield the best prediction of the values of the dependent variable, y; to develop some idea of the possible etiology of the values of y by unearthing which of the group of variables $(x_1, x_2,$ etc.), when taken together, has the most influence on these y values; and possibly to rate the predictor variables in the order of their importance.

LINEAR REGRESSION WITH CHANGE OF ORIGIN OF THE INDEPENDENT VARIABLE

When the straight line was considered in Chapter 8, the equation used was

$$Y = a + bx,$$

where the origin of x was the real origin at 0. This gave rise to two simultaneous normal equations which could be solved by "sheer force" to yield a and b.

$$a \text{ equation: } Na + b\Sigma x = \Sigma y$$

$$b \text{ equation: } a\Sigma x + b\Sigma x^2 = \Sigma xy.$$

The general solution of the two simultaneous equations was

$$b = SP_{xy}/SS_x, \text{ and } a = \bar{y} - bx.$$

The equation of the line is often written with the origin of x at $\bar{x}$ as

$$Y = m + b(x - \bar{x}).$$

In this simpler form, the two simultaneous or normal equations become

$$m \text{ equation: } Nm = \Sigma y, \text{ and}$$
$$b \text{ equation: } bSS_x = SP_{xy}.$$

Immediately,

$$m = \bar{y} \text{ and } b = SP_{xy}/SS_x,$$

so that, when x = 0,

$$Y = m + b(-\bar{x}) = \bar{y} - b\bar{x} = a.$$

The Residual SS for variation around the line,

$$Q = \Sigma(y - Y)^2$$

can always be calculated in a direct form by computing every individual $(y - Y)$, but this is tedious and produces considerable round off errors. A general way of calculating Q is to calculate the SS due to the model, and to subtract this value from the uncorrected Σy^2. The SS due to the model for the first formulation of the line is

$$a\Sigma y + b\Sigma xy.$$

For the second formulation of the line, the SS due to the model is

$$m\Sigma y + bSP_{xy}.$$

Note that the SS due to the model is the sum of the right-hand sides of the normal equations multiplied by the computed coefficients.

Then,

$$Q = \Sigma y^2 - (a\Sigma y + b\Sigma xy), \text{ or also}$$
$$Q = \Sigma y^2 - m\Sigma y - bSP_{xy}$$

It should be noted that, in this second form, since $m\Sigma y = CT$,

$$Q = SS_y - bSP_{xy} = SS_y - \text{Regression SS}$$

a form for calculating Q which has already been used in Chapter 8. The SS due to the model is greater than the Regression SS since it includes the effect of the intercept, i.e., CT.

MULTIPLE REGRESSION WITH ORIGIN OF THE INDEPENDENT VARIABLES x_1, x_2 AT 0.

In the case of multiple regression with two independent variables, x_1 and x_2, the multiple regression equation represents a plane and can be written as

$$Y = a + b_1 x_1 + b_2 x_2,$$

where a is the intercept with the origin of x_1, x_2 taken as the real 0, i.e., a is the height of the plane at $x_1 = 0$ and $x_2 = 0$; and b_1 is the slope of the plane with respect to the x_1 axis, i.e., the change in y per unit change in x_1, and b_2 is the slope of the plane with respect to the x_2 axis, i.e., the change in y per unit change in x_2. b_1 and b_2 are often called the *Partial Regression Coefficients*, whereas in the straight line discussion there was only one slope, merely called the Regression Coefficient or, sometimes, the *Total Regression Coefficient*.

As an illustrative example, data are presented in Table 9.1 for the control group of 40 patients from a study by Menaker et al.[1] Patients with a history of appreciable plaque formation, were given a complete dental prophylaxis. Following this, they pursued their normal oral hygiene procedures for four weeks to provide a normalization period for plaque growth. At that time, plaque (*preplaque*) was scored for all teeth using the Turesky modification of the Quigley-Hein Index,[2] a dimensionless score after the patients had rinsed with a solution of Fast Green. A complete dental prophylaxis was again performed after which all patients were given a nonmedicated placebo mouthrinse to use twice daily, but refrained from other oral hygiene procedures except for their usual brushing habits

TABLE 9.1
Pre- and Postplaque Scores and Weight (in 10 lb. Units) for 40 Control Patients

Patient Number	Preplaque (x_1)	Weight (lb/10) (x_2)	Postplaque (y)	Patient Number	Preplaque (x_1)	Weight (lb/10) (x_2)	Postplaque (y)
1	2.52	14.0	2.43	21	1.83	19.0	1.81
2	1.66	14.0	1.84	22	2.12	12.2	2.65
3	0.65	9.8	0.53	23	2.78	13.3	2.81
4	1.72	14.0	2.02	24	2.88	13.2	3.33
5	1.89	18.5	1.89	25	1.21	10.5	1.27
6	2.58	15.5	3.00	26	1.67	13.5	1.32
7	2.45	17.5	2.23	27	1.91	18.0	1.68
8	1.85	13.5	2.57	28	2.44	12.2	2.38
9	1.60	9.7	1.85	29	0.54	19.0	0.86
10	2.34	16.0	2.09	30	1.68	15.5	1.82
11	1.00	10.9	1.42	31	1.91	13.5	1.71
12	2.21	12.5	2.32	32	2.62	10.8	2.23
13	2.38	19.0	2.21	33	2.42	16.0	2.85
14	1.02	13.7	1.00	34	1.28	15.4	1.36
15	1.61	13.6	1.61	35	2.39	11.5	2.17
16	1.46	16.5	1.35	36	1.48	11.6	2.02
17	1.25	15.0	0.95	37	2.03	17.0	2.20
18	1.52	15.0	1.20	38	2.17	12.9	2.33
19	1.92	19.0	2.04	39	2.02	15.2	2.52
20	1.64	19.0	1.61	40	2.25	17.0	2.10
				Average	1.8725	14.6000	1.9395

with a new toothbrush and a standard toothpaste. Three weeks later, they were scored for plaque (*postplaque*) in the same manner as the preplaque scoring. The patient's weight was obtained in a standard manner,* since the view had been expressed that heavier patients might conceivably eat more and, therefore, tend to have more plaque. Appropriate summary values of the data are given below.

Summary of Data in Table 9.1

Preplaque (x_1):	$\Sigma x_1 = 74.9000$	$\Sigma x_1^2 = 152.4548$	$\Sigma x_1 x_2 = 1{,}097.5750$
Weight (x_2):	$\Sigma x_2 = 584.0000$	$\Sigma x_2^2 = 8{,}819.9600$	$\Sigma x_1 y = 157.2079$
Postplaque (y):	$\Sigma y = 77.5800$	$\Sigma y^2 = 165.2514$	$\Sigma x_2 y = 1{,}132.3540$
	$SS_y = 14.784990$	$SS_{x1} = 12.204550$	$SS_{x2} = 293.560000$
	$SS_{yx1} = 11.939500$	$SP_{yx2} = -0.314000$	$SP_{x1 x2} = 4.035000$

According to the method of Least Squares, the best estimates of a, b_1, and b_2 are obtained by minimizing the SS of the points about the plane, i.e., minimizing $Q = \Sigma (y - Y)^2$. We are assuming that the variance of y about the plane is constant for all x_1, x_2, i.e., homoscedasticity. This minimization gives rise to three simultaneous (normal) equations, namely

$$a \text{ equation: } Na + b_1 \Sigma x_1 + b_2 \Sigma x_2 = \Sigma y\dagger$$
$$b_1 \text{ equation: } a\Sigma x_1 + b_1 \Sigma x_1^2 + b_2 \Sigma x_1 x_2 = \Sigma x_1 y$$
$$b_2 \text{ equation: } a\Sigma x_2 + b_1 \Sigma x_1 x_2 + b_2 \Sigma x_2^2 = \Sigma x_2 y.$$

From the summary of the data of Table 9.1, these equations can be filled in, giving the numerical equations:

a equation: (1) $40a + 74.9000b_1 + 584.0000b_2 = 77.5800$:
$$a = 0.311562$$

b_1 equation: (2) $74.9000a + 152.4548b_1 + 1{,}097.5750b_2$
$$= 157.2079: b_1 = 0.983092$$

b_2 equation: (3) $5{,}840.0000a + 157.2079b_1 + 8{,}819.9600b_2$
$$= 1{,}132.3540: b_2 = -0.0145823$$

---

*The weights are recorded in 10-pound units in order to make the SS_{x2} more similar in magnitude to SS_{x1} so that the simultaneous equations can be solved more easily.

†The first equation shows that the plane passes through the mean point $\bar{y}$, $\bar{x}_1, \bar{x}_2$.

The solution of these three simultaneous equations to obtain the estimates of a, b_1, and b_2, to obtain the multiple regression equation, proceeds in a standard algebraic manner, which is an extension of the method already illustrated for the straight line (Chapter 8).[3] *

Plaque score represents an average of scores over a number of teeth but has no dimension. Consequently a is dimensionless. b_1 represents the change in postplaque, y, score per unit change in pre-plaque score, x_1 (assumed to be the same for all values of x_2). b_1 is dimensionless. However, b_2 represents the change in postplaque score per change of 10 pounds in weight and is obviously not a pure number. The importance of x_1 and x_2 in the prediction of y can evidently not be assessed by a direct comparison of the partial regression coefficients unless some adjustment is made for the difference in dimension.

The plane has now been fitted:

$$Y = a + b_1x_1 + b_2x_2.$$

The Residual variation, $Q = \Sigma(y - Y)^2$ around this plane, can be calculated in direct form by computing every individual $(y - Y)$ for every x_1, x_2 combination. This is very tedious, unless there are only a few points. The Residual variation can also be computed as:

$$Q = \Sigma(y - Y)^2 = \Sigma y^2 - \text{SS due to the Model},$$

where,

$$\text{SS due to the Model} = a\Sigma y + b_1\Sigma x_1 y + b_2\Sigma x_2 y$$
$$= 77.5800(0.311562)$$
$$+ 157.2079(0.983092) + 1{,}132.3540(-0.0145823) = 162.2085$$

so that

$$Q = 165.2514 - 162.2085 = 3.0429.$$

The number of degrees of freedom for Q is $(N - 3)$ because there are three simultaneous equations involved. In the series of 40 values of $(y - Y)$, there are three restrictions, namely,

---

*In the interest of accuracy to six significant figures, the equations were solved using a program for a pocket calculator (HP 41C). Throughout this chapter, an excessive number of significant figures and decimals have been retained in order to show numerically the equivalence of various procedures.

$$\Sigma(y - Y) = 0; \Sigma x_1(y - Y) = 0; \text{and } \Sigma x_2(y - Y) = 0.$$

If 37 values of $(y - Y)$ are available, the rest of these values can readily be obtained. If $Q = \Sigma(y - Y)^2$ is divided by $(N - 3)$, the variance about the plane would be obtained as $s^2_{y.x_1x_2}$, the square of the Standard Error of Estimate around the plane,

$$s^2_{y.x_1x_2} = 3.0429/37 = 0.08224.$$

$s^2_{y.x_1x_2}$ is an estimate of $\sigma^2_{y.x_1x_2}$, the assumed constant variation of the distributions of y about the plane.

MULTIPLE REGRESSION WITH ORIGIN AT THE MEAN, $\bar{x}_1, \bar{x}_2$

A more convenient formulation of the plane which will be used from now on is

$$Y = m + b_1(x_1 - \bar{x}_1) + b_2(x_2 - \bar{x}_2),$$

where the origin is taken as $\bar{x}_1, \bar{x}_2$, and m stands for the height of the plane at $\bar{x}_1\bar{x}_2$. Because $\Sigma(x_1 - \bar{x}_1) = 0$ and $\Sigma(x_2 - \bar{x}_2) = 0$, the three simultaneous equations become:

m equation: (1) $Nm = \Sigma y$

b_1 equation: (2) $b_1 SS_{x_1} + b_2 SP_{x_1x_2} = SP_{yx_1}$

b_2 equation: (3) $b_1 SP_{x_1x_2} + b_2 SS_{x_2} = SP_{yx_2}$.

Using the summary of the data of Table 9.1, the following numerical equations are obtained:

m equation: (1) $40m = 77.580000; m = \bar{y} = 1.939500$

b_1 equation: (2) $12.204550b_1 + 4.035000b_2 = 11.939500;$
$\quad b_1 = 0.983091$

b_2 equation: (3) $4.035000b_1 + 293.560000b_2 = -0.314000;$
$\quad b_2 = -0.0145823.$

Equation (1) is solved directly, to give

$$m = \bar{y} = 1.939500.$$

Solving Equations (2) and (3) by the ordinary method used to solve the two simultaneous equations in Chapter 8, the values of $b_1 = 0.983091$ and $b_2 = -0.00145823$ are obtained, the same as those obtained from solving the equations in the previous form, showing that the values of the slopes remain the same regardless of the shift of origin. m, the new intercept at $\bar{x}_1$, $\bar{x}_2$ comes out merely as $\bar{y}$. The old intercept taken at the origin is:

$$a = \bar{y} - b_1\bar{x}_1 - b_2\bar{x}_2$$
$$= 1.939500 - (0.983091)(1.872500) - (-0.0145823)(14.600000)$$
$$= 0.311564.$$

This is the same as the intercept already given in the first formulation of the plane.

The residual variation about the plane is

$$Q = \Sigma y^2 - \text{SS due to the model} = \Sigma y^2 - m\Sigma y - b_1 SP_{x_1 y} - b_2 SP_{x_2 y}$$
$$= SS_y - (b_1 SP_{x_1 y} + b_2 SP_{x_2 y}),$$

which, in this form, resembles the method of calculating Q for the straight line. The part involving b_1 and b_2 is called the Regression SS, and is less than what was previously called the SS due to the Model, by the correction for the intercept (CT).

$$Q = 14.784990 - [(0.983091)(11.939500)$$
$$+ (-0.0145823)(-0.314000)]$$
$$= 14.784990 - 11.742194 = 3.042796.$$

Except for rounding, Q is the same value previously obtained.

The value of b_1 and b_2 are not the values obtained by fitting two separate lines of y on x_1 and y on x_2 because x_1 and x_2 are not independent of each other. In fact, it is seen that $SP_{x_1 x_2} = 4.035000$ rather than 0, so that x_1 and x_2 are correlated with each other. If x_1 and x_2 were uncorrelated, so that $SP_{x_1 x_2} = 0$, the normal equations would have been much simpler since the term $SP_{x_1 x_2}$ would have dropped out and both b_1 and b_2 would have been obtained immediately and would be the same as the b_1 and b_2 of two straight lines. This almost never happens in practice with the customary variables used.

TABLE 9.2
Analysis of Variance for Multiple Regression for Data in Table 9.1

Source of Variation	df	SS	MS
Regression on x_1, x_2	2	$11.742194 = b_1 SP_{x_1 y} + b_2 SP_{x_2 y}$	5.8711
Deviations from Plane	37	$3.042796 = \Sigma(y - Y)^2$	$0.082238 = s_{y.x_1 x_2}$
Total	39	14.784990	

SIGNIFICANCE OF REGRESSION

In terms of testing the significance of the regression, the ANOVA table is employed — an extension of that already shown in the case of the straight line in Chapter 8. The total variation of y can be sub-divided as shown in Table 9.2.

The significance of the Regression SS with df = 2, obviously cannot be tested by the t-test. Under the null hypothesis that the true value of b_1 and $b_2 = 0$, the Regression MS is estimating the same parameter as $s^2_{y.x_1 x_2}$, namely, $\sigma^2_{y.x_1 x_2}$. If, however, the plane has real slopes, i.e., if the true regression coefficients are not equal to zero, then it would be expected that the Regression MS would be greater than $s^2_{y.x_1 x_2}$, so that under the null hypothesis, the ratio

$$\frac{\text{Regression Mean Square}}{\text{Deviations Mean Square}}$$

should follow the F-distribution:*

$$F_{2,37} = \frac{5.8711}{0.082238} = 71.3916,$$

which is statistically very significant (P is much less than .01). Thus, the relationship between the postplaque and weight and preplaque scores taken together is significant. This does not say that both of these independent variables contribute significantly to the post-plaque score. That is another question which should be explored.

---

*This assumes that y at each x_1, x_2 combination is normally distributed, a reasonable assumption since y is a mean of a number of elementary scores.

COEFFICIENT OF DETERMINATION;
MULTIPLE CORRELATION COEFFICIENT

The ratio, Regression SS/Total SS, is often called the *Coefficient of Determination*, R^2.

$$R^2 = \text{Regression SS/Total SS} = 11.742194/14.78499 = .794197.$$

In the case of the straight line regression, there was an equivalent definition of the Coefficient of Determination as

$$r^2 = \text{Regression SS/Total SS.}$$

It was pointed out that for a bivariate surface, r^2 was the square of the coefficient of correlation and was an estimate of a parameter of that surface. r^2 or its square root, r, is not apt to be thought of as an estimate of a parameter unless there is a correlation problem (bivariate surface) involved. In addition to being called the Coefficient of Determination, R^2 is also called the square of the Multiple Correlation Coefficient between y and x_1, x_2, $R^2_{y.x_1x_2}$, even if x_1, x_2 are fixed variables so that a pure regression problem is involved. $R_{y.x_1x_2}$ would be an estimate of some parameter if there were a correlation problem involved with an appropriate trivariate surface. In that case, of course, there would be three values of R^2, namely, $R^2_{y.x_1x_2}$, $R^2_{x_1.yx_2}$, and $R^2_{x_2.yx_1}$.

The F-test just proposed to test the significance of the Regression is, at the same time, the test of significance of R^2. For a problem with p variables (p – 1 independent variables),

$$F_{(p-1),(N-p)} = \frac{R^2(N-p)}{(p-1)(1-R^2)} = \frac{(0.794197)(37)}{2(0.205803)} = 71.3918,$$

the same as from the ANOVA. The formula for testing R^2 by means of F appears to be a simple extension of the test of significance of r by means of the t-test previously presented on page 203.

SIGNIFICANCE OF SEPARATE INDEPENDENT VARIABLES

While it has been shown that a significant relation exists between the postplaque score, and preplaque score and weight, this summary statement is not very illuminating, any more than the F-test in the usual ANOVA where more than two treatments are compared. It is desired to know which of the treatments may be producing the effect, which is the motivation for the use of multiple comparison methods.

If the importance of x_1 and x_2 could be assessed by comparing b_1 and b_2, (0.983091 and -0.0145823), it would appear that x_2 is much less important than x_1. b_1 and b_2 should not be compared, however, because they are not dimensionless, as has already been pointed out. Standardized coefficients (the so-called *beta coefficients*) are often calculated as:

$$b_1 s_1 / s_y = 0.983091\sqrt{12.204550/14.784990} = 0.893190,$$

and

$$b_2 s_2 / s_y = -0.0145823\sqrt{293.560000/14.784990} = -0.0649776.$$

It is evident that weight is a far less important variable than pre-plaque score. In fact, it will be shown that the effect of weight is not statistically significant.

The coefficients, b_1 and b_2, should be tested separately for significance from zero. A direct way of doing this is to obtain a separate standard error for b_1 and b_2 and then perform a t-test on b_1 vs. 0, and of b_2 vs. 0, using the respective standard errors with an $s_{y.x_1 x_2}$ based on 37 degrees of freedom. These standard errors are not so easily calculated, involving the inversion of a matrix.

A very general and appealing alternative procedure is to fit the regression line of y on x_1, ignoring x_2, and then compare the Regression SS when only x_1 is used, with that when both x_1 and x_2 are used. When only x_1 is used,

Regression SS accounted for by x_1 (ignoring x_2) = $(SP_{x_1 y})^2 / SS_{x_1}$

$$= 11.680206.$$

Notice that this accounts for almost all of the Regression SS given by the model that uses x_1 and x_2 (the plane) which was 11.742194. The difference is 11.742194 - 11.680206 = 0.061988 with df = 1. This is the Regression SS of y on x_2 beyond x_1, i.e., the extra SS accounted for by x_2 once x_1 is in the formula. A significance test is performed to find out whether anything is gained by introducing x_2.

$$F_{1,37} = \frac{\text{SS due to } x_2 \text{ after } x_1}{s^2_{y.x_1 x_2}} = \frac{0.061988}{0.082238} = 0.7538.$$

TABLE 9.3
Tests of Significance of Partial Regression Coefficients[a]

Source of Variation	df	SS	MS	F	df
Deviations from					
Plane	37	3.042796	0.082238		
Regression on $x_1 x_2$	2	11.742194	5.8711	71.3916	2,37
Regression on x_1					
(ignoring x_2)	1	11.680206	11.680206		
Regression on x_2					
(beyond x_1)	1	0.061988	0.061988	0.7538	1,37
Regression on x_2					
(ignoring x_1)	1	0.000336	0.000336		
Regression on x_1					
(beyond x_2)	1	11.741858	11.741858	142.7790	1,37

[a]Possibly a penalty for multiple comparisons might be invoked here, e.g., making each test at the 2.5% level, in order to obtain an overall level of 5%[4].

P is much greater than .05.

Evidently, it may not be necessary to ask the other question: What is the effect of preplaque score once weight is brought into the formula? — but the same procedure can be followed:

Regression SS for postplaque on weight ignoring x_1

$$= (SP_{x_2 y})^2/(SS_{x_2})^2 = (-0.31400)^2/293.5600 = 0.000336.$$

What is left over for the preplaque score is almost the whole Regression SS,* i.e.,

$$11.742194 - 0.000336 = 11.741858$$

$$F_{1,37} = 11.741858/0.082238 = 142.7790.$$

The whole testing procedure can be summarized in an ANOVA table (Table 9.3). It is noted that in our example

$$\text{SS due to } x_1 \text{ (ignoring } x_2) + \text{SS due to } x_2 \text{ (ignoring } x_1) =$$
$$11.680206 + 0.000336 = 11.680542.$$

---

*This is due to the small effect of weight and also explains why the $F_{1,37}$ for testing the extra effect of preplaque score is almost twice the $F_{2,37}$ for testing the whole regression on x_1, x_2.

In our example, this is less than

$$\text{SS due to } x_1 \text{ (beyond } x_2) + \text{SS due to } x_2 \text{ (beyond } x_1) =$$
$$11.741858 + 0.061988 = 11.803846.$$

Both of the above sums differ from the Regression SS due to x_1 and x_2 (11.742194) because the correlation between x_1 and x_2 ($SP_{x_1 x_2}$) is not zero. The difference in the three quantities and the direction of the inequality depend on the various correlations, r_{yx_1}, r_{yx_2}, and $r_{x_1 x_2}$.

Since weight seems unimportant, the line relating y to x_1, i.e., postplaque to preplaque scores, whose slope is

$$b = SP_{yx_1}/SS_{x_1} = 0.978283$$

might be adequate for predicting y. This b is not equal to the partial regression coefficient when weight is included in the model (0.983091), although the difference is small because weight was so unimportant. The slope, b, is close to 1, because y and x_1 are the same variable (plaque score) at different times.

PARTIAL CORRELATION COEFFICIENT

There is another way of viewing this problem of the extra effect of x_1 or x_2, in terms of partial correlation coefficients. The question of whether x_2 adds anything beyond x_1 (or whether x_1 adds anything beyond x_2) can be answered by computing the partial correlation coefficient $r_{yx_2 . x_1}$ of y and x_2 given x_1, or "holding x_1 constant" (and the partial correlation coefficient $r_{yx_1 . x_2}$ of y on x_1 holding x_2 constant). In essence, what is done is to adjust y for its linear relation to x_1, and x_2 for its linear relation to x_1. This results in an adjusted y and an adjusted x_2, having removed the influence of x_1. The correlation between the adjusted y and the adjusted x_2 is computed.

Under the assumption of linearity of the relationships, the partial correlation coefficients can be computed from the simple or total correlation coefficients:

$$r_{yx_1} = .888822; r_{yx_2} = -.004766; r_{x_1 x_2} = 0.67412.$$

Thus,

$$r_{yx_2 \cdot x_1} = \frac{r_{yx_2} - (r_{yx_1})(r_{x_1 x_2})}{\sqrt{(1 - r^2_{yx_1})(1 - r^2_{x_1 x_2})}}$$

$$= \frac{-.004766 - (.888822)(.067412)}{\sqrt{[1 - (.888822)^2][1 - (.067412)^2]}}$$

$$= -.141489.$$

We see that the correlation between preplaque score and weight (-.004766) is changed to (-.141489) when the influence of post-plaque is removed. It is still small, however. The significance test of $r_{yx_1 \cdot x_2}$ is a t-test similar to that for the usual r, (p. 203) except that the N and df are reduced by 1.

$$t_{37} = \frac{r_{yx_2 \cdot x_1}\sqrt{(N-3)}}{\sqrt{1 - r^2_{yx_1 \cdot x_2}}} = \frac{-.141489\sqrt{37}}{\sqrt{1 - (.141489)^2}} = -0.869390.$$

It should be noted that $t^2 = 0.7558$. Except for rounding, this is the same value which was obtained for F when testing the Regression SS for x_2 beyond x_1.

Similarly, $r_{yx_1 \cdot x_2}$ may be computed:

$$r_{yx_1 \cdot x_2} = \frac{r_{yx_1} - (r_{yx_2})(r_{x_1 x_2})}{\sqrt{(1 - r^2_{yx_2})(1 - r^2_{x_1 x_2})}}$$

$$= \frac{(.888822) - (-.004766)(.067412)}{\sqrt{[1 - (-.004766)^2][(1 - (.067412)^2]}}$$

$$= .891180.$$

Notice that this correlation coefficient is almost exactly the same as the correlation between y and x_1 when x_2 was completely ignored, showing what a very small role is played by x_2.

$$t_{37} = r\sqrt{N-3}/\sqrt{(1 - r^2)} = (.891180)(6.082763)/\sqrt{[1 - (.891180)^2}$$

$$= 11.949382$$

$$F_{1,37} = t^2_{37} = 142.7877.$$

This test of significance of the partial correlation coefficient is testing the regression on x_1 beyond x_2 (performed previously on the ANOVA in Table 9.3).

MULTIPLE LINEAR REGRESSION WITH
MORE THAN TWO INDEPENDENT VARIABLES

For simplicity, we have taken the case of two independent variables because then the calculations can be made with a pocket calculator without too much difficulty.* Even in that case, the calculations of the various sums of squares and products and the solution of three simultaneous equations are tedious. Especially tedious would be the calculations of the separate $(y - Y)$'s if the residuals from the plane were to be examined. Some of the tedium is removed if a change of origin is made, because then there are only two simultaneous equations to be solved. This still entails some tedious calculations, e.g., SS and SP. With more than two independent variables,† it is very laborious to perform the necessary computations even if the model were changed so that the mean were the origin. In this case, computer programs can be of inestimable help, as shown in the Appendix. A study of multiple regression, including some of the hand calculations (tedious though they may be) should have been done previously in one or more problems if one hopes to understand the material printed out by the computer. The printout generated by these computer programs corresponds to the various procedures described above. It would be a mistake to run a computer program as soon as a multiple regression problem arises without knowing anything about multiple regression, and hope that the computer output can be interpreted properly.

MULTIPLE LINEAR REGRESSION WITH
DUMMY VARIABLES

In the usual multiple regression problem, all of the independent variables (as well as the dependent variable) are quantitative. The usual regression procedures can, however, be employed when one or more of the independent variables are dichotomous because, in that case, they can be scaled as 0 and 1 and thus correspond to a numerical

---

*Note that if x_2 is taken as $(x_1)^2$, the multiple regression equation will correspond to that of a parabola.

†For example, the third independent variable (x_3), might be the product $x_1 x_2$ with a partial regression coefficient b_3. A significance test performed on b_3 would then be testing the assumption of an additive model, i.e., a constant effect of x_1 whatever the value of x_2 (or a constant effect of x_2 whatever the value of x_1). Such a test is, in fact, equivalent to the ANOVA test of interaction.

value. Such variables are usually called *indicator* or *dummy* variables. For example, treatment I and treatment II could be called 0 and 1 in terms of the variable, treatment, or male and female could be called 0 and 1. Obviously, if there were more than two treatments, it would be necessary to break them up into sets of dummy variables. Thus, if there were four treatments, three dummy variables would have to be used to encompass the variable, treatment.

The multiple regression procedure is really a very general procedure which encompasses many other procedures in statistics, e.g., the ANOVA is a multiple regression problem where all of the independent variables are dummy variables. In Chapter 10 (Analysis of Covariance), an example will be discussed of the analysis of covariance. The analysis actually corresponds to a case where some of the independent variables are quantitative and some are dummy variables. The most general computer programs make little or no distinction in their printout between ANOVA problems and ANOCOVA problems and multiple regression problems.*

REFERENCES

1. Menaker, L., Weatherford, T. W., Pitts, G., Ross, N. M., and Lamm, R.: The effects of Listerine antiseptic on dental plaque, Alabama Journal of Medical Sciences, 16:71, 1979.

2. Turesky, S., Gilmore, N. D., and Glickman, I.: Reduced plaque formation by the chloromethyl analogue of victamine C, J Periodontal, 41:41, 1970.

3. Dixon, W. J., and Massey, F. J., Jr.: Introduction to Statistical Analysis, 3rd ed. McGraw-Hill, New York, 1969.

4. Miller, R. G.: Simultaneous Statistical Inference, 2nd ed., New York, Springer-Verlag, 1981.

5. Snedecor, G. W., and Cochrane, W. G.: Statistical Methods, 7th ed. Iowa State Univ. Press, Ames, Iowa, 1980.

6. Armitage, P.: Statistical Methods in Medical Research, Oxford, U.K., Blackwell Scientific Publications, 1971.

7. Draper, N. R., and Smith, H.: Applied Regression Analysis, 2nd ed., New York, Wiley, 1981.

---

*For further discussion of multiple regression, the reader is referred to texts by Snedecor and Cochran[5], Armitage,[6] and Draper and Smith[7]. See Appendix for illustration of the use of computer programs (SAS and SPSS) for the multiple linear regression problem discussed in this chapter.

10
Analysis of Covariance

The comparison of means of two independent samples was discussed in Chapter 5 (t-test) and of more than two samples in Chapter 7 (one-way analysis of variance). In such problems, at the start of the experiment the samples are assumed to be similar with respect to all variables, tangible and intangible, that may influence the main variable under consideration. The extraneous variables, often called *concomitant variables*, are presumably unaffected by the treatments under investigation. To ensure uniformity with respect to the concomitant variables, the experimental subjects should be assigned to the various groups in some random manner. While random allocation of the subjects will ensure that the groups will be alike in their average values with respect to any concomitant variable within the limits of chance fluctuation, they may not be precisely alike.

Sometimes it is felt that the variable under study is correlated with one of the concomitant variables to such an extent that it would be advantageous to have the average value of this concomitant variable equal in all samples. There is a statistical technique used to neutralize sample differences in a concomitant variable when comparing the average values of the variable of interest. This technique is the analysis of covariance with one concomitant variable in a one-way layout of data.[1] Essentially, the method amounts to a combination of regression methods (Chapter 8) and analysis of variance (Chapter 7).

The analysis of covariance is a refinement of the analysis of variance. In its simplest application, it is used to compare the means of independent samples after statistically eliminating the random sampling differences of a variable, x, concomitant to the main variable, y, under study. In addition, the variation in y is reduced by the elimination of the effect of the variation in x within a sample. In certain instances, this increases the possibility of establishing statistical significance among the means of y if a true difference exists.

This chapter illustrates the analysis of covariance in its simplest form, as a technique to compare the means of independent samples after adjusting for discrepancies in the sample averages of a concomitant variable, when those discrepancies are due solely to random fluctuations. Certain tests utilizing covariance will also be mentioned, such as the test of the dependence of one variable on another and the test of the parallelism of lines, i.e., equality of slopes. These tests, by themselves, are not classical examples of the analysis of covariance, although often they are so labeled. It should be noted that the procedures of the analysis of covariance for the type of layout (one-way) described here are not restricted to equal sample sizes.

A double-blind clinical evaluation of a new analgesic agent for postoperative oral pain was run to determine whether there was any effect on artificially induced pain when the medication was administered in advance. Accordingly, 60 patients were studied, age 21 to 57 years, from the student body and dental clinic of Temple University School of Dentistry. A number of measurements, including pulse rate (left radial artery) while in a sitting position and pulp test of the maxillary left central incisor, were taken and are reported here.[2,3] Other variables — such as blood pressure and pressure pain threshold — were recorded but are not reported here. The pulse rate was taken as a possible indication of the level of the patient's general reflex excitability, and the pulp test, the main variable under consideration, as an indication of the pain response level of the patient. The Burton Vitalometer was used as the pulp tester, with the stimulus applied to the middle of the dried labial aspect of the tooth, with toothpaste as the conductor. The patient was instructed to signify the minimal stimulus, increasing from 0 to 10 in 0.5 units.

After these determinations were made, each patient received a pink capsule designated only by code number, 1 through 60. The capsules were assigned by a predetermined random allocation. Three treatments were employed: Drug A, a widely used nonnarcotic agent stated to be similar to codeine in its analgesic potential; Drug B, a new drug of similar characteristics; and Drug P, a placebo capsule. The study was conducted in a double-blind manner, the patients being told merely that a test was being performed with analgesic agents. One and one-half hours after taking the capsule, the same measurements were made on the patient as were made initially. The data of the 60 patients — i.e., drug taken, initial pulse rate (x), and the difference (y), between initial and final pulp test readings, appear in Table 10.1.

TABLE 10.1
Initial Pulse Rates (x) and Increments (y) in Pulp Test Readings of 60 Patients According to Medication

	Drug A		Drug B		Placebo	
	x	y	x	y	x	y
	88	-1.0	84	0.0	76	0.5
	80	0.0	84	0.5	88	1.0
	80	0.5	68	-0.5	76	0.0
	76	0.0	80	-0.5	90	0.5
	90	0.5	80	1.0	68	0.5
	88	1.0	76	0.5	80	1.5
	72	-0.5	92	0.5	68	-0.5
	80	0.5	112	-0.5	80	0.0
	80	0.5	84	1.0	80	1.0
	80	1.0	68	-2.0	84	-0.5
	72	-0.5	96	-4.0	76	-0.5
	88	0.0	112	-1.0	100	0.5
	68	-3.0	74	-0.5	96	-0.5
	68	0.0	88	0.0	92	0.5
	72	-0.5	96	0.0	72	-0.5
	80	-1.0	96	0.0	72	1.0
	76	-1.0	100	0.5	96	0.0
	82	0.0	100	0.0	84	-1.5
	76	-1.0	76	-5.0	76	-1.0
	88	-1.0	72	2.0	96	0.5
Means:	79.20	-0.275	86.90	- .400	82.50	+ .125

The experiment was designed to answer the question: Are the three treatments equal in their average effect on pain threshold? The effect is measured by the difference (y) in final pulp test reading and initial pulp test reading. The assumption has evidently been made that y is the proper way to take care of the influence of the initial reading on the final reading. The average values of x and y are given in Table 10.1.

ANALYSIS OF VARIANCE

The basic calculations for computing the various Sums of Squares (SS) and Products (SP) necessary for the Analysis of Covariance, are given in Table 10.2.

The one-way analysis of variance in Table 10.3 is used to test the differences among the mean changes in pulp test reading of the three treatment groups. The appropriate F test is

TABLE 10.2
Computations for Constructing Analysis of Covariance in Table 10.4.

	Drug A	Drug B	Drug P	All Measurements (A + B + P)
N	20	20	20	60
Σx	1,584	1,738	1,650	4,972
$\bar{x}$	$79.20 = \bar{x}_A$	$86.90 = \bar{x}_B$	$82.50 = \bar{x}_P$	$82.87 = \bar{x}_0$
Σx^2	126,328	154,372	137,988	418,688
$(\Sigma x)^2/N$	125,452.80	151,032.20	136,125.00	412,013.07
Σy	-5.5	-8.0	+2.5	-11.0
$\bar{y}$	$-0.275 = \bar{y}_A$	$-0.400 = \bar{y}_B$	$+0.125 = \bar{y}_P$	$-0.183 = \bar{y}_0$
Σy^2	17.75	54.00	11.25	83.00
$(\Sigma y)^2/N$	1.51	3.20	0.31	2.02
Σxy	-387.00	-695.00	+221.00	-861.00
$(\Sigma x)(\Sigma y)/N$	-435.60	-695.20	+206.25	911.53

TABLE 10.3
Analysis of Variance Table for Comparing Mean Changes in Pulp Test Reading for Drugs A, B, and Placebo

Source of Variation	df	Sum of Squares for y(SS_y)	Mean Square
Within treatments	57	77.98	1.37
Between treatments	2	3.00	1.50
Total	59	80.98	

$$F_{2,57} = \frac{\text{Between Treatments MS}}{\text{Within Treatments MS}} = \frac{1.50}{1.37} = 1.09,$$

indicating that, as far as can be demonstrated, the three treatments may be alike, on the average, in their effects on pain threshold.

There is a possibility that change in pain threshold (y) is related to initial pulse rate (x). For example, the effectiveness of treatment may be greater for subjects with a high pulse rate. Although the initial pulse rate is unaffected by treatment, the random allocation of the 60 individuals to the three treatment groups does not ensure that the average pulse rates will be exactly the same (Table 10.1). If the change in pulp test reading (y) is related to initial pulse rate (x), then the comparison of the average changes ($\bar{y}$) may be influenced by the differences in the average pulse rates ($\bar{x}$). To compare $\bar{y}$'s for the three treatment groups, first "adjust" them to a common $\bar{x}$ and then make the comparison of the adjusted averages. This is accomplished by the analysis of covariance.

It is assumed that the dependent variable y is linearly related to the independent or concomitant variable x and that x is unaffected by the treatments under investigation. From the ANOVA in Table 10.4 (page 228), we find

$$F_{2,57} = \frac{\text{Between Treatments MS}}{\text{Within Treatments MS}} = \frac{596.93 \div 2}{6{,}078.00 \div 57} = \frac{298.47}{106.63} = 2.80.$$

The $\bar{x}$'s for the various treatments do not differ from each other, — nor should they under randomization (except α percent of the time).

ANALYSIS OF COVARIANCE TABLE

Table 10.4 is the standard analysis of covariance table and contains all the data of the experiments summarized in a form amenable to performing the necessary F tests. The Sum of Squares for x (SS_x) and for y (SS_y) are calculated as explained in Chapter 7. The Sum of Products for x and y(SP_{xy}) for each treatment group, e.g., Treatment A, is calculated as illustrated in Chapter 8:

$$SP_{xy} = \overset{20}{\Sigma}(x - \bar{x}_A)(y - \bar{y}_A) = \overset{20}{\Sigma}xy - \frac{(\overset{20}{\Sigma}x)(\overset{20}{\Sigma}y)}{20} = \overset{20}{\Sigma}xy - CT_{xy}.$$

SP_{xy} is similarly computed for Treatments B and P. Pooling of these SP_{xy} values for three treatments gives the Within Treatments SP_{xy}.

The Total SP_{xy} is calculated from all 60 pairs of values without regard to treatment:

$$SP_{xy} = \overset{60}{\Sigma}(x - \bar{x}_0)(y - \bar{y}_0) = \overset{60}{\Sigma}xy - \frac{(\overset{60}{\Sigma}x)(\overset{60}{\Sigma}y)}{60} = \overset{60}{\Sigma}xy - CT_{xy},$$

where x_0 and y_0 are the means of all 60 readings.

The Between Treatments SP_{xy} may be calculated by subtracting the Within Treatments SP_{xy} from the Total SP_{xy}. It may also be calculated separately as:

$$SP_{xy} = 20(\bar{x}_A - \bar{x}_0)(\bar{y}_A - \bar{y}_0) + 20(\bar{x}_B - \bar{x}_0)(\bar{y}_B - \bar{y}_0)$$
$$+ 20(\bar{x}_P - \bar{x}_0)(\bar{y}_P - \bar{y}_0).$$

TABLE 10.4

Analysis of Covariance Table for Comparing Mean Changes in Pulp Test Reading — Drugs A, B, and Placebo — Using Pulse Rate as the Concomitant Variable*

Source of Variation	df	Sum of Squares (SS_x)	Sum of Products (SP_{xy})	Sum of Squares (SS_y)	Slope SP_{xy}/SS_x	SS_y Due to Slope	df	Reduced SS_y	df
Within Treatment A	19	875.20	46.80	16.24	0.05553	2.6988	1	13.5412	18
Within Treatment B	19	3,339.80	0.20	50.80	0.00006	0.0000	1	50.8000	18
Within Treatment P	19	1,863.00	14.75	10.94	0.00790	0.1168	1	10.8232	18
					Total	2.8156	3	75.1622	54
Within Treatments	57	6,078.00	63.55	77.98	0.01046	0.6645	1	77.3155	56
Between Treatments	2	596.93	-13.02	3.00	Adjusted Between Treats			3.2820	2
Total	59	6,674.93	50.53	80.98	0.00757	0.3825	1	80.5975	58

*y = Final – Initial Pulp Test Reading; x = Pulse Rate.

A shortcut method for calculating the Between Treatments SP_{xy} would be:

$$SP_{xy} = \frac{(\Sigma x_A)(\Sigma y_A)}{20} + \frac{(\Sigma x_B)(\Sigma y_B)}{20} + \frac{(\Sigma x_P)(\Sigma y_P)}{20} - \frac{\overset{60}{(\Sigma x)}\overset{60}{(\Sigma y)}}{60}$$

$$= CT_A + CT_B + CT_P - CT.$$

It will be noted that

Total SP_{xy} = Within Treatments SP_{xy} + Between Treatments SP_{xy},

so that the Total Sum of Products has been subdivided in exactly the same way as the Total Sum of Squares in the analysis of variance. In effect, the same formulas are used in calculating the SP as in calculating the SS, except that the SS is actually an SP using the same variable twice, e.g., $SS_x = SP_{xx}$.

REGRESSION LINES

Using the SS_x, SP_{xy}, and SS_y values within a given treatment, one can determine the equation of the line relating y to x and how much of the fluctuation of individual y values about their mean (SS_y) is due to the slope and how much to the deviation of y's about the straight line relating y to x. As in any regression (Chapter 8), the assumption is made that the variation about the line is normal and homoscedastic). For example, under Treatment A,

$$b = \frac{SP_{xy}}{SS_x} = \frac{48.60}{875.20} = 0.05553 \text{ units of change per beat}$$

$$a = \bar{y} - b\bar{x} = -4.6730.$$

Graphically, the 20 (x, y) points of Treatment A and their regression line may be presented as in Figure 10.1. The part of SS_y that is accounted for by the slope is

$$\text{Regression SS} = \frac{(SP_{xy})^2}{SS_x} = \frac{(48.60)^2}{875.20} = 2.6988,$$

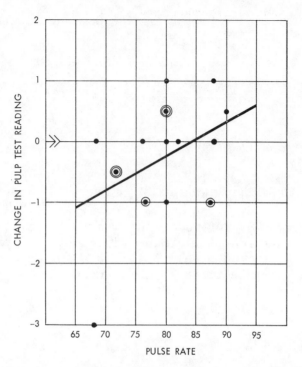

FIG. 10.1 Linear Regression of Change in Pulp Test Reading on Pulse Rate (Drug A).

and the part due to the variation of the y's about the line:

$$\text{Residual SS}_y \text{ about the line} = \text{Reduced SS}_y = \text{SS}_y - \frac{(\text{SP}_{xy})^2}{\text{SS}_x}$$

$$= 16.24 - 2.6988 = 13.5412, \text{ with df} = 18.$$

$$s_{y.x}^2 = 13.5412/18 = 0.7523.$$

A test of significance for the slope is given by:

$$F_{1,18} = 2.6988/0.7523 = 3.59; \text{ this is statistically not significant at the 5\% level.}$$

The regression lines for Treatments B and P can be summarized similarly. The regression coefficients for the three treatments separately are given in Table 10.4. The Regression SS and the Reduced

SS_y are also given for the three treatments. Analysis of covariance assumes equality of the true residual variances ($\sigma^2_{y.x}$), estimated by $s^2_{y.x}$.

It is reasonable, under the null hypothesis, to assume that the true slopes for the three treatments are the same. Even if the treatments have different effects on the pain threshold, the effect (y) may well be constant for all pulse rate values, i.e., no interaction between the treatment and pulse rate, so that the regression lines would have the same slopes but different intercepts. The lines would be parallel but at different heights. It is possible, in fact, to test the assumption of parallelism using information in Table 10.4 by an extension of the method given in Chapter 8.

The best estimate of the common slope is a weighted average of the three separate estimates, given by

$$b = \frac{\text{Within Treatments } SP_{xy}}{\text{Within Treatments } SS_x} = 0.01046.$$

Thus, there are three true regression lines assumed to have the same slope, estimated as equal to 0.01046, and having possibly different intercepts.

Test for Parallelism

The pooled SS_y around the three separate lines with 54 degrees of freedom is 75.1622, so that

$$s^2_{y.x} = 75.1622/54 = 1.3919.$$

The SS_y around the three parallel lines is 77.3155 with 56 df. The difference in the two (77.3155 − 75.1622 = 2.1533) measure the difference between the slopes with 2 df. A test of parallelism is

$$F_{2,54} = (2.1533/2)/1.3919 = 0.77.$$

F is not statistically significant at the 5% level, so that the lines may be parallel with a common slope of 0.01046.

The pooled Regression SS around the three separate lines is 2.8156 with 3 df, and around the three parallel lines is 0.6645 with 1 df. The difference is also 2.1533, which was obtained by comparing residual variations.

Equations of Parallel Lines

For Treatment A, the estimate of the intercept is:

$$a_A = \bar{y}_A - b(\bar{x}_A) = -1.1034$$

Similarly,

$$a_B = \bar{y}_B - b(\bar{x}_B) = -1.3090$$
$$a_P = \bar{y}_P - b(\bar{x}_P) = -0.7380.$$

The equations of the three parallel lines are

$$A: \quad Y = a_A + bx = -1.1034 + 0.01046x$$
$$B: \quad Y = a_B + bx = -1.3090 + 0.01046x$$
$$P: \quad Y = a_P + bx = -0.7380 + 0.01046x.$$

The three parallel lines for the three treatments are given in Figure 10.2.

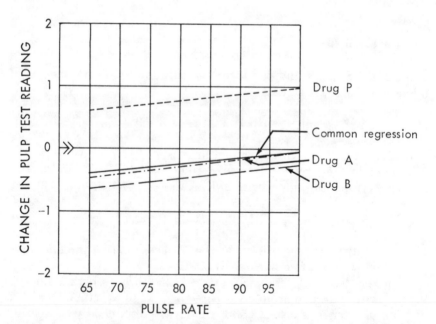

FIG. 10.2 Parallel Linear Regressions of Change in Pulp Test Reading on Pulse Rate (Drugs A, B, and Placebo) and Common Linear Regression.

Significance of Common Slope

Within Treatments SS_y can now be subdivided into SS_y due to the assumed common slope,

$$\frac{(SP_{xy})^2}{SS_y} = 0.6645,$$

with one degree of freedom, as given in Table 10.4 and into the pooled variation of individual y's about their three respective parallel lines, computed as

$$\text{Within Treatments Reduced } SS_y = SS_y - \frac{(SP_{xy})^2}{SS_x} = 77.3155,$$

with 56 degrees of freedom, as shown in Table 10.4. The variance of y's around the lines is then

$$s_{y.x}^2 = \frac{77.3155}{56} = 1.3806,$$

the Reduced Mean Square Within Treatments.

It is often common practice to test the original assumption that y is related to x, i.e., to test the statistical significance of the difference of the slope, b, from zero (as in Chapter 8).

$$SE_b = \frac{s_{y.x}}{\sqrt{SS_x}} = \frac{\sqrt{77.3155 \div 56}}{\sqrt{6,078.00}} = 0.01507$$

$$t = \frac{0.01046 - 0}{0.01507} = 0.694.$$

This is not statistically significant at the .05 level. A convenient alternative form of this test is

$$F_{1,56} = \frac{SS_y \text{ due to slope} \div 1}{\text{Reduced MS Within Treatments}} = \frac{0.6645}{77.3145 \div 56} = 0.48 = t^2.$$

Adjusted Means

Although it has not been definitely demonstrated that y is related to x, the rationale for such a relation exists, and consequently there is still merit in using the analysis of covariance to compare the three mean changes in pulp test reading adjusted to a common $\bar{x}$ value. The adjusted $\bar{y}$'s are:

Adjusted $\bar{y}_A = \bar{y}_A - b(\bar{x}_A - \bar{x}_0) = -0.275 - 0.01046(79.20 - 82.87)$
$$= -0.2387$$

Adjusted $\bar{y}_B = \bar{y}_B - b(\bar{x}_B - \bar{x}_0) = -0.400 - 0.01046(86.90 - 82.87)$
$$= -0.4422$$

Adjusted $\bar{y}_P = \bar{y}_P - b(\bar{x}_P - \bar{x}_0) = +0.125 - 0.01046(82.50 - 82.87)$
$$= +0.1289.$$

The three adjusted values are the heights at $\bar{x}_0$ of the three parallel lines in Figure 10.2. The differences among the adjusted $\bar{y}$'s are merely the vertical distances between the parallel lines. If the $\bar{y}$'s were adjusted to any x value other than $\bar{x}_0$, the differences in the adjusted $\bar{y}$'s would be the same, by virtue of parallelism, and are, in fact, the same as the differences in the intercepts.

Comparing Adjusted Means — Analysis of Covariance

The comparison of the adjusted mean changes in pulp test reading is complicated by their lack of independence, caused by using the same b in computing all three adjusted averages. If the three treatments are equally effective with respect to influencing pulp test reading, then the three regression lines should coincide. There should be a single regression line whose estimated slope, (Total SP_{xy})/(Total SS_x), equals 0.00757 as shown in Table 10.4. The estimated common regression line is depicted in Figure 10.2. The variation of all 60 values of y around this single line, with 58 degrees of freedom, is

$$\text{Total Reduced } SS_y = SS_y - \frac{(SP_{xy})^2}{SS_x} = 80.5975,$$

as shown in Table 10.4. The variation of the y's about the three separate parallel lines and the variation of the y's about the one common line should be the same, under the null hypothesis, when the degrees of freedom are taken into account, except for the sampling errors. If the three treatments are not equally effective, the Total Reduced SS_y should be larger than the Within Treatments Reduced SS_y after adjustment for inequalities in degrees of freedom. To compare the two Reduced SS_y's:

$$F_{2,56} = \frac{(\text{Total Reduced SS}_y - \text{Within Treatments Reduced SS}_y)/2}{(\text{Within Treatments Reduced SS}_y)/56}$$

$$= \frac{(80.5975 - 77.3155)/2}{77.3155/56} = 1.19.$$

Consequently, after adjusting for differences in average initial pulse rate, it cannot be established that the three treatment mean changes in pulp test reading are statistically significantly different at the .05 level.

All of the procedures discussed thus far, i.e., separate regressions, SS due to slope, Reduced SS, tests of parallelism, tests of significance of slopes, tests of adjusted means, are often referred to as the *Analysis of Covariance* since they use covariances in the arithmetic. Classically, it is only the last step, that of comparing adjusted means, that was the original purpose of the analysis of covariance.*

It should be emphasized that all of the preliminary steps, i.e., parallelism, etc., are taken in a sense, to justify the model. Unfortunately, this justification in terms of significance tests has some rather unknown effects on our control of the significance level in the final step, i.e., comparing adjusted means. While it might seem appropriate to avoid some of these difficulties by proceeding directly to the final step, assuming parallelism, etc., many investigators would rather check the model and lose some control of significance levels, rather than get the "right answer to the wrong model."

Comparing Two Selected Treatments

In originally setting up the experiment, we were not confined to asking the single question: Are the three analgesic agents equal in their average effects on pain threshold? Other pertinent questions might have been: (1) Are two of the analgesics — e.g., A and B — equal in their effect? (2) If two of the treatments — e.g., A and B — are equally effective in their influence on pain threshold, does the effect differ from that of the third treatment, P? If more than one significance test were made in an experiment, each at the .05 level, then the overall significance level of the experiment may be greater than .05. In other words, some penalty for making multiple compari-

---

*See Appendix for illustration of a computer program (BMDP IV) for this analysis of covariance. This is an adaptation of multiple linear regression with a mixture of dummy and measured variables.

TABLE 10.5
Modification of Table 10.4 for Comparing Mean Changes in Pulp Test
Reading for Drugs A and B*

Source of Vairation	df	SS_x	SP_{xy}	SS_y	Slope SP_{xy}/SS_x	SS_y Due to Slope	df	Reduced SS_y	df
Within Treatments	57	6,078.00	63.55	77.98	.010	0.6645	1	77.3155	56
Between Treatments A and B	1	592.90	– 9.625	0.15					
Total	58	6,670.90	53.93	78.13	.008	0.4360	1	77.6940	57

*y = final – initial pulp test reading; x = pulse rate.

sons may be called for, such as dividing α = .05 by the number of tests if the comparisons were decided upon beforehand.

The mechanics of comparing two adjusted means, say $\bar{y}_A$ = –0.2387 and $\bar{y}_B$ = –0.4422 (see page 235), may be handled in various ways, including a direct t-test on the adjusted means:

$$\text{Est. SE}_{\bar{y}_A - \bar{y}_B} = s_{y.x}\sqrt{1/N_A + 1/N_B + (\bar{x}_A - \bar{x}_B)^2/SS_x}$$
$$= 1.1750\sqrt{1/20 + 1/20 + (-7.70)^2/6,078} = 0.3893,$$

where $s_{y.x}$ is the reduced standard deviation, using all the data with 56 df, and SS_x is the Within Treatments SS_x, using all of the data.

$$t_{56} = (\text{adj. } \bar{y}_A - \text{adj. } \bar{y}_B)/\text{est. SE}_{\bar{y}_A - \bar{y}_B} = 0.2035/0.3893 = 0.523.$$

Alternatively, the test may be made through a modification of the analysis of covariance table.

To test the significance of the difference in the average change under A and under B, the necessary analysis of covariance table is Table 10.5. Here the values on the line Within Treatments are exactly the same as those in Table 10.4. Although Placebo's effect on pain threshold is not involved in the test of the difference in the mean change in pulp test reading for Treatments A and B, we do use the 20 (x, y) values of the sample treated with Placebo to help estimate the common slope of the regression lines for A and B, because the slope is assumed to be unaffected by treatment. In this way, we also obtain a better estimate (i.e., one with more degrees of freedom) of the Within Treatments Reduced SS_y. The SS and SP for Between Treatments A and B are calculated from the 40 pairs of values for these treatments as

$$CT_A + CT_B - CT_{A+B}.$$

The SS and SP on the Total line are obtained by addition of the values Within Treatments and Between Treatments A and B. The slope, the SS_y due to the slope, and the Reduced SS_y on the Total lines are computed in the same way as the corresponding figures in Table 10.4, and have a similar interpretation. If Treatments A and B are equally effective, there is a single regression line whose slope is

$$\frac{\text{Total SP}_{xy}}{\text{Total SS}_x} = \frac{53.93}{6,670.90} = 0.008.$$

The variation of individual y's about this line is the Total Reduced $SS_y = 77.6940$. If A and B are not equally effective, the Within Treatments Reduced SS_y should be smaller than the Total Reduced SS_y after adjusting for the difference in degrees of freedom. The statistical test to compare the two Reduced SS_y's is

$$F_{1,56} = \frac{(\text{Total Reduced SS}_y - \text{Within Treatments Reduced SS}_y) \div 1}{(\text{Within Treatments Reduced SS}_y) \div 56}$$

$$= \frac{(77.6940 - 77.3155) \div 1}{77.3155 \div 56} = 0.27 = t^2.$$

The Case of Nonparallelism

When the lines are not taken to be parallel, the adj. $\bar{y}$ of a treatment depends on what x is used in the equation of the line. If some x must be chosen, a reasonable choice is $\bar{x}_0$ for all the data. Then

$$\text{adj. } \bar{y}_A = \bar{y}_A - b_A(\bar{x}_A - \bar{x}_0) = -0.275 - 0.05553(79.20 - 82.87)$$
$$= -0.0712$$

$$\text{adj. } \bar{y}_B = \bar{y}_B - b_B(\bar{x}_B - \bar{x}_0) = -0.400 - 0.00006(86.90 - 82.87)$$
$$= -0.4002$$

$$\text{adj. } \bar{y}_P = \bar{y}_P - b_P(\bar{x}_P - \bar{x}_0) = +0.125 - 0.00790(82.50 - 82.87)$$
$$= +0.1279.$$

The est. SE of each y is given by:

$$\text{Est. SE}_{y_A} = \sqrt{s_{y \cdot x}\left(\frac{1}{N_A} + \frac{(\bar{x}_A - \bar{x}_0)^2}{SS_x(A)}\right)}$$

$$= \sqrt{1.3919\left(\frac{1}{20} + \frac{(-3.67)^2}{875.20}\right)} = 0.3015$$

$$\text{Est. SE}_{y_B} = \sqrt{s_{y \cdot x}\left(\frac{1}{N_B} + \frac{(\bar{x}_B - \bar{x}_0)^2}{SS_x(B)}\right)}$$

$$= \sqrt{1.3919\left(\frac{1}{20} + \frac{(4.03)^2}{3339.80}\right)} = 0.2762$$

$$\text{Est. SE}_{y_P} = \sqrt{s_{y \cdot x}\left(\frac{1}{N_P} + \frac{(\bar{x}_P - \bar{x}_0)^2}{SS_x(P)}\right)}$$

$$= \sqrt{1.3919\left(\frac{1}{20} + \frac{(-0.37)^2}{1863.00}\right)} = 0.2640.$$

$s_{y \cdot x}$ is the pooled residual variation around three nonparallel lines with 54 df. From Table 10.4,

$$s_{y \cdot x} = \frac{75.1622}{54} = 1.3919.$$

We are assuming, of course, that the true residual variation is the same around each line.

To compare two adj. $\bar{y}$'s, say $\bar{y}_A$ and $\bar{y}_B$, we may construct a t-test:

$$t_{54} = \frac{(\text{adj. } \bar{y}_A - \text{adj. } \bar{y}_B)}{\text{est. SE}} = \frac{(-0.0712 - 0.4002)}{\sqrt{(0.3015)^2 + (0.2762)^2}} = \frac{0.3290}{0.4089} = 0.80.$$

Obviously, the value of t differs somewhat from that when parallelism was assumed. Also, the value of t would differ if some other x were used in the adjustment.

The method suggested is equivalent to the test of main effects in a two-way ANOVA where there is interaction between the two factors. In that case, the main effect tested is an average effect corresponding to an "average stratum", i.e., x. In such a situation, the test of main effects is not very useful if there is a lot of non-parallelism, including, for example, an intersection of the lines within the observed range of x.

To compare the adj. $\bar{y}$'s for more than two treatments when parallelism is not assumed, one could construct an appropriate F-test based on the variation among the various adj. $\bar{y}$'s.

USING THE INITIAL VALUE
AS THE CONCOMITANT VARIABLE

A frequent problem arises when comparing average changes in a measurement since there is a possibility that a change in the measurement is related to the initial measurement. This implies that taking account of the relation between the final and initial measurements by a difference does not completely adjust for the relationship. If the difference were adequate, the slope of the regression of the difference on the initial measurement would be zero. In that case, the regression of the final on the initial value would yield a slope of one.

In a study of the effect of a rubber tip for gingival stimulation, Chilton and Maher[4] measured the average number of bleeding points (score of 2 or 3 in the Löe-Silness Gingival Index) per surface for a group of subjects using the tip and for a group which did not use it. The data for 20 patients in each group are presented in Table 10.6. (See page 240.)

Using the increment as the response variable in this study, the change (increment) in the average number of bleeding points may be related to the initial average number of bleeding points. Perhaps the effectiveness of the interdental massage may be greater in those individuals with a relatively high average number of bleeding points before the start of the study. The use of the analysis of covariance to compare two "treatment" mean changes adjusted for initial reading is illustrated by comparing mean change in bleeding points for Group A and Group B. The basic calculations necessary for computing the various Sums of Squares (SS) and Products (SP) necessary for the Analysis of Covariance, are given in Table 10.7. (See page 241.)

Table 10.8 (see page 242) is the appropriate analysis of covariance table. The calculations are similar to those of Table 10.4, except that there are only two samples, rather than three. The slope of the two lines assumed to be parallel, is

$$b = \frac{\text{Within Treatments SP}_{xd}}{\text{Within Treatments SS}_d} = \frac{-14.8097}{29.1890} = -0.5074.$$

The significance test for the slope is

$$F_{1,37} = \frac{(\text{SS}_{xd} \text{ due to slope)MS}}{(\text{SS}_d \text{ Reduced)MS}} = \frac{7.5140 \div 1}{18.4125 \div 37} = 15.10.$$

TABLE 10.6
Average Number of Bleeding Points Per Surface for 20 Patients in Group A and 20 in Group B at the Initial (x), and Final (y) Examinations, and the Incremental Values (d = y – x)

	Group A			Group B		
	(x)	(y)	(d)	(x)	(y)	(d)
	2.82	1.75	-1.07	2.04	2.57	+0.53
	1.89	1.75	-0.14	2.25	2.57	+0.29
	0.88	0.13	-0.75	1.11	1.11	0.00
	0.96	1.25	+0.29	1.11	0.32	-0.79
	1.89	0.21	-1.68	1.82	0.93	-0.89
	1.36	1.64	+0.28	1.29	1.25	-0.04
	3.25	2.04	-1.21	1.14	1.14	0.00
	3.42	1.92	-1.50	2.61	1.04	-1.57
	0.86	0.96	+0.10	1.82	0.79	-1.03
	2.04	1.32	-0.72	1.93	1.04	-0.89
	1.50	0.25	-1.25	1.48	0.67	-0.81
	1.42	0.54	-0.88	2.25	0.96	-1.29
	1.39	1.07	-0.32	3.14	2.21	-0.93
	0.64	0.00	-0.64	0.61	1.07	+0.46
	3.50	0.89	-2.61	1.32	0.54	-0.78
	2.00	0.86	-1.14	1.32	0.25	-1.07
	2.00	0.19	-1.81	3.61	4.32	+0.71
	2.79	0.75	-2.04	3.11	1.32	-1.79
	3.39	0.82	-2.57	1.79	0.50	-1.39
	3.39	1.00	-2.39	1.86	0.64	-1.22
Means:	2.0695	0.9670	-1.1025	1.8855	1.2605	-0.6250

The difference of this b from 0 is statistically highly significant, showing that the difference is not an adequate method of taking account of the relation of bleeding points at the final examination to the bleeding points at the initial examination. The fluctuation of individual d values around the two parallel lines is measured by Within Treatments Reduced SS_d = 18.4125.

The mean changes in average bleeding points for Groups A and B adjusted to the same average initial bleeding point scores are:

$$\text{adj. } \bar{d}_A = \bar{d}_A - b(\bar{x}_A - \bar{x}_0) = -1.1025 - (-.5074)(2.0695 - 1.9775)$$
$$= -1.0558$$

$$\text{adj. } \bar{d}_B = \bar{d}_B - b(\bar{x}_B - \bar{x}_0) = -0.6250 - (-.5074)(1.8855 - 1.9775)$$
$$= -0.6717.$$

The test of significance of the difference between the adjusted means is:

TABLE 10.7

Computations for Constructing Analysis of Covariance in Tables 10.8 and 10.9

	Group A	Group B	All Measurements (A + B)
N	20	20	40
Σx	41.39	37.71	79.10
$\bar{x}$	$2.0695 = \bar{x}_A$	$1.8855 = \bar{x}_B$	$1.9775 = \bar{x}_0$
Σx^2	103.4287	82.5191	185.9478
$(\Sigma x)^2/N$	85.6566	71.1022	156.4203
Σy	19.34	25.21	44.55
$\bar{y}$	$0.9670 = \bar{y}_A$	$1.2605 = \bar{y}_B$	$1.1138 = \bar{y}_0$
Σy^2	26.2518	49.7233	75.9751
$(\Sigma y)^2/N$	18.7018	31.7772	94.6769
Σxy	45.0054	56.9315	101.9369
$(\Sigma x)(\Sigma y)/N$	40.0241	47.5335	88.0976
Σd	-22.05	-12.50	-34.55
$\bar{d}$	$-1.1025 = \bar{d}_A$	$-0.6250 = \bar{d}_B$	$-0.8638 = \bar{d}_0$
Σd^2	39.6697	18.3794	58.0491
$(\Sigma d)^2/N$	24.3101	7.8125	29.8426
Σxd	-58.4233	-25.5876	84.0109
$(\Sigma x)(\Sigma d)/N$	-45.6325	-23.5688	-68.3226

$$F_{1,37} = \frac{(\text{Total Reduced SS}_d - \text{Within Treatments Reduced SS}_d)/1}{(\text{Within Treatments Reduced SS}_d)/37}$$

$$= \frac{(19.8708 - 18.4125)/1}{18.4125/37} = 2.93.$$

$$t_{37} = \frac{(\text{adj. } \bar{d}_A - \text{adj. } \bar{d}_B) - 0}{\sqrt{s_{dx}^2 \left(\dfrac{1}{N_A} + \dfrac{1}{N_B} + \dfrac{(\bar{x}_A - \bar{x}_B)^2}{SS_x} \right)}}$$

$$= \frac{-1.0558 - (-0.6717) - 0}{\sqrt{0.4976[2/20 + (2.0695 - 1.8855)^2/29.1890]}}$$

$$= \frac{0.3841}{0.2244} = 1.712.$$

Using the Final Reading as the Response Variable

If we were to compare the mean number of bleeding points at the final evaluation (y) for each group, adjusted for the initial score,

TABLE 10.8

Analysis of Covariance Table for Comparing Mean Changes in Number of Bleeding Points Per Tooth Surface — Groups A and B Using Initial Scores as the Concomitant Variable*

Source of Variation	df	SS_x	SP_{xd}	SS_d	Slope	SS_d Due to Slope	df	SS_d Reduced	df
Within Groups	38	29.1890	−14.8097	25.9265	−.5074	7.5140	1	18.4125	37
Between Groups	1	0.3386	−0.8786	2.2801				1.4583	1
Total	39	29.5276	−15.6883	28.2061	−0.5313	8.3353	1	19.8708	38

*d = final – initial average bleeding points; x = initial average bleeding points.

TABLE 10.9

Analysis of Covariance Table for Comparing the Mean Final Number of Bleeding Points Per Tooth Surface — Groups A and B Using the Initial Scores as the Concomitant Variable*

Source of Variation	df	SS_x	SP_{xy}	SS_y	Slope	SS_y Due to Slope	df	SS_y Reduced	df
Within Groups	38	29.1890	14.3793	25.4961	0.4926	7.0836	1	18.4125	37
Between Groups	1	0.3386	−0.5400	0.8614				1.4587	1
Total	39	29.5276	13.8393	26.3575	0.4687	6.4863	1	19.8712	38

*x = initial average bleeding points; y = final average bleeding points.

the appropriate analysis of covariance table would be Table 10.9. The slope relating the final to the initial reading is

$$B = \frac{14.3793}{29.1890} = 0.4926.$$

In the previous anlaysis of d, b = -0.5074. We note that b = B - 1. B is just as statistically significantly different from 1 as b was from 0. The fact that B is not equal to 1 emphasizes the fact that the increment is not a sufficient description of the relationship of the final to the initial reading.

The adjusted final mean values of bleeding points, using the mean initial value for all the data ($\bar{x}_0$) are:

adj. $\bar{y}_A = \bar{y}_A - B(\bar{x}_A - \bar{x}_0) = 0.9670 - (.4926)(2.0695 - 1.9775)$
$$= 0.9217$$

adj. $\bar{y}_B = \bar{y}_B - B(\bar{x}_B - \bar{x}_0) = 1.2605 - (.4926)(1.8855 - 1.9775)$
$$= 1.3058.$$

To compare the adjusted means, we go through the same procedure as in Table 10.8, computing the Reduced SS_y for the Within Groups and for the Total. We note that the Residual SS is identical with that of Table 10.8. The total Reduced SS is also the same as that of Table 10.8 except for rounding. The same test of significance of the adjusted means results, namely, $F_{1,37} = 1.4587/(18.4125/37)$ = 2.93.

Many analysts, when confronted with this problem of an analysis of covariance with initial and final values, have used the second form of analysis of covariance shown in Table 10.9. While this is certainly correct, many other investigators prefer to see the adjusted increment rather than the adjusted final value. These can, of course, be obtained from the adjusted final values by subtracting $\bar{x}_0 = 1.9775$:

$$\text{adj. } \bar{d}_A = \text{adj. } \bar{y}_A - \bar{x}_0 = -1.0558$$
$$\text{adj. } \bar{d}_B = \text{adj. } \bar{y}_B - \bar{x}_0 = -0.6717.$$

It should be noted that the adjusted $\bar{d}$'s differ by the same amount as the adjusted $\bar{y}$'s.

COMMENTS ON THE USE OF
THE ANALYSIS OF COVARIANCE

It is assumed that the dependent variable is linearly related to the independent or concomitant variable, and that the latter is unaffected by the treatments under investigation. The appropriate F-tests in the analysis of covariance require the same assumptions concerning normality and equality of variance necessary to make the F-tests in the parallel analysis of variance.[5]

It is possible to use an extension of the principles discussed in this chapter to investigate the differences in the average of some response variable, y, after simultaneously adjusting for sample differences in two or more covariates. The analysis of covariance with two or more concomitant variables would be the statistical technique.[1]

Attrition of the subjects may occur during the experimental period. When this attrition appears to be random, as judged by its effect on the concomitant variable, the analysis of variance or covariance may be performed, just as with no attrition. If the loss of subjects appears to be nonrandom and to disturb seriously the initial similarity of the groups with respect to the concomitant variable, the comparison of means of the sample by the analysis of variance may be misleading. The analysis of covariance technique may be used to equalize the concomitant variable throughout all the samples. However, it must be used with caution, because the concomitant variable *is* affected by the treatment, and the use of the technique amounts to a projection beyond the known facts since it may not be possible for the samples to have the same average with respect to the concomitant variable.[5]

On occasion, the experimenter is unable to assign subjects randomly to the various samples and is forced instead to work with intact groups. In these instances, it is difficult to conceive of any sample differences in the concomitant variable as random differences, and, in fact, the differences may at times be distressingly large. As in the case of nonrandom attrition, the analysis of covariance technique is often used to equalize the samples with respect to a concomitant variable. This amounts to an artificial comparison of the means of y's, since the groups are not alike with respect to the variable x and also, coincidentally, not alike in many other respects.

In some experimental situations, the concomitant variable, x, may be controlled experimentally rather than statistically. For example, blocks may be formed consisting of subjects very nearly alike, if not exactly alike, with respect to x. The number of subjects per block is some multiple of the number of treatments at issue.

Oftentimes, the multiple is 1. The x differs from block to block (stratum to stratum). These blocks may occur naturally, e.g., animal litters, and, in such a circumstance, a whole series of concomitant variables is equalized by nature. The statistical analysis is the analysis of variance with two criteria of classification or in a two-way layout of data (Chapter 7). This analysis is often preferable to the analysis of covariance as a method for controlling differences in a concomitant variable because fewer assumptions are required to satisfy the statistical model, e.g., linearity of relation of the response variable to the concomitant variable (the covariate).[6] For practical reasons, however, the formation of blocks or strata is not always convenient and sometimes is not possible. Furthermore, in the case of attrition, one runs into the problem of unequal number of readings in the cell or even of missing values in a two-way analysis of variance, resulting in laborious arithmetic. Where intact groups are used in the experiment, it is generally not feasible to form blocks by such devices as pairing subjects of one intact group with subjects of another.[3]

REFERENCES

1. Snedecor, G. W., and Cochran, W. G.: Statistical Methods, 7th ed., Ames, Iowa State Univ. Press, 1980.

2. Chilton, N. W., and Berger, A.: Unpublished data, Temple Univ. School of Dentistry.

3. Michelsen, P. B., and Chilton, N. W.: Studies in the Design and Analysis of Dental Experiments. 8. Application of analysis of covariance to dental research, J Dent Res 44:321, 1965.

4. Chilton, N. W., and Maher, T.: The clinical effectiveness of interdental massage on gingival inflammation, Abstract No. 206, 60th General Session, Inter. Assn. Dent. Res., 1982.

5. Cochran, W. G.: Analysis of Covariance. Its nature and uses, Biometrics 13:277, 1957.

6. Cox, D. R.: Planning of Experiments, New York, Wiley, 1958.

11

Chance Variation
(Relative Frequencies)

The analysis of measurement data in terms of measures of centering and variation was presented in Chapter 2. The analysis of enumeration data — i.e., data according to a qualitative scale of classification — was briefly discussed in terms of relative frequencies. The subsequent chapters developed the concept of chance variation for measurement data, especially in terms of means, and its role in statistical inferences. Such matters were considered as comparing a mean with a standard, comparing two means, comparing more than two means. Corresponding methods for enumeration data will be presented in Chapters 11 through 14.

This chapter will develop the chance variation of relative frequencies and illustrate its role in comparing a relative frequency with a standard. The methods will be primarily those appropriate for the one sample problem with a dichotomous scale.

As a hypothetical problem, in a sample of 10 chimpanzees infected with the herpes simplex virus and given a particular drug, 60% remain symptom-free and do not develop oral manifestations. In a universe of similarly infected chimps not given this treatment, it is known that only 40% are asymptomatic. The question is whether this sample of 10 treated chimps can be thought of as coming from a different universe with respect to the frequency of asymptomatics. If repeated groups or samples of 10 infected chimps not given this drug are observed, how often will it be noted that 60% are asymptomatic? The answer to this question will help us to decide whether the observed 60% in the unique sample of 10 could easily be explained by the standard untreated universe with 40% asymptomatic, or whether a different universe has to be hypothesized. The question can be answered either by doing a certain amount of empirical sampling or by utilizing some aspects of probability theory.

Empirical Sampling

A universe of a very large number of chips was constructed, 40% white and 60% (i.e., 100% – 40%) colored. In other words, the probability that a randomly drawn chip will be white is 0.4 or 40%, and that the chip will be colored is 0.6 or 60%. From this universe, 1,150 samples of 10 chips each (= n) were drawn. The distribution of the percent of white chips in these samples is shown in Table 11.1. As one might expect, the relative frequency of white chips (p) that occurs with the greatest frequency is 40%, which is the true value (p') in the universe of reference. Around this value, the percentage of white chips (asymptomatics) varies greatly, going from 0% to 80%. In fact, all but 12 of the 1,150 samples, or 1%, fall within the range 10% to 70%, which might be referred to as the *sampling range*.

The sampling distribution of the percentage of white chips is also the sampling distribution of the number white (x), of the number of colored chips (n – x), and the percentage of colored chips (q = 100 – p). Thus, if the chance distribution is centered at 40% white, it is also centered at 4 whites, 6 colored, and at 60% colored.

When, in another sampling experiment from the same universe, the size of the samples was increased to 20 chips, there was less variability in the percentage of white chips. These percentages varied from 15% to 70%, with most of the percentages falling in the "sampling range" 20% to 60%. Thus the experience of empirical sampling confirms the intuitive feeling that increasing the sample size decreases the variability of the relative frequency.

TABLE 11.1

Chance Distribution of Relative Frequencies for 1,150 Samples of n = 10 Drawn from a Universe of True Relative Frequency 40%

Number White (x)	Number Colored (n – x)	Percentage White (p)	Percentage Colored (q)	Number of Samples (f)
0	10	0	100	5
1	9	10	90	45
2	8	20	80	149
3	7	30	70	245
4	6	40	60	282
5	5	50	50	240
6	4	60	40	129
7	3	70	30	48
8	2	80	20	7
9	1	90	10	0
10	0	100	0	0
Total				1150

If, in a new sample of 10 chips not known to arise from the reference universe, 0% or 80% were observed, there would be a good reason to suspect that the sample came from another universe. In the sample of chimpanzees used here, 60% were asymptomatic (white). This value falls comfortably within the sampling range, so that the treated chimps may very well belong to the untreated universe. In other words, the observed 60% does not differ significantly from the hypothetical universe 40%. While there may be an effect of the treatment, it has not been demonstrated.

The estimated probability of a deviation of 20% or more (60% - 40%) from the universe value of 40% may be calculated from Table 11.1. Negative deviations of 20% or more occur when there are 0%, 10%, or 20% white chips. There are 5 + 45 + 149 = 199 such samples. Positive deviations of 20% or more occur when the percentage white is 60%, 70%, 80%, 90% or 100%. There are 129 + 48 + 7 = 184 such samples. Consequently, a deviation of 20% or more is obtained in 383 samples out of 1,150, a probability (P) of 33.3%. Since this probability is not small, the deviation of 20% is called not statistically significant. In other words, the 60% of the treated sample does not deviate significantly from the control universe value of 40%, since such a difference can readily be obtained through the action of chance factors alone. If, on the other hand, 0% of the chimps in the sample of 10 treated animals were asymptomatic, significance could be asserted, since such a deviation of 40% - 0% or 40% could be equaled or exceeded only 5% or 1% of the time, a rather infrequent occurrence. As was discussed in Chapter 4, a decision of "statistical significance" is made whenever the sample value is such that samples as rare or rarer occur only 5% or 1% of the time or less. Any small probability could serve as the critical value, although customarily either $P = 0.05$, as just mentioned, or $P = 0.01$ is chosen. The choice should be made during the planning phase of the experiment, keeping in mind that the smaller the critical value of P chosen, the more difficult it is to attribute the observed fluctuation to something other than chance. This critical value of P is often called α, as mentioned before.

SOME ASPECTS OF PROBABILITY THEORY

While probability concepts have been utilized in all of the discussions of statistical inference referring to means, differences in means, slopes, etc., it did not seem necessary to discuss certain fundamental aspects of probability theory at that time. It does seem appropriate to discuss some of these more formal aspects in connection with the development of the concept of chance variation for relative frequencies. Rigorous mathematical development will be avoided.

Definitions

A great incentive to theoretical investigations of probability came from attempts to determine the outcome of games of chance. Since this goal is of great interest to most people, it can serve as a springboard for the discussion here. From a well-shuffled deck of playing cards (52 cards, 13 cards in each of four suits), the probability that a randomly drawn card would be an ace is readily calculable. Of the 52 cards, 4 are aces and 48 are not aces, so that the probability of drawing an ace is $4/(4 + 48) = 4/52 = 1/13$, assuming that good shuffling makes each of these 52 cards equally likely to be drawn. If one actually constructed a universe (an infinite number) of draws, 1/13th of the draws should be aces i.e., 1/13 or 7.7% of the time the draw should be an ace. The probability of obtaining a particular outcome of a trial in examples such as card drawing, or coin tossing, or throwing a die can be determined a priori. Thus, the probability of obtaining tails when freely tossing a coin is 1/2, if indeed it is equally likely that heads or tails will be face up on a particular toss. It is in these special situations, where the events can be analyzed into equally likely possibilities, that the probability of success, p', and the probability of failure, q', can be determined on an a priori basis.

In most cases, the probability of success, p', in the universe cannot be determined a priori. In such instances, the probability is taken as the relative frequency in a very large sample from that universe. The larger the sample, the more closely will the relative frequency represent p'. This is an *a posteriori* definition of the probability of success.

Two Fundamental Theorems

In the empirical sampling problem discussed, samples of 10 chips were drawn from a universe in which 40% of the chips were white (W) and 60% were colored (C). It is assumed that the chips are independent of each other in the sense that the outcome of one chip has no influence on the outcome of another chip. The number of white chips (x) drawn can vary from 0 to 10, so that the percentage of white chips would go from 0% to 100%. In order that no chips from the sample of 10 be white, all 10 must be colored (C). The probability that the first chip would be C is 60% or .6, that the second chip would be C is also 60% or .6, that the third chip would be C is .6, and so on for all the 10 chips. The probability of all the 10 chips being C is then .6 × .6 × .6 × .6 × .6 × .6 × .6 × .6 × .6 × .6 = $(.6)^{10}$ = .006 or .6%. This follows from the theorem on *Mutually Independent Events:* "If two or more events are mutually independent so that the occurrence of one does not influence the occurrence of the others, the probability of all occurring is the product of their separate probabilities."

To illustrate this theorem further, if two coins are tossed independently of each other, the probability of two tails coming up is 1 in 4, since there are four equally likely ways in which two coins may come up (HH, HT, TH, and TT) and only one of these is favorable to two tails. This probability can also be obtained as the probability of tails with the first coin times the probability of tails with the second coin, or $1/2 \times 1/2 = 1/4$. If 80% of all cases of periodontal disease have subgingival deposits present and 50% of all cases have occlusal traumatism, then .8 × .5 = .4 or 40% of all cases should have both factors present, if there is no relation between the occurrence of these two factors.

In another instance, one of the 10 chips in the sample is to be white (W). For example, suppose that the white chip were number 3, and the nine other chips were colored (C). The probability of that chip being W is .4 and the probability for each of the other nine being C is .6. Thus the probability of such an occurrence is $(0.4)(.6)^9$. This situation will also occur if a different chip, say number 5, were W and the others C. The probability of this event is also $(0.4)(0.6).^9$ In fact, there are 10 *mutually exclusive ways* in which one chip may be W and 9 chips C. The probability for each of these 10 ways is $(.4)(.6)^9$ and thus the probability of any of the 10 ways is the sum of these 10 terms, or $10(.4)(.6)^9$ = .004 = 0.40%. This is in accord with the theorem of *Mutually Exclusive Events:* "If two or more events are mutually exclusive so that when one occurs the other cannot occur, the probability of one or the other occurring is the sum of their separate probabilities."

To illustrate this theorem further, the probability of drawing an ace from a well-shuffled bridge deck is 1/13, and of drawing a king is also 1/13. These are obviously mutually exclusive events. The probability of drawing an ace or a king is obviously 8 cards out of the deck of 52 = 8/52 = 1/13 + 1/13. If 10% of the population are under age 5 and 8% between age 5 and 9, then obviously 18% are under age 10.

Binomial

In the case where 2 of the 10 chips are to be W, 8 are to be C. For example, chips number 1 and number 2 are to be W and the next 8 are to be C. The probability of this is $(.4)^2(.6)^8$. There are actually, however, 45 mutually exclusive ways of selecting the 2 chips that are to be W. This follows from the fact that the first W chip can be chosen from 10 and the next W chip from the 9 remaining chips. The order of choosing the chips is not pertinent, however, and there are two orders in which the particular 2 chips may be drawn. Therefore, the number of ways in which 2 chips can be picked from 10 is $(10)(9)/2 = 45$. The probability of drawing 2 white chips is then $45(.4)^2(.6)^8 = .121 = 12.1\%$.

The probability of any 3 particular chips being W and the other 7 C is $(0.4)^3(0.6)^7$. There are $(10)(9)(8)/(2)(3) = 120$ ways of selecting 3 chips in the sample of 10. The denominator $(2)(3) = 6$ follows from the fact that the 3 particular chips chosen can be chosen in 6 orders, just as the letters a, b, and c can be arranged in 6 orders (abc, acb, bac, bca, cab, and cba). Thus, the probability of 3W and 7C chips is $120(.4)^3(.6)^7 = .215 = 21.5\%$.

The coefficient of 120 in this case of 3W and 7C is the combination of 10 things taken 3 at a time, $_{10}C_3$ or $\binom{10}{3}$. When 3 things are picked from 10, the 7 things that remain also represent a selection from the 10, so that the combination of 10 things taken 7 at a time, $_{10}C_7$, is equal to $_{10}C_3$. The number of combinations can easily be evaluated as

$$_{10}C_3 = {}_{10}C_7 = \frac{10!}{7!3!} = \frac{(10)(9)(8)(7)(6)(5)(4)(3)(2)(1)}{[(7)(6)(5)(4)(3)(2)(1)][(3)(2)(1)]} = 120.$$

Generalizing, the number of ways in which x things can be selected from n things is

$$_nC_x \text{ or } \binom{n}{x} = \frac{n!}{x!(n-x)!}, \text{ or in the illustration} = \frac{10!}{7!(10-7)!}$$

where n! is factorial n and represents the products of all the integers from 1 through $n\binom{n}{x}$ is frequently called the *binomial coefficient*.

When the probability is calculated for further numbers of white and colored chips, the theoretical chance distribution in Table 11.2 is obtained. The theoretical chance distribution is in excellent agreement with the empirical distribution of Table 11.1. The probability of obtaining 60%W (and 40%C) chips is 11.2% from the theoretical distribution and also 11.2% from the empirical distribution based on 1,150 samples from the specified universe.

The probabilities of the various kinds of samples in terms of x or p in Table 11.2 can be derived from the expansion of the expression $(a + b)^{10}$, where $a = .6$ and $b = .4$. This is known as the *binomial distribution*.

$$(a + b)^{10} = a^{10} + 10a^9b + 45a^8b^2 + 120a^7b^3 + 210a^6b^4$$
$$+ 252a^5b^5 + 210a^4b^6 + 120a^3b^7 + 45a^2b^8 + 10ab^9 + b^{10}.$$

The exponent of a declines steadily while the exponent of b increases. The coefficient of each term is the appropriate combination term. It can be obtained from the coefficient of the preceding term in the following manner: the coefficient of the *fourth* term is that of the *third* term (45) times 8 (the decreasing exponent of a in the *third* term) divided by 3 (the third term). Thus, $(45 \times 8)/3 = 120$. Similarly, the coefficient of the fifth term is $(120 \times 7)/4 = 120$. As a check, the sum of all the coefficients in the expansion is 2^n, so that for $n = 10$,

$$2^n = 2^{10} = 1 + 10 + 45 + 120 + 210 + \ldots + 1 = 1{,}024.$$

TABLE 11.2
Chance Distribution of Number White and Percentage White in Random Samples of 10 Drawn From a Universe of 40% White

x No. W	$(n - x)_p$ No. C	p %W	q %C	Probability in Percent	
				By theorem	By experiment*
0	10	0	100	1 $\quad(.6)^{10} =$ 0.6	0.7
1	9	10	90	$10(.4)^1 (.6)^9 =$ 4.0	3.9
2	8	20	80	$45(.4)^2 (.6)^8 =$ 12.1	12.9
3	7	30	70	$120(.4)^3 (.6)^7 =$ 21.5	21.3
4	6	40	60	$210(.4)^4 (.6)^6 -$ 25.1	24.5
5	5	50	50	$252(.4)^5 (.6)^5 =$ 20.1	20.8
6	4	60	40	$210(.4)^6 (.6)^4 =$ 11.2	11.2
7	3	70	30	$120(.4)^7 (.6)^3 =$ 4.2	4.2
8	2	80	20	$45(.4)^8 (.6)^2 =$ 1.1	0.6
9	1	90	10	$10(.4)^9 (.6)^1 =$ 0.2	—
10	0	100	0	$1(.4)^{10} \qquad =$ 0.0	—
Total				100.1	100.1

*Percentage based on 1,150 samples from Table 11.1.

In terms of success and failures (favorable and unfavorable results of the trial), there are (n + 1) terms in the expansion of the binomial $(q' + p')^n$, corresponding to the number of successes (x) from 0 to n. The general term denoting the probability of x successes and (n - x) failures may be denoted as

$$\frac{n!}{x!(n - x)!} (p')^x (q')^{n-x}.$$

The general theorem relating to the probabilities of the various possible numbers of successes and failures may be stated: "when drawing random samples of size n from a universe whose relative frequency of success is p' and of failure q', the probabilities of obtaining 0, 1, 2, . . . , n successes (relative frequencies of success 0/n, 1/n, 2/n, . . . , n/n) are given by successive terms of the binomial $(q' + p')^n$." It should be noted that the successive terms of the expansion of the binomial $(p' + q')^n$ yield the probability of n, n - 1, n - 2, . . . , 1, 0 successes. The terms are the same as of the expansion $(q' + p')^n$ except that they are in *reverse order*.

The probabilities calculated from the sum of the terms in the tails of the binomial expansion should agree well with the probability, P, of a deviation of 20% or more (in either direction) from the universe value of 40% is 0.6 + 4.0 + 12.1 + 11.2 + 4.2 + 1.1 + 0.2 = 33.4%, as compared with the previously obtained empirical value of 33.5% seen in Table 11.1.

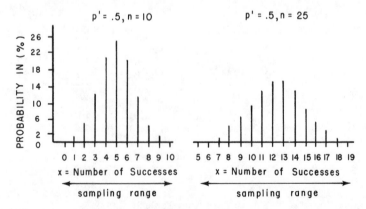

FIG. 11.1 Binomial Expansions for p' = 1/2 and n Varying.

Normal Curve Approximation

When both p' and q' are $1/2$, then the binomial distribution is always symmetrical, regardless of the value of n. Figure 11.1 depicts the expansions of the two binomials $\left(\frac{1}{2}+\frac{1}{2}\right)^{10}$ and $\left(\frac{1}{2}+\frac{1}{2}\right)^{25}$, both of which are symmetrical. These would be the binomials corresponding to tossing 10 or 25 coins, respectively. When p' is not equal to $1/2$, the expansion of the binomial is not symmetrical, unless n is sufficiently large. When we look at the graphs depicting the expansion for $p' = 1/6$ and $q' = 5/6$, for $n = 10$ and $n = 30$ (Fig. 11.2), we see this more clearly. For $n = 10$, the expansion is markedly asymmetrical, and for $n = 30$, fairly symmetrical. A useful rule of thumb is that the binomial expansion is essentially symmetrical when the expected number of successes (np') is 5 or more and the expected number of failures (nq') is also 5 or more. When $p' = 1/6$, then for $n = 10$, $np' = (1/6)(10) = 1.67$, while for $n = 30$, $np' = (1/6)(30) = 5$. When p' is close to 0 or 1, somewhat larger expected numbers would improve the symmetry.

The mean and standard deviation of the binomial, as can be demonstrated algebraically, are given by:

$$\text{in terms of p: } \mu_p = p' \quad SE_p = \sigma_p = \sqrt{\frac{p'q'}{n}}$$

$$\text{in terms of x: } \mu_x = np'; \quad SE_x = \sigma_x = \sqrt{np'q'}.$$

BINOMIAL EXPANSIONS FOR $p'=1/6$ AND n VARYING

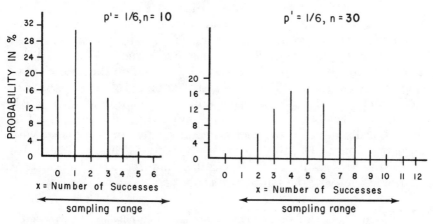

FIG. 11.2 Binomial Expansions for $p' = 1/6$ and n Varying.

When the binomial is symmetrical, a normal curve with the same mean and standard deviation should fit the binomial very well. The discrepancies would for the most part be due to the fact that the scale of the x or p values for the binomial is discrete while the normal curve presupposes continuity.

Single Sample Compared with a Standard (Dichotomous Scale)

The simplest type of problem involving enumeration data consists of comparing a sample of n independent items, each classified into one of two mutually exclusive categories (dichotomous qualitative scales of classification), with a corresponding hypothesized universe. For example, from dental surveys of a very large number of 11-year-old New Jersey children, it was found that 5% of those with fluoride-free public water supplies had no dental caries experience. This figure may be considered a universe value (p'). When 110 children, 11 years of age, living in communities with 1-2 ppm naturally occurring fluoride in the public water supply but otherwise similar to the universe group, were surveyed, 31 children or 28.2% (= p) were found to be free of dental caries experience. The problem then is whether the sample of 110 children from a fluoride-rich area with 28.2% of them caries free, could have been obtained from a universe in which 5% of the children were similarly caries free (the null hypothesis, H_0). The alternative hypothesis (H_1) is that the sample of 110 children is derived from a universe in which p' is not equal to 5% (p' $\neq$ 5%). This null hypothesis will be tested at the 1% level, i.e., the critical value of P is 1%.

The chance distribution of p in successive samples of size 110 drawn from the hypothesized universe is given by the expansion of the binomial* $(.95 + .05)^{110}$, as illustrated in Figure 11.3 and Table 11.3. It is possible to use the binomial distribution thus obtained to determine whether p = 28.2% lies in the zone of significance or non-significance (P = .01). Adding the terms of the binomial for x $\geqslant$ 31, it is obvious that the sum is zero to more than five decimals. This sum is usually doubled to yield a two-tailed test in accordance with the expression of H_1, the alternative hypothesis. It is still zero. We ask for the probability of x $\geqslant$ 31 rather than for x > 31 because of the discontinuity of the sampling distribution.

---

*Extensive tables of the binomial expansion are available.[2] Shorter tables are also available.[3]

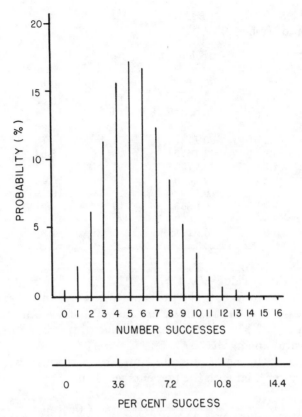

FIG. 11.3 Expansion of Binomial $(.95 + .05)^{110}$

From Figure 11.3, the binomial distribution is fairly symmetrical. Also, np' and nq' are 5.5 and 104.5, respectively. This binomial can be well approximated by a normal curve with a mean = $p' = 5\%$ and a standard deviation

$$\sigma_p = SE_p = \sqrt{\frac{p'q'}{n}} = \sqrt{\frac{(5\%)(95\%)}{110}} = 2.08\%.$$

Converting the observed value of p = 28.2% to standard normal curve units,

$$z = \frac{28.2\% - 5.0\%}{2.08\%} = 11.2.$$

TABLE 11.3
Expansion of $(.95 + .05)^{110}$

No. Successes (x)	% Successes (p)	Probability of Successes (p)	No. Successes (x)	% Successes (p)	Probability of Successes (p)
0	0.00	0.00354	11	10.00	0.01297
1	0.91	0.02053	12	10.91	0.00564
2	1.82	0.05887	13	11.82	0.00223
3	2.73	0.11153	14	12.73	0.00082
4	3.64	0.15704	15	13.64	0.00027
5	4.55	0.17522	16	14.54	0.00009
6	5.45	0.16138	17	15.45	0.00002
7	6.36	0.12620	18	16.36	0.00001
8	7.27	0.08551	19	17.27	0.00000
9	8.18	0.05101	20	18.18	0.00000
10	9.09	0.02712			
				Total	1.00000

Since the critical value of z for $\alpha = .01$ is 2.58, the null hypothesis, H_0, is rejected. In fact, P, the probability of equalling or exceeding z, is much less than .01. It can be concluded that the universe generatin the sample of 110 does not have a value of $p' = 5\%$ for caries-free, the implication being that $p' > 5\%$.

Of course, the significance test may be performed with the proportions rather than with the percentages. Thus,

$$p = .282; p' = .05; \sigma_p = \sqrt{\frac{p'q'}{n}} = \sqrt{\frac{(.05)(.95)}{110}} = 0.0208$$

$$z = \frac{.282 - .05}{0.0208} = 11.2.$$

The significance test may also be performed by comparing the observed number of caries-free children (x = 31) with the number expected to be caries-free under the null hypothesis (np' = 5.5). The standard deviation of the binomial in terms of x is

$$\sigma_x = SE_x = \sqrt{np'q'} = \sqrt{(110)(.05)(.95)} = 2.286.$$

Then,

$$z = \frac{(31 - 5.5)}{2.286} = 11.2.$$

This is the same value of z as the obtained when using percentages of caries-free children.

It is important to note that in some problems involving relative frequencies, the rate is expressed per 1,000, or per 100,000 e.g., neoplastic disease. Thus, if a death rate from all causes of 11.3 per 1000 population is to be compared with a theoretical death rate of 8 per 1000, in terms of rates, $\sigma_p = \sqrt{\dfrac{(8)(992)}{n}}$.

Continuity Correction

When it is possible to use the normal curve as the approximate sampling distribution of relative frequencies, the test of p vs. p′ can be refined by making a correction for continuity. The scale of variation of the observed p's as represented by the binomial is discrete, whereas the approximating normal curve assumes continuous variation. The approximation can be improved by making a continuity correction. This amounts to calculating the observed sample proportion p, as

$$\frac{\text{Number of Successes} \pm \frac{1}{2}}{n} = p \pm \frac{1}{2n},$$

where the (+) sign is used if p is greater than p′. If p is expressed in percent, the corrected value is $p \pm \dfrac{50}{n}$. In terms of the number of successes, the number corrected for continuity is $x \pm \frac{1}{2}$. In the fluoride problem just discussed,

$$p' = 5\%, \ p = \frac{31 - \frac{1}{2}}{110} = 0.277 \text{ or } 27.7\% \text{ and } z = \frac{27.7 - 5.0}{2.08} = 10.9$$

employing the correction for continuity. It is obvious that in this example the result is still highly significant statistically. The continuity correction will make little difference when n is large. Exactly how large n should be depends on the closeness of p′ to 0% or 100%. If the basic binomial distribution is not symmetrical in the first place, then the continuity correction may not be useful. In that case, the binomial should be used as the chance distribution rather than the normal curve approximation.

Alternate Method Using Z^2

There is another way of performing the arithmetic for testing an observed relative frequency against a universe or population relative frequency — different computationally, but yielding the same result. Instead of focusing on the number or relative frequency of success, it uses the number of successes and failures. The observed frequencies are compared with the theoretical frequencies expected under the null hypothesis. In the fluoride example, 31 of the 110 children had no caries and $(110 - 31) = 79$ children had caries. If the sample had been drawn from a universe with 5% caries-free 11-year-old children (the null hypothesis) then in a sample of 110 children, theoretically $(.05)(110) = 5.5$ would be expected to be caries free and $(.95)(110) = 104.5$ would be expected to have caries. The values are summarized in Table 11.4.

The number of observed children who have had caries experience is too small by 25.5, but this is compensated for by an excess of 25.5 in the observed caries-free children, so that the sum of the discrepancies between the observed (O) and theoretical (T) frequencies is zero. The theoretical values can include a fraction or decimal part of an individual, while, obviously, the observed values cannot.

The deviation of the observed from the theoretical frequencies is measured by squaring each discrepancy $(O - T)$, dividing by the appropriate theoretical frequency (T), and adding the resulting values. Thus,

$$\sum \left[\frac{(O - T)^2}{T} \right] = \frac{(79 - 104.5)^2}{104.5} + \frac{(31 - 5.5)^2}{5.5} = \frac{(-25.5)^2}{104.5} + \frac{(25.5)^2}{5.5}$$

$$= 6.22 + 118.23 = 124.45.$$

This sum, 124.45, is actually z^2, where z is the value on the standard normal curve.* Note that $\sqrt{124.45} = 11.2$, the value of z previously found.

If there were perfect agreement between the observed and the theoretical frequencies, z^2 would be zero. When the agreement is good, z^2 will be small; when the agreement is poor, z^2 will be large. Even if a sample of 110 cases had been drawn from the universe in question, some discrepancy between the observed and the theoretical universe frequencies could be expected merely through the action

---

*As will be seen in Chapter 13, z^2 is actually χ^2 (lowercase Greek letter Chi square) with one degree of freedom.

TABLE 11.4

110 Children, 11 Years Old, From Fluoride-Rich Areas, by Caries Experience, Compared with the Expected Experience, Assuming 5% Caries Free[1]

Caries Experience	Observed Frequency (O)	Theoretical Frequency (T)	Discrepancy (O - T)
Caries	79	104.5	-25.5
Caries-free	31	5.5	+25.5
Total	110	110	0

of chance factors alone. To decide whether the value of z^2 obtained is larger than might be expected merely through the action of chance factors, the square root is taken to obtain z, which is then evaluated in terms of the standard normal curve.*

Continuity Correction Using Z^2

The continuity correction can be incorporated into the calculation of z^2. Each observed frequency value is brought closer to the corresponding theoretical frequency by 1/2 unit, and then z^2 is computed as before (see Table 11.5 on page 262), giving $z^2 = 119.62$. The value of z = 10.9 is the same as before.

Confidence Limits

A sample is usually taken to estimate a characteristic of the universe from which it was drawn. The sample of 110 children from fluoride-rich areas in New Jersey can be used to estimate the true relative frequency of caries-free children. The estimate of this parameter is the observed relative frequency, namely, 31 out of 110 = 28.2%. Because of chance errors, the true value may be different from this estimate, of course. The significance test has already shown that the true value could not be 5%. A range of values can be established that would include the true value of the parent universe (p') with a measurable degree of certainty. This range is called the *confidence range*.

---

*The value of z^2 may be referred directly to tables of z^2 which are tables of χ^2 with one degree of freedom. The upper tail of the distribution of z^2 (of χ^2) is, of course, equivalent to the lower and upper tails of the distribution of z, since $(\pm z)^2 = z^2$.

TABLE 11.5
110 Children, 11 Years Old, From Fluoride-Rich Areas, by Caries Experience, Compared with the Expected Experience, Assuming 5% Caries Immunity, Using the Correction for Continuity[1]

Caries Experience	Observed Frequency, Corrected for Continuity (O)	Theoretical Frequency (T)	Discrepancy (O - T)
Caries	79.5	104.5	−25.0
Caries-free	30.5	5.5	+25.0
Total	110.0	110.0	0

$$z^2 = \sum \frac{(O - T)^2}{T} = \frac{(-25.0)^2}{104.5} + \frac{(25.0)^2}{5.5} = 5.98 + 113.64 = 119.62.$$

If it is desired to obtain the 99% confidence range, then the sample value of 28.2% is regarded as differing from the true value by as much as $2.58 SE_p$ in either direction at the most. The SE_p can be computed approximately as $SE_p = \sqrt{\frac{pq}{n}} = \sqrt{\frac{(28.2\%)(71.8\%)}{110}} = 4.29\%$, so that $2.58 SE_p = 11.1\%$. The "minimum" value of p' may be taken as 28.2% − 11.1% and the "maximum" value as 28.2% + 11.1%, giving a range from 17.1% to 39.3%. These limits are called the 99% *confidence limits.* The fact that the confidence range does not include 5% is another way of demonstrating that p = 28.2% is significantly different from 5%, as already demonstrated by the significance test. The confidence limits on p' and the significance test of p vs. p' are not exactly complementary since in the one case p is used to compute an approximate SE_p while in the other case, p' is used to compute SE_p. There are methods available for calculating the confidence interval that do not involve the approximation to SE_p occasioned by substituting p for p'.

REFERENCES

1. Wisan, J.M.: Dental caries and fluorine water, Pub Health News, N.J. Dept. of Health, 27:139, 1944.
2. National Bureau of Standards: Tables of the Binomial Probability Distribution, Applied Mathematics Series #6, Washington, D.C., U.S. Dept. of Commerce, 1952.
3. Dixon, W.J., and Massey, F.J., Jr.: Introduction to Statistical Analysis, 3rd ed., New York, Wiley, 1969.

12
Comparison of Two Relative Frequencies

It is unusual to find an experimental situation in which a sample and a universe relative frequency or standard of reference are compared, as in Chapter 11. In oral biological research, it is unlikely that any sizeable body of data has been accumulated relating to a particular universe and its parameter; as a result, we have no experience with the universe in question. If, for example, we are investigating the effect of feeding rats a certain chemical to protect the teeth from caries, we must know the normal occurrence of caries in such animals. Even if we had some data on this normal caries experience, they might not refer to the particular strain of animals being studied, or the exact dietary intake may differ, or the living conditions of the animals may not be comparable. It is therefore quite unlikely that a truly comparable standard would be available in a particular experiment.

TWO INDEPENDENT SAMPLES
(FOURFOLD TABLE)

In the usual experimental problem, a sine qua non is that a control sample, similar in all respects to the experimental sample, must be taken. In the simplest type of design, the control and experimental samples should differ only with respect to the one factor under investigation. In the experiment selected here, 46 rats of the same strain were studied in terms of whether they remained caries-free or not when a special diet was fed to them during the period of tooth calcification. One group, consisting of 15 rats, ate a standard diet ad libitum and were considered as a *control*. The other group, 31 rats, ate the same diet to which 0.004% cadmium chloride had been added.

This was the *experimental* group.[1] Other than in the number of animals in each group, these two samples presumably differ only in the presence of $CdCl_2$ in the diet. If the two groups were not constituted in the same way with respect to various relevant factors, then all of our statistical reasoning and manipulations would be unable to help us decide whether cadmium feeding inhibited caries. In such a case, it might still be possible, however, to subdivide the samples with respect to these secondary factors and make the comparison separately for each subgroup, or at least to make some appropriate adjustment to rule out the inequalities. It is not necessary that both groups be of the same size in order to make a valid comparison, although such an arrangement would make the analysis much simpler. Furthermore, an experimental design striving for groups of equal size would usually result in a more efficient experiment. For a given total number of animals, the standard error would be less for groups of equal size than for groups of unequal size, thus making it easier to detect statistical significance.

One should make sure that the groups being compared are comparable before the treatments are applied. Unrestricted randomization, as suggested in Chapter 5, would ensure that the two groups are alike within chance variation. From a table of random numbers, the first 15 numbers between 1 and 46 would identify the 15 rats assigned to the standard diet with the remainder being put on the experimental diet. Of course, it would be more efficient, as a rule, to allocate the same number of individuals to each group.

When the results of this experiment were examined, it was found that 7 of 15 rats (46.7%) in the control group and 18 of 31 rats (58.1%) in the experimental group remained caries-free. There was a difference of (58.1% – 46.7% =) 11.4% more caries-free animals in the $CdCl_2$ experimental group. The question can then be posed, "Could a difference of 11.4% in one direction or the other have readily occurred through chance action or could it have been related to the presence of $CdCl_2$ in the diet?"

In this experiment, we take as the null hypothesis that there is no real difference in the percentage of caries-free animals (or caries inhibition) in the two groups, and that any difference observed can be explained through the action of chance factors. If our statistical analysis casts doubt on the veracity of this hypothesis, then an alternative hypothesis (previously postulated), that cadmium feeding had produced a change in freedom from caries, might reasonably be accepted.

The first thing to do after obtaining the final data in this experiment is to summarize the data in tabular form. In Chapter 2, different methods of tabulation of data were presented, and Table 2.4 illus-

TABLE 12.1
The Effect of Cadmium on the Production of Dental Caries in the Rat[1]

Group Studied	Caries-Free Animals	Animals with Caries	Total	% Caries-Free Animals
Experimental (CdCl$_2$)	18	13	31 (n_1)	58.1% (p_1)
Control	7	8	15 (n_2)	46.7% (p_2)
Total	25	21	46	54.3% (p_0)

trated the summarization of double dichotomy data into a fourfold table. The data for the cadmium feeding study have been summarized in Table 12.1.

In this table, the findings in each dietary group are quickly discernible by reading across from left to right. Thus, in the experimental diet sample, 18 rats were caries-free and 13 had caries, out of a total of 31 animals (n_1), for a percentage of 58.1% caries-free rats. This 58.1% may be designated as p_1, so that q_1, the percentage of rats with caries, is (100.0% - 58.1% =) 41.9%. Similarly, for the control group, 7 out of 15 (n_2) animals, or 46.7% remained caries-free, so that p_2 = 46.7% and q_2, the percentage of rats with caries in the control group, would be (100.0% - 46.7% =) 53.3%. The overall percentage of rats in both groups together that remained caries-free is obtained by totaling the number of caries-free rats and dividing by the total number of rats. Thus, 25 rats out of 46, or 54.3%, remained caries-free. This overall percentage is designated as p_0, while the overall percentage of rats with caries, q_0, is (100.0% - 54.3% =) 45.7%. It may be noted that 54.3% is a *weighted average* of the two separate percentages, 58.1% and 46.7%. Thus 58.1% applies for 31 rats, whereas 46.7% applies for only 15. The weighted average is then computed as

$$\frac{58.1\% \times 31 + 46.7\% \times 15}{31 + 15} = 54.3\%.$$

The result is, of course, the same as that obtained from the "Total" row in Table 12.1.

Significance Test

The investigator can proceed to test the null hypothesis that the difference between p_1 and p_2 of 11.4% can be explained as a chance occurrence. The method of analysis illustrated in Chapter 11 is not applicable to this study, however, since the number of animals in the control group (n_2) is not large enough for p_2 to be considered as the universe percentage of caries-free rats. As a sample of limited size, the relative frequency of the control group is subject to sampling fluctuation similar to that of the experimental group. In accordance with the null hypothesis that both control and experimental groups do not really differ in the percentage of caries-free rats, it follows that both groups could be considered as samples of 15 and 31 rats drawn from a universe having the same relative frequency or probability of caries. If pairs of samples of size 15 and 31, respectively, were drawn repeatedly from the same universe of caries-susceptible rats, the difference in the two respective percentages of caries-free animals would not necessarily always be zero. The differences might sometimes be greater than and sometimes less than zero. If pairs of samples were repeatedly drawn from the same universe, however, the average difference between the proportion of caries-free rats in each pair of samples would, of necessity, be zero.

It is necessary to know the nature of the variation of these differences ($p_1 - p_2$). The proportions or percentages (p_1) of caries-free rats occurring in repeated samples of 31 rats (n_1) would, in most cases, be distributed approximately according to a normal curve whose center would be at the true (universe) percentage of caries-free rats (p'), with a standard deviation:

$$\sigma_{p_1} = SE_{p_1} = \sqrt{\frac{p'q'}{31}}.$$

Similarly, the percentage of caries-free rats (p_2) in successive samples of size 15 (n_2) will be distributed, in most cases, approximately in a normal curve centered about the true percentage (p') with a standard deviation

$$\sigma_{p_2} = SE_{p_2} = \sqrt{\frac{p'q'}{15}}.$$

The difference between the two percentages ($p_1 - p_2$) will be distributed in a normal curve centered at the true difference, zero, with a standard deviation

$$\sigma_{p_1 - p_2} = SE_{p_1 - p_2} = \sqrt{SE_{p_1}^2 + SE_{p_2}^2}.$$

In the formulas for SE_{p_1} and SE_{p_2}, the values of p' and q' (percentage of rats with caries) are called for. Unfortunately, these values are unknown. Since we are assuming, at this stage, that no real difference exists between p_1 and p_2 (and q_1 and q_2), we can pool the two samples and regard the result as a larger sample from the universe. The percentage of caries-free rats in this pooled sample (p_0 = 25/46 = 54.3%) is the best estimate we have of the percentage of caries-free rats in the universe. Similarly, q_0 = 21/46 = 45.7% is the best estimate of the percentage of rats with caries in the universe. Thus p_0 and q_0 are substituted in the formulas*:

$$\sigma_{p_1} = SE_{p_1} = \sqrt{\frac{p_0 q_0}{n_1}} = \sqrt{\frac{(54.3\%)(45.7\%)}{31}} = \sqrt{80.0\%} = 8.9\%.$$

$$\sigma_{p_2} = SE_{p_2} = \sqrt{\frac{p_0 q_0}{n_2}} = \sqrt{\frac{(54.3\%)(45.7\%)}{15}} = \sqrt{165.4\%} = 12.9\%.$$

SE_{p_1} (= 8.9%) is a measure of the chance error in p_1 for the cadmium experimental group, and SE_{p_2} (= 12.9%) is a measure of the chance error in p_2 for the control group.

The normal curve representing the chance distribution of differences between these two percentages is centered at zero, with a standard deviation:

$$\sigma_{p_1 - p_2} = SE_{p_1 - p_2} = \sqrt{SE_{p_1}{}^2 + SE_{p_2}{}^2}$$
$$= \sqrt{80.0\% + 165.4\%} = \sqrt{245.4\%} = 15.7\%.$$

The appropriate normal curve of differences in percentages of caries-free rats is therefore centered at zero and has a standard deviation of 15.7%. If we are operating at a 5% level of significance (α), then differences up to 1.96 standard deviations on either side of the mean $-(1.96)(15.7\%)$ to $+(1.96)(15.7\%)$ = -30.8% to $+30.8\%$ are regarded as being within the sampling zone, i.e., not statistically significant. Differences greater than $\pm 30.8\%$ would be statistically significant. If we were operating at the 1% level (α = 1%), the difference would have to exceed 2.58 SE in order to be statistically significant, i.e., less than -40.5% or greater than $+40.5\%$. An investigator will occasionally hedge and term differences between 1.96 and 2.58 standard deviations from zero of "borderline significance."

In the problem under discussion, the difference between the percentage of rats remaining caries-free in the experimental diet

---

*The replacement of p' and q' by p_0 and q_0 means that attention is being focused on only those fourfold tables that have the same marginal totals as the observed fourfold table.

group and in the control group is 11.4%, i.e., $p_1 - p_2 = 58.1\% - 46.7\%$ = 11.4%. This difference is less than 30.8% and may be called not statistically significant using the 5% level. The difference we have just found falls only 0.73 standard deviations away from zero, since

$$z = \frac{(p_1 - p_2) - 0}{SE_{p_1 - p_2}} = \frac{11.4\%}{15.7\%} = 0.73.*$$

The probability (P) of equaling or exceeding a z of 0.73, i.e., of exceeding a difference of 11.4%, is approximately 0.47 (see Table 3.1). This means that about 47% of the time we would get a difference as large as 11.4% or larger in either direction, when drawing samples from the same universe. The same value of z would be obtained of course, by comparing q_1 and q_2, the proportion of rats with caries in each sample. Note that we ask for the probability of equaling or exceeding the observed z, because of the discontinuity of the sampling distribution (the hypergeometric distribution).

From the analysis, one may conclude that the difference of 11.4% between the percentages of caries-free rats on a diet supplemented with 0.004% $CdCl_2$ during the period of calcification of the teeth and those on a control diet can readily occur through chance action alone. The original null hypothesis, that cadmium produces no change in the occurrence of rat caries as determined under the conditions of this experiment, has therefore not been disproved, and can tentatively be accepted.

Just because the null hypothesis has not been disproved does not necessarily mean that no difference exists between the two universes sampled. This analysis shows merely that the data do not warrant the conclusion that a real difference exists between the results of each treatment.

One-Tailed Test

If, in the planning stage of the experiment, the investigator decided that he was interested only in whether $CdCl_2$ dietary supplementation increased the percentage of caries-free rats (i.e., afforded greater

---

*Although p' and q' are replaced by p_0, q_0 in the evaluation of the standard error, the ratio still follows the standard normal curve.

protection), a one-tailed rather than a two-tailed test would be called for. In that case, the null hypothesis (H_0) remains the same, but the alternative hypothesis (H_1) is that the true difference is greater than zero $[(p_1' - p_2') > 0]$ rather than that the true difference is not equal to zero $[(p_1' - p_2') \neq 0]$. The zone of significance would then be in the upper tail only, corresponding to 1% or 5% of the area of the curve. The appropriate critical values of z are +2.32 or +1.64. Such a statistical test is a one-tailed (or one-sided) test. Obviously, the observed difference of +11.4% is not statistically significant even when using this one-tailed test.

The decision to utilize a one-tailed test must be made in advance — in the planning phase of the experiment, certainly before viewing the data. In the majority of experiments, it is safer practice to specify a two-tailed test — i.e., $\frac{1}{2}P$ in the lower tail and $\frac{1}{2}P$ in the upper tail of the sampling curve.

Limitations on the Use of Normal Curve Techniques

In order for the normal curve analysis to be employed freely for the fourfold table, it is necessary that both samples be sufficiently large to satisfy certain theoretical considerations. Since the chance distribution of relative frequencies is fundamentally a point binomial, this distribution has to be symmetrical before the normal curve can be used safely for significance tests. This symmetry requires that each of four products — $n_1 p_0$, $n_2 p_0$, $n_1 q_0$, and $n_2 q_0$ — must be 5 or more. Thus, the use of the normal curve was justified in the cadmium feeding problem, since:

$$n_1 p_0 = (31)(.543) = 16.8 \qquad n_1 q_0 = (31)(.457) = 14.2$$

$$n_2 p_0 = (15)(.543) = 8.1 \qquad n_2 q_0 = (15)(.457) = 6.9$$

If the value of any of the four expressions — $n_1 p_0$, $n_2 p_0$, etc. — is less than 5, the normal curve test must be used with caution. In such a situation, it may be useful to utilize the idea of a borderline significance zone within which decision can be reserved. Undoubtedly the best way to handle such situations would be to use the exact sampling distribution of differences in relative frequencies, which is the hypergeometric distribution. Extensive tables of the hypergeometric distribution are available.[2] This test is often referred to as Fisher's Exact test.[3]

Continuity Correction

The scale of $(p_1 - p_2)$ in the chance distribution of relative frequencies is discontinuous. The probability, P, attached to the difference, as given by the normal curve, can be improved on when n_1 and n_2 are only moderately large by making a continuity correction. This correction amounts to measuring the difference between the relative frequencies, expressed in proportions as $p_1 - p_2 \pm \dfrac{1}{2} \left(\dfrac{1}{n_1} + \dfrac{1}{n_2} \right)$. The (+) is used if $(p_1 - p_2)$ is negative and the (-) if $(p_1 - p_2)$ is positive. For p_1 and p_2 expressed as percent, the correction is $\pm \dfrac{100}{2} \left(\dfrac{1}{n_1} + \dfrac{1}{n_2} \right)$.

In Table 12.1 the $(p_1 - p_2)$ of +11.4% is reduced by $\dfrac{100}{2} \left(\dfrac{1}{31} + \dfrac{1}{15} \right)$ = 4.9%. This yields 11.4% – 4.9% = 6.5% as the adjusted difference. $z = \dfrac{6.5\% - 0\%}{15.7\%} = 0.41$, and P = 68%. Without this continuity correction, $z = 0.73$ and P = 47%. The effect of the correction is always to lower the magnitude of z.

The continuity correction for the fourfold table is useful for moderate values of n_1 and n_2. When the difference $(p_1 - p_2)$ is very small, the application of the continuity correction may change the sign of the difference. In such a case, the correction should not be used. When n_1 and n_2 are so small that symmetry does not exist, the normal curve cannot be used safely. The use of the continuity correction does not help make the normal curve more applicable in such a case either.

Confidence Interval on $(p_1' - p_2')$.

After a significance test on $(p_1' - p_2')$ vs. 0 has been performed, whether or not the difference is significant, we may want to establish an interval which should cover the true value of the parameter $(p_1' - p_2')$. In fact, very often the purpose of the study is to establish this interval, rather than to do a significance test. Since we do not necessarily accept the hypothesis that $(p_1' = p_2')$, we do not use a common estimate in the evaluation of the standard error of $p_1 - p_2$. In fact, an approximate standard error is used which uses p_1 and p_2, respectively, as

$$\text{est. } SE_{p_1 - p_2} = \sqrt{p_1 q_1 / n_1 + p_2 q_2 / n_2}.$$

It is still true that

$$[(p_1 - p_2) - (p_1' - p_2')] \text{ est. } SE(p_1 - p_2)$$

is distributed asymptotically as z. Consequently, the 95% confidence interval for $(p_1' - p_2')$ extends from

$$\left[(p_1' - p_2') - 1.96 \sqrt{p_1 q_1 / n_1 + p_2 q_2 / n_2} \right]$$

up to

$$\left[(p_1 - p_2) + 1.96 \sqrt{p_1 q_1 / n_1 + p_2 q_2 / n_2} \right].$$

While this interval is approximately the same whether $p_1 q_1$ and $p_2 q_2$ or $p_0 q_0$ are used, nevertheless it seems more reasonable to use $p_1 q_1$ and $p_2 q_2$.

In the problem under discussion, $(p_1 - p_2) = 11.4\%$, and

$$\text{est. } SE(p_1 - p_2) = \sqrt{\frac{(58.1)(41.9)}{31} + \frac{(46.7)(53.3)}{15}} = 15.6\%.$$

This value is not very different from the standard error when $p_0 q_0$ was used (15.7%). In fact, this is usually the case. The 95% confidence interval is the interval from

$$11.4\% - 1.96(15.6\%) = -19.2\% \text{ up to } 11.4\% + 1.96(15.6\%) = 42.0\%.$$

This interval includes 0, agreeing with the significance test on page 268 ($z = 0.73$). When z is computed using p_1 and p_2 for the est. $SE_{p_1 - p_2}$, $z = 0.74$. While the confidence interval and the significance test are in agreement, the confidence interval is not exactly the complement of the significance test because the standard errors are calculated using a different p.

Alternate Method Using z^2

The significance test for the fourfold table is often performed in a different way arithmetically. The deviations of the observed from the theoretical frequencies determined under the assumption of the null

TABLE 12.2

Observed Results of Root Canal Fillings of 197 Cases, According to Culture or Nonculture of Canal Contents Before Filling[4]

	O			
	Normal	*Failure*	*Total*	*% Failure*
Cultured	110	11	121	9.1
Noncultured	59	17	76	22.4
Total	169	28	197	14.2

hypothesis are measured and assessed. For example, in a study of the importance of culturing the contents of root canals before final obturation,[4] it was found that of a total of 121 cases in which negative cultures had been obtained, the results of 110 cases were classified as "normal" and 11 as "failures" on follow-up examination. In a group of 76 cases in which the canal contents were not cultured before obturation, 59 were classified as "normal" and 17 as "failures" on follow-up, using the same criterion of classification for "normal" and "failure" as for the cultured canal cases. The problem involved is to determine whether culturing the canals before final obturation produced a percentage of failures significantly different from that of the relatively simpler procedure of obturation without prior negative cultures.

The two frequency distributions can be summarized by a four-fold table (Table 12.2). The null hypothesis to be tested is that there is no difference in clinical results obtained by obturating root canals with or without prior negative cultures of the canal contents. If no difference existed between the follow-up findings after culturing and nonculturing endodontic techniques, then the overall percentage of

TABLE 12.3

Theoretical Results of Root Canal Fillings of 197 Cases, According to Culture or Nonculture of Canal Contents Before Filling, Assuming no Difference in Failure Rate

	T			
	Normal	*Failure*	*Total*	*% Failure*
Cultured	103.8	17.2	121.0	14.2
Noncultured	65.2	10.8	76.0	14.2
Total	169.0	28.0	197.0	14.2

TABLE 12.4
Table of Discrepancies

	(O – T)		
	Normal	*Failure*	*Total*
Cultured	(110 – 103.8) = +6.2	(11 – 17.2) = –6.2	0
Noncultured	(59 – 65.2) = –6.2	(17 – 10.8) = +6.2	0
Total	0	0	

failure (14.2%) or normal (100.0% – 14.2% = 85.8%) would occur in both the cultured and noncultured cases. We can therefore construct a fourfold table of theoretical frequencies in which no differences exist between the results in both groups (Table 12.3). The numbers in the cells of this table of no difference or of no relation are obtained by applying the overall percentage of failure to the respective totals (14.2% × 121 = 17.2; 14.2% × 76 = 10.8) and the overall percentage of normal (or "success") to the respective totals (85.8% × 121 = 103.8; 85.8% × 76 = 65.2).

Having the four observed (O) and theoretical (T) values, we can proceed to evaluate the discrepancies between them. To illustrate the necessary computation, a table of (O – T) values has been constructed (Table 12.4). Theoretically, (O – T) values add up to zero both horizontally (row-wise) and vertically (column-wise). We can thus see, at this point, that knowing one (O – T) value, we can readily calculate the values in all of the other cells in this table. In the fourfold table, all the values are the same, except for sign. Each (O – T) value is squared and then divided by the corresponding T value, as shown in Table 12.5. The summary value of the four discrepancies between O and T is obtained by adding these four $(O – T)^2/T$ contributions, 0.37 + 0.59 + 2.23 + 3.56 = 6.75.

TABLE 12.5
Contributions to $\sum \left[\dfrac{(O – T)^2}{T} \right]$

	$\dfrac{(O – T)^2}{T}$	
	Normal	*Failure*
Cultured	$(+6.2)^2/103.8 = 0.37$	$(-6.2)^2/17.2 = 2.23$
Noncultured	$(-6.2)^2/ 65.2 = 0.59$	$(+6.2)^2/10.8 = 3.56$

TABLE 12.6
Table of Discrepancies of Table 12.4 Modified by Continuity Correction

	$(O - T)$		
	Normal	Failure	Total
Cultured	+5.7	-5.7	0
Noncultured	-5.7	+5.7	0
Total	0	0	0

It can be shown algebraically, in the case of the fourfold table, that the $\sum \left[\dfrac{(O - T)^2}{T} \right] = z^2$.* To assess the significance of z^2, the square root is extracted and referred to the standard normal curve. Thus, $z = \sqrt{6.75} = 2.60$. This is the same value of z as if the data had been analyzed by using the standard error approach. A z value of 2.60 can be equaled or exceeded less than 1% of the time by chance alone. If an α of 1% is the previously chosen level of significance, the result of the experiment (i.e., the difference between the results with and without culturing) may be called statistically significant. The null hypothesis, that there is no difference between the results of obturating root canals with and without prior culturing of the canal contents, is therefore rejected, and an alternative hypothesis that the failure rates are different can be embraced. Evidently, then, fewer failures occur when the canals are cultured prior to obturation.

Continuity Correction

The theoretical frequencies are calculated as before, but the observed frequencies are all adjusted by half a unit to bring them into closer agreement with the theoretical frequencies: all the discrepancies are reduced numerically by half a unit. The table of discrepancies in Table 12.4 is modified as in Table 12.6, and the values of Table 12.5 will appear as in Table 12.7, yielding a z^2 value of 5.71, as compared with the previously computed $z^2 = 6.75$. The effect of the correction is always to lower the magnitude of z^2. The correction is not em-

---

*z^2 for the foufold table is the simplest example of the χ^2 (chi-square) test of association or homogeneity. In this case, χ^2 has one degree of freedom. Examples of the χ^2 test of association or homogeneity for more than one degree of freedom are presented in Chapter 13.

TABLE 12.7
Table of Contributions to $\Sigma\left[\dfrac{(O - T)^2}{T}\right]$ **of Table 12.5 Modified by**
Continuity Correction

	$\dfrac{(O - T)^2}{T}$	
	Normal	*Failure*
Cultured	$(+5.7)^2/103.8 = 0.31$	$(-5.7)^2/17.2 = 1.89$
Noncultured	$(-5.7)^2/\ 65.2 = 0.50$	$(+5.7)^2/10.8 = 3.01$

ployed if the discrepancy $(O - T)$ is so small that an alteration by half a unit would change its sign.

Shortcut Calculation Method

$$\Sigma\left[\frac{(O - T)^2}{T}\right]$$ or z^2 for the fourfold table can also be calculated in a shortcut way by using a different algebraic formulation. If the cells are denoted by letters (a, b, c, and d) as seen in Table 12.8, the computations are then:

$$z^2 = \frac{(ad - bc)^2(a + b + c + d)}{(a + c)(b + d)(a + b)(c + d)}$$

$$= \frac{[(110)(17) - (11)(59)]^2(110 + 11 + 59 + 17)}{(110 + 59)(11 + 17)(110 + 11)(59 + 17)}$$

$$= \frac{(1221)^2(197)}{(169)(28)(121)(76)} = \frac{293{,}695{,}677}{43{,}515{,}472} = 6.75.$$

This is the same result as previously obtained.

TABLE 12.8
Table for Calculating $\Sigma\left[\dfrac{(O - T)^2}{T}\right]$ **by Shortcut Algebraic Formula**

	Normal	*Failure*	*Total*
Cultured	110 (a)	11 (b)	121
Noncultured	59 (c)	17 (d)	76
Total	169	28	197

The continuity correction can be made directly using this formula:

$$z^2 = \frac{[\,|ad - bc| - 1/2(a + b + c + d)^2\,](a + b + c + d)}{(a + c)(b + d)(a + b)(c + d)},$$

where $|ad - bc|$ refers to the difference $ad - bc$ without regard to sign.

Examination of the Relation Between Two Measured Variables by Grouping the Data into a Fourfold Table

In studying the relation between two simultaneously obtained measurements in Chapter 8, the data on calcium solubility in saliva and ptyalin activity of Table 8.5 were divided into two equal groups, according to a high ($\geqslant$ 14 mg%) or low salivary calcium solubility (Table 8.6) and a comparison of means test (t-test) performed on the means of ptyalin activity. That is, the scale of calcium solubility was dichotomized and the resulting two means of the other variable were compared.

Another way of examining the relation between the two variables is to regroup the data into a fourfold table — i.e., dichotomize both scales. The data in Table 8.5 are divided into two approximately equal groups according to high or low amylolytic index values by drawing a vertical line at x = 2.6 in Figure 8.6. We can thus summarize the swarm of points into a fourfold table, since the two lines we have drawn divide the points into four parts: (1) an upper left quadrant, which is *high* in calcium dissolved and *low* in amylolytic index; (2) a lower left quadrant, which is *low* in calcium dissolved and *low* in amylolytic index; (3) an upper right quadrant, which is *high* in calcium dissolved and *high* in amylolytic index; and (4) a lower right quadrant, which is *low* in calcium dissolved and *high* in amylolytic index. Adding the number of points for each of the four quadrants, one obtains Table 12.9. Examining this table, we can see immediately that there is some tendency for the amylolytic index and calcium dissolved values both to be high or both to be low. This tendency does not seem to be very marked, but it can be tested for significiance by comparing this table of observed frequencies (O) with a table of theoretical frequencies (T).

The theoretical table is readily constructed. With the data subdivided, half of the 34 persons have low calcium dissolved. Consequently, of these 15 with an amylolytic index value above 2.6, we would expect half to be high for calcium dissolved and half to be

TABLE 12.9

Simultaneous Measurement of Amylolytic Index and Calcium Solubility of 34 Individuals, Classified as High or Low Groups

		Observed Values (O) Amylolytic Index		
		Low	High	Total
Calcium	High	7	10	17
dissolved	Low	12	5	17
	Total	19	15	34

low. Similarly, for the 19 below the dividing value for the amylolytic index, we would expect an equal division with respect to the values of calcium dissolved in saliva. The theoretical fourfold table would then appear as Table 12.10. The value z^2, corrected for continuity, is 1.91, so that $z = 1.38$. Referring this value to the standard normal curve, such discrepancies are found to be equaled or exceeded more than 5% of the time by chance. Although we have observed a positive relationship between these two variables, it is not strong enough to be significant when the data are grouped into a fourfold table. Unless the relationship is strong, the significance may not be detected by coarse grouping into a fourfold table.

The scatter diagram (Figure 12.1) of another problem — in which 28 individuals were measured for dental height in occlusion and dental height in physiologic rest — shows that a strong positive relationship exists between these two variables.[5] When these points are condensed into a fourfold table as indicated in the graph, Table 12.11 is obtained.

Correcting for continuity, $z^2 = 7.04$, so that $z = 2.65$. P, the probability of equaling or exceeding z, is less than 1%. There is, therefore, a definite tendency for the dental height in physiological rest to be associated positively with the dental height in occlusion — i.e., if one is high, the other tends to be high, and if one is low, the

TABLE 12.10

Theoretical Frequencies (T)

		Amylolytic Index		
		Low	High	Total
Calcium	High	9.5	7.5	17.0
dissolved	Low	9.5	7.5	17.0
	Total	19.0	15.0	34.0

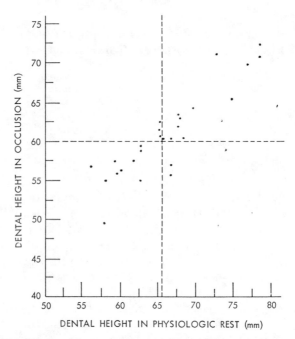

FIG. 12.1 Scatter Diagram of 28 Individuals According to Their Dental Height at Physiological Rest and in Occlusion.

other tends to be low. Thus, the examination of the relationship between the two variables by the fourfold table, high-low grouping, will detect the presence of a strong relationship.

TWO CORRELATED (PAIRED) SAMPLES

In the usual fourfold table, it is assumed that the two samples are drawn independently of each other. The samples would not be independent if the choice of the individuals to be included in the first sample somehow determined which ones should be included in the second sample. Such a situation would exist if each individual in the second sample were paired with one in the first sample, or if the same individual could be used in both samples. This latter situation obviously could not occur if the question of fatality (i.e., outcome expressed as death or survival) were being investigated, but could arise if, say, two methods of testing of salivary samples were being compared, or if two treatments were being compared for frequency of reactions, both on the same individual.

TABLE 12.11
Simultaneous Measurement of Dental Height in Occlusion and Dental Height in Physiologic Rest of 28 Individuals, Classified as High or Low Groups[5]

| | | Observed Values (O) Dental Height in Physiologic Rest | | |
		Low	High	Total
Dental height	High	3	12	15
in occlusion	Low	11	2	13
	Total	14	14	28

The table of theoretical frequencies would be:

| | | Theoretical Frequencies (T) Physiologic Rest | | |
		Low	High	Total
Occlusion	High	7.5	7.4	15.0
	Low	6.5	6.5	13.0
	Total	14.0	14.0	28.0

A clinical study of the effectiveness of two topical anesthetic preparations, tetracaine 2% and Sq 2636 (here referred to as tetracaine and Sq), was performed.[6] These two preparations were applied in a random sequence to the lower jaw of 52 subjects, with one isolated quadrant receiving one drug and the other isolated quadrant the other drug. As a result of the randomization, about half the time one drug was applied to the right side and half the time to the left side of the subjects. The presence (plus) or absence (minus) of anesthesia was noted at 10 minutes after the application of the drugs. The results of a study of this type can be summarized, in general terms, as in Table 12.12A. The specific data from this study are presented in Table 12.12B. What we wish to compare in Table 12.12 is the proportion of the 52 individuals who show a positive reaction with tetracaine (p_1 = 86.5%) with the proportion of the same 52 individuals who show a positive response with Sq (p_2 = 69.2%). These proportions are displayed in the total column and in the total row of Table 12.12B — i.e., they are the marginal proportions. Because of the design of the experiment, using each individual as his own control, these proportions of positives cannot be compared by the procedure previously presented in this chapter, which assumes that there are two independent samples of size 52.

The difference between the two marginal proportions in Table

TABLE 12.12
Fourfold Table for Two Correlated Samples

A. Schematic Fourfold Table

		Treatment B		
		+	−	Total
Treatment A	+	a	b	a + b
	−	c	d	c + d	$p_1 = (a + b)/n$
Total		a + c	b + d	n

$$p_2 = (a + c)/n$$
$$p_1 - p_2 = [(a + b)/n] - [(a + c)/n] = (b - c)/n$$

B. Individuals Classified According to Response to Topical Anesthetics
At 10 Minutes After Application

		Sq 2636		
		+	−	Total
Tetracaine	+	33	12	45
	−	3	4	7	$p_1 = (45/52) = 86.5\%$
Total		36	16	52

$$p_2 = (36/52) = 69.2\%$$
$$p_1 - p_2 = (45/52) = (36/52) = (12 - 3)/52 = 17.3\%$$

12.12B is determined entirely by the fact that the number of individuals who were positive with tetracaine and negative with Sq (b = 12) is not the same as the number who were positive with Sq and negative with tetracaine (c = 3). These 15 individuals will be referred to as having "untied responses." The number positive with respect to both drugs (a = 33) appears in both of the marginal proportions. These individuals (and the four whose responses were both negative) will be referred to as having "tied responses."

The null hypothesis that the true marginal proportions are equal is equivalent to the null hypothesis that the number of individuals with untied responses are equally divided. Consequently, the pertinent analysis is to determine whether the division of the b + c (12 + 3 = 15 in this case) individuals with untied responses differs significantly from an even split, i.e., a 50:50 division. This test is referred to as the *McNemar test*.[3] In effect, by considering only the untied pairs, the problem will be resolved by the methods already described in Chapter 11. It is actually a special case in which $p' = 1/2$.

Exact Test

To test whether the division of the 15 untied individuals — namely, 12 and 3 — differs significantly from a 50:50 division, the binomial $(1/2 + 1/2)^{15}$ may be expanded. P, the probability of 3 or less, or 12 or more, individuals in one of the cells on the "untied" diagonal of the fourfold table — say, the lower left corner, c — is obtained by adding the first four and the last four terms of the binomial expansion,

$$P = (1/2)^{15} + (15)(1/2)^{15} + (105)(1/2)^{15} + (455)(1/2)^{15}$$
$$+(455)(1/2)^{15} + (105)(1/2)^{15} + (15)(1/2)^{15} + (1/2)^{15}$$
$$= 1{,}152/(2)^{15} = 0.0352.$$

Thus, the observed distribution (12, 3) differs significantly from a 50:50 distribution at the 5% level. In other words, the proportion of pluses with tetracaine (86.5%) differs significantly from the proportion of pluses with Sq (69.2%) at the 5% level. Tables of the binomial expansion are available in various sources.[7] Tables for the special case of the binomial where $p' = 1/2$, as in this case, are even more readily available.[8,9]

The normal curve approximation can be employed, because of the symmetry of the binomial. To test whether a sample of size 15 with a $p = \dfrac{3}{15} \times 100 = 20.0\%$ could readily have been drawn from a universe with a $p' = 50.0\%$, p can be located on the unit normal curve. Thus,

$$z = \frac{(p - p')}{\sqrt{\dfrac{p'q'}{N}}} = \frac{(20 - 50)}{\sqrt{\dfrac{(50)(50)}{15}}} = \frac{-30}{12.91} = -2.32.$$

The probability of exceeding z without regard to sign — i.e., the probability of a sample as rare or rarer drawn under the conditions of the null hypothesis — is 2.0%, and hence the difference is statistically significant at the .05 level of significance.

Utilizing the continuity correction, as discussed in Chapter 11, to obtain a result closer to that of the exact binomial test, corrected $p = \dfrac{3.5}{15} = 23.33\%$, and corrected $z = \dfrac{(23.33 - 50.0)}{12.9} = \dfrac{26.67}{12.91} = 2.07$, and P = 3.9%. This P is close to the exact P = 3.52% resulting from the use of the binomial.

TABLE 12.13
Observed and Theoretical Frequencies of 15 Untied Pairs of Responses
to Two Topical Anesthetics at 10 Minutes After Application (Null
Hypothesis States a 50:50 Division)

Sq	Tetracaine	Observed (O)	Theoretical (T)
+	−	3	7.5
−	+	12	7.5
Total		15	15.00

The approximation to the binomial may also be carried out by
evaluating the fluctuations of the observed from the theoretical frequencies set up under the null hypothesis (Table 12.13). Thus,

$$z^2 = \sum \left[\frac{(O - T)^2}{T} \right] = \frac{(3 - 7.5)^2}{7.5} + \frac{(12 - 7.5)^2}{7.5} = 2.70 + 2.70 = 5.40.$$

Then, $z = \sqrt{5.40} = 2.32$ so that P = 2.0%. In this case of a theoretical
50:50 division, z^2 (or χ^2 with one degree of freedom) can be computed simply as

$$z^2 = \frac{(12 - 3)^2}{(12 + 3)} = \frac{81}{15} = 5.40.$$

z^2 can be corrected for continuity very simply in this case where
$p' = 1/2$. That is,

$$\text{Corrected } z^2 = \frac{(|12 - 3| - 1)^2}{12 + 3} = \frac{64}{15} = 4.27,$$

and $\sqrt{4.27} = 2.07 = $ corrected z.

Independent Sample Approach

The experiment cited here, in which each individual was used as his
own control, was designed to reduce the variations of response to the
two different treatments. If, however, the data in Table 12.12B were
analyzed erroneously, as though they pertained to two independent
groups of 52 patients each, they would be summarized as in Table
12.14. The two rows in Table 12.14 are merely the two margins of

TABLE 12.14
Responses of 52 Individuals to Two Topical Anesthetics Classified in a Fourfold Table as if the Two Samples Were Independent

Treatment	+	−	Total	
Tetracaine	45	7	52	$p_1 = 36/52 = 69.2\%$
Sq	36	16	52	$p_2 = 45/52 = 86.5\%$
Total	81	23	104	

Response column spans + and −.

Corrected $z^2 = 3.57$.

Table 12.12B. The comparison of interest in this fourfold table is still that between the proportion of pluses for one treatment and the proportion of pluses for the other treatment. The results of many experiments indeed pertain to independent samples and appear in exactly this form.

The test of significance of the difference in proportions of pluses for this type of fourfold table can be performed by calculating the z or z^2 presented at the beginning of this chapter. Employing the simplified computing formula with the correction for continuity, as given previously,

$$\text{Corrected } z^2 = \frac{104 \left(|(36)(7) - (16)(45)| - \frac{104}{2} \right)^2}{(81)(23)(52)(52)} = 3.57.$$

$z = \sqrt{3.57} = 1.89$ and $P = 5.9\%$. The P value is greater than the $P = 3.8\%$ obtained from the correct test. The fact that the correct P value is less than the P value derived from the analysis of the sample as though they were independent, emphasizes the need for, and the efficiency of, utilizing the relationship between the two samples in the final test of significance.

REFERENCES

1. Leicester, H.M.: The effect of cadmium on the production of dental caries in the rat, J Dent Res 25:337, 1946.
2. Lieberman, C., and Owen, D.: Tables of the Hypergeometric Probability Distribution, Stanford, Stanford Univ. Press, 1961.
3. Siegel, S.: Nonparametric Statistics, New York, McGraw-Hill, 1956.
4. Buchbinder, M.: A statistical comparison of cultured and non-cultured root canal cases, J Dent Res 20:93, 1941.

5. Wylie, W. L.: Overbite and vertical facial dimensions in terms of muscle balance, Angle Orthodont 14:13, 1944.

6. Kutscher, A. H., and Chilton, N. W.: Unpublished data, Columbia Univ. School of Dental and Oral Surgery.

7. National Bureau of Standards: Tables of the Binomial Probability Distribution, Applied Mathematics Series #6, Washington (D.C.). U.S. Dept. of Commerce, 1952.

8. Dixon, W. J., and Massey, F. J., Jr.: Introduction to Statistical Analysis, 3rd ed., New York, McGraw-Hill, 1969.

9. Walker, H., and Lev, J.: Statistical Inference, New York, Holt, 1953.

13
Chi Square

An understanding of a distribution called the chi square (lowercase Greek letter χ^2) distribution is prerequisite to any further discussion of the analysis of enumeration data (proportions or relative frequencies). The χ^2 distribution was developed by Karl Pearson for various types of problems involving enumeration data.[1] These were goodness of fit problems in which observed and theoretical distributions were compared, and problems in which two or more observed frequency distributions were compared. The observed (O) and theoretical (T) frequencies in the various cells of a table were compared and the discrepancies summarized as $\chi^2 = \sum \left[\dfrac{(O - T)^2}{T} \right]$. In repeated experiments of the same type, this quantity follows a distribution known as the χ^2 distribution (when the null hypothesis is true). An important parameter of the χ^2 distribution is known as the *number of degrees of freedom*. The number of degrees of freedom depends on the number of discrepancies being summarized, and on the number of restrictions imposed on them. There is, in fact, a family of χ^2 distributions with each number of degrees of freedom determining a different curve.

Pearson was using the χ^2 distribution as an approximation to binomials and multinomials. It was not until later that Fisher pointed out that Pearson's resolution applied to the solution of a large number of problems in the field of measurements involving standard deviations (or variances).[2] In fact, the χ^2 distribution is basic and underlies the theory of the t-test, F-test, etc.

Let us assume that x is distributed in a normal curve with mean, μ, and standard deviation, σ. If repeat values of x are drawn independently at random from this distribution, then the quantity $z^2 = \dfrac{(x - \mu)^2}{\sigma^2}$, which will be computed for each value of x, will follow the χ^2 distribution with one degree of freedom. This curve is depicted in Figure 13.1, and is, of course, the distribution of z^2; χ^2 ranges from 0 to ∞. The value of χ^2 exceeded 5% of the time is 3.84, and the value exceeded 1% of the time is 6.66, which is depicted on the graph in Figure 13.1. These numbers are, of course, the squares of z = 1.96 and z = 2.58.

If the x's are taken at random in groups of N, say 10, from the normal distribution and the following quantities formed,

$$\overset{N}{\underset{\Sigma}{}} \left[\frac{(x - \mu)^2}{\sigma^2} \right] = \overset{N}{\underset{\Sigma}{}} z^2,$$

these quantities are also distributed as χ^2 but with N degrees of freedom, in this case, 10. The appropriate curve is depicted in Figure 13.2. The values of χ^2 exceeded 5% and 1% of the time for this curve, 18.31 and 21.16 are, of course, much larger than the corresponding values for one degree of freedom.

The shape of the χ^2 curve depends entirely on the number of

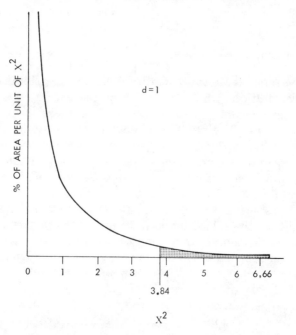

FIG. 13.1 Chance Distribution of χ^2 for One Degree of Freedom.

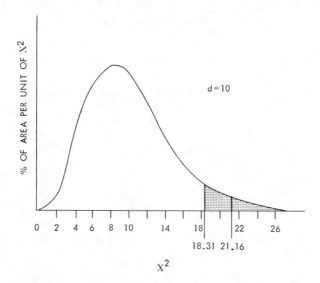

FIG. 13.2 Chance Distribution of χ^2 for Ten Degrees of Freedom.

degrees of freedom. Curves for various numbers of degrees of freedom are given in Figure 13.3. For a small number of degrees of
freedom, the curve is very skewed. For a large number of degrees of
freedom, e.g., 30, the distribution is not too dissimilar from a normal
curve. The mean value of χ^2 is equal to the degrees of freedom and

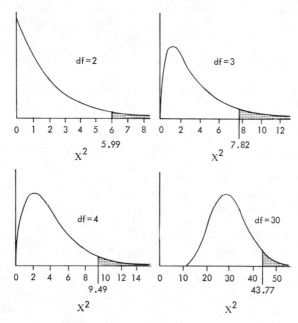

FIG. 13.3 Chance Distribution of χ^2 for 2, 3, 4 and 30 Degrees of
Freedom.

287

TABLE 13.1
Table of χ^2 Corresponding to Different Levels of Significance

	P in Percentages				
df	50	10	5	2	1
1	0.45	2.71	3.84	5.41	6.64
2	1.39	4.61	5.99	7.82	9.21
3	2.37	6.25	7.82	9.84	11.34
4	3.36	7.78	9.49	11.67	13.28
5	4.35	9.24	11.07	13.39	15.09
6	5.35	10.64	12.57	15.03	16.81
7	6.35	12.02	14.07	16.62	18.48
8	7.34	13.36	15.51	18.17	20.09
9	8.34	14.68	16.92	19.68	21.67
10	9.34	15.99	18.31	21.16	23.21
11	10.34	17.28	19.68	22.62	24.72
12	11.34	18.55	21.03	24.05	26.22
13	12.34	19.81	22.36	25.47	27.69
14	13.34	21.06	23.68	26.87	29.14
15	14.34	22.31	25.00	28.26	30.58
16	15.34	23.54	26.30	29.63	32.00
17	16.34	24.77	27.59	31.00	33.41
18	17.34	25.99	28.87	32.35	34.80
19	18.34	27.20	30.14	33.69	36.19
20	19.34	28.41	31.41	35.02	37.57
21	20.34	29.62	32.67	36.34	38.93
22	21.34	30.81	33.92	37.66	40.29
23	22.34	32.01	35.17	38.97	41.64
24	23.24	33.20	36.42	40.27	42.98
25	24.34	34.38	37.65	41.57	44.31
26	25.34	35.56	38.88	42.86	45.64
27	26.34	36.74	40.11	44.14	46.96
28	27.34	37.92	41.34	45.42	48.28
29	28.34	39.09	42.56	46.69	49.59
30	29.34	40.26	43.77	47.96	50.89

P = probability of getting a larger value of χ^2 by chance alone; df = number of degrees of freedom.

The values of χ^2 which are equaled or exceeded just P% of the time are given in the body of the table. Thus, for df = 10, a value of χ^2 of 18.31 is exceeded 5% of the time. On the chance distribution of χ^2 for df = 10, the tail area to the right of 18.31 is 5% of the whole area of the curve.

Note: When there are more than 30 degrees of freedom, the expression $\sqrt{2\chi^2} - \sqrt{2df - 1}$ may be used as z and referred to normal curve tables (the probability desired is the whole area of the normal curve to the right of z).

[Table 13.1 is abridged from Table III of Fisher: *Statistical Methods for Research Workers*, published by Oliver and Boyd, Ltd., Edinburgh, by permission.]

the variance of χ^2 is equal to twice the degrees of freedom. Table 13.1 gives the values of χ^2 exceeded P% of the time for various numbers of degrees of freedom. As the number of degrees of freedom increases, the value of χ^2 exceeded 50% of the time approaches the number of degrees of freedom.

If random samples of size N, say 10, are drawn from the normal distribution, the mean $\bar{x}$ of each sample computed, and the quantities $\sum \left[\dfrac{(x - \bar{x})^2}{\sigma^2} \right]$ formed, these quantities are also distributed as χ^2, not with N degrees of freedom, but with (N - 1) degrees of freedom, in this case, 9. The reduction of one degree of freedom is occasioned by the restraint introduced in using $\bar{x}$ instead of μ. $\Sigma(x - \bar{x}) = 0$, so that only (N - 1) of the deviations $(x - \bar{x})$ need to be known to describe the whole series of N deviations. This particular aspect of the χ^2 distribution can be used to compare an observed standard deviation, $s = \Sigma\sqrt{(x - \bar{x})^2/(N - 1)}$ for a sample drawn from a normally distributed universe, with a standard deviation, σ. In fact, the quantity $\dfrac{(N - 1)(s^2)}{\sigma^2}$ is distributed as χ^2 with df = (N - 1) under the null hypothesis that the standard deviation of the universe is σ. The χ^2 test for variance problems uses the upper (or lower) tail of the curve, and very commonly both tails.

To summarize then, the χ^2 test and the associated χ^2 distribution were evolved for problems with enumeration data. In these problems, its use represents a certain amount of approximation. The use of χ^2 for variance problems when sampling normal distributions is, however, exact. This chapter illustrates the use of χ^2 in problems involving enumeration data.

χ^2 TEST OF GOODNESS OF FIT

The oldest use of χ^2 is the so-called Goodness of Fit test in which an observed distribution according to a qualitative or quantitative scale is compared with that specified by some hypothesis. There was little need in the past for this application of χ^2 in the analysis of oral biological data, but with the recent increase in research in genetics applied to this area, this test in various forms has proved to be a statistical tool of practical importance. The discussion is subdivided according to the way in which the hypothesis specifies the theoretical frequencies.

TABLE 13.2

Comparison of Frequencies of the Three Blood Groups A, AB, and B Among 151 Children from AB × AB Marriages with a Theoretical Distribution[3]

Frequencies	Blood Groups			Total
	A	AB	B	
Observed	39	70	42	151
Theoretical (1:2:1)	37.75	75.50	37.75	151.00
(O – T)	+1.25	–5.50	+ 4.25	0.00

$$\chi^2 = \sum \left[\frac{(O - T)^2}{T} \right] = \frac{(1.25)^2}{37.75} + \frac{(-5.50)^2}{75.50} + \frac{(4.25)^2}{37.75} = 0.920.$$

Proportions in Categories Explicitly Given

Some research has been done on the relationship of blood groupings and caries susceptibility. An example involving blood groups may, therefore, be of interest. Stern states[3]: "progeny from marriages between two parents of the genotype $I^A I^B$ belong to three blood groups: A, AB, and B. They are expected in the proportion 1:2:1, and we may want to compare a specific observation with this expectation." As an example of this type of problem, he presents the data in Table 13.2.

The only restriction on the theoretical frequencies arises from the fact that their total must be the same as the total of the observed frequencies, since this number is fixed at 151. Therefore, the df in this example are the number of categories less one, i.e., $3 - 1 = 2$. Referring the χ^2 value obtained in this case, 0.920, with df = 2, to the tables of the χ^2 distribution, it is noted that the probability of equaling or exceeding* 0.920 is greater than 0.50. The difference between the observed and the expected distributions is, therefore, not significant. In this sense the proportions predicted from Mendelian considerations do indeed fit the distribution of the three blood groups in 151 children.

There are other proportions that can be predicted from Mendel's

---

*We need the notation "equaling or exceeding" since the exact distribution is a discontinuous multinomial. We note that significance can be asserted only by being far out in the upper tail.

laws. When genes exhibiting simple dominance are on different chromosomes and double hybrids are crossed, the proportions of offspring of such matings showing the four phenotypes should be in the ratio 9:3:3:1. This assumes independent segregation of the genes. For example, in rats the agouti or normal gray coloring (A) is dominant to nonagouti (a) and the nonwaltzing behavior (R) is dominant to waltzing (r). Gasic presents data on 115 offspring of double hybrid matings with respect to these two characteristics.[4] His data as well as the theoretical frequencies are given in Table 13.3.

There is one restriction, since the totals of the observed and theoretical distributions are equal. Thus, df = 3 corresponding to P > .50. Thus, the observed distribution does not deviate significantly from the theoretical distribution based upon independent segregation, i.e., the genes of coat color and waltzing behavior may well be located on different chromosomes.

In some instances, the proportions for the categories are divided into subsets within each of which they add up to one, i.e., 100%. Haldane pointed out a type of *amelogenesis imperfecta* that is sex-linked, compared with most types, which are autosomal dominant.[5] In the sex-linked (the gene is in the X chromosome) dominant inheritance, if the female has the gene, 50% of the sons and 50% of the daughters are affected. This would also be true for the case of an autosomal dominant. If the male has the gene, however, *all* the daughters but none of the sons inherit the condition. By combining several pedigrees, Gorlin observed 18 affected daughters and 10 non-affected sons.[6] If the mother contributes the defective gene or if it is an autosomal dominant, 50% of the 18 daughters and 50% of the

TABLE 13.3
Observed and Theoretical (9:3:3:1) Frequencies of Offspring from Double Hybrid Crossing[4]

Phenotype	Number of Offspring		(O – T)
	Observed (O)	Theoretical (T)	
AR	61	64.7	-3.7
Ar	24	21.6	+2.4
aR	22	21.6	+0.4
ar	8	7.2	+0.8
Total	115	115.1	-0.1

$$\chi^2 = \sum \left[\frac{(O - T)^2}{T} \right] = \frac{(-3.7)^2}{64.6} + \frac{(2.4)^2}{21.5} + \frac{(0.4)^2}{21.5} + \frac{(0.8)^2}{7.2} = 0.57$$

TABLE 13.4

Distribution of Amelogenesis Imperfecta of 28 Offspring and Theoretical Distribution Based Upon Autosomal Dominance[8]

Offspring	Number Observed (O)	Number Expected (T)
Affected daughters	18	9
Nonaffected daughters	0	9
Total daughters	18	18
Affected sons	0	5
Nonaffected sons	10	5
Total sons	10	10
Total offspring	28	28

10 sons should be affected. Gorlin's data as well as the theoretical frequencies based on this hypothesis, appear in Table 13.4.

In this case, the theoretical distribution is deduced from two statements of the 1:1 ratio, one for the daughters and one for the sons. The totals are specified for both the daughters and the sons, so that there are two restrictions instead of one, giving a df of 2, i.e., categories -2. The χ^2 is calculated as

$$\chi^2 = \frac{(9)^2}{9} + \frac{(-9)^2}{9} + \frac{(-5)^2}{5} + \frac{(5)^2}{5} = 28, \text{ with P} < .01,$$

yielding high statistical significance. The observed cases do not fit the theoretical distribution based upon autosomal dominance, so that the alternate hypothesis, that of a sex-linked inheritance, can be embraced with the defective gene coming from the male.

Actually, χ^2 of 28 is the sum of two separate χ^2 values that can be calculated from these data, each with 1 df: for the daughters, $\chi^2 = (18 - 9)^2/9 + (0 - 9)^2/9 = 18$; for the sons, $\chi^2 = (6 - 5)^2/5 + (10 - 5)^2/5 = 10$. This is an illustration of the additive nature of χ^2.

Theoretical Distribution Given by a Function with all Parameters Stated

One frequent application of the χ^2 Goodness of Fit test is in the fit of an observed distribution by a theoretical one where the theoretical distribution is completely specified by some function, e.g., bi-

TABLE 13.5

Chance Distribution of Number of White Chips in 1150 Random Samples of Size 10, Drawn From a Universe of 40% White

Number White Chips	Observed Distribution (O)	Expected Distribution (T)	(O - T)
0	5	7.0	-2.0
1	45	46.4	-1.4
2	149	139.1	+9.9
3	245	247.2	-2.2
4	282	288.4	-6.4
5	240	230.8	+9.2
6	129	128.2	+0.8
7	48	48.8	+0.8
8	7 ⎫	12.2 ⎫	
9	0 ⎬ 7	1.8 ⎬ 14.1	
10	0 ⎭	0.1 ⎭	-7.1
Total	1,150	1,150.0	0.0

nomial. Such an example appears in Table 13.5, in which the chance distribution of the number of white (and black) chips in samples of size 10 is given for an actual sampling experiment. The theoretical distribution is given by the binomial $(.6 + .4)^{10}$.

The value of chi square is calculated as

$$\chi^2 = \frac{(-2.0)^2}{7.0} + \frac{(-1.4)^2}{46.4} + \frac{(9.9)^2}{139.1} + \frac{(-2.2)^2}{247.2} + \frac{(-6.4)^2}{288.4} + \frac{(9.2)^2}{230.8} + \frac{(0.8)^2}{128.2}$$

$$+ \frac{(-0.8)^2}{48.8} + \frac{(-7.1)^2}{14.1} = 5.423, \text{ with df} = 8.$$

It was necessary to combine several terminal groups in order that the theoretical frequencies be 5 or more. In order to refer the computed χ^2 to the available tables of χ^2, the theoretical frequencies should not be too small. One convenient rule is that the frequencies should be 5 or more. This χ^2 of 5.423 has only one restriction on the degrees of freedom, since the totals are fixed at 1,150, so that there are 8 degrees of freedom. The probability of equaling or exceeding a χ^2 of 5.423 with 8 df is greater than 50%, showing that the theoretical distribution certainly fits the empirical sampling distribution. "Pooling" of the frequencies to obtain a minimum of 5, causes the test to lose some of its sensitivity. Unfortunately, it is precisely in the tails of the distribution that discrepancies from the null hypothesis are expected to arise.

Theoretical Distribution Given by a Function
with Estimated Parameters

Binomial

Motivated by data presented by Kraus[7] on the frequency of occurrence of the cusp of Carabelli in different racial and ethnic groups, Goodman obtained a theoretical distribution.[8] He stated, "If random mating exists, in a population at equilibrium one may expect the three genotypes in a two-allele system to occur in the proportions $p^2(CC) + 2pq(Cc) + q^2(cc)$, where p is the frequency of the gene C and q is the frequency of its allele c."

The value of p in Goodman's formulation has to be estimated from Kraus' observed data as $p = [2(CC) + 1(Cc)]/2(274) = .4872$. Using this p, the theoretical frequency can be obtained as given in Table 13.6:

$$\chi^2 = \sum \left[\frac{(O - T)^2}{T} \right] = \frac{(28.1)^2}{64.9} + \frac{(-56.0)^2}{137.0} + \frac{(28.0)^2}{72.0} = 46.0.$$

There are two restrictions (p and the total) so that there is only one df. For $\chi^2 = 46.0$, $P < .001$, so that the observed distribution differs significantly from the theoretical distribution, thus leading to the rejection of Goodman's theory.

Normal Curve

Occasionally, one tests the fit of an observed distribution, like that of blood inorganic phosphorus levels of 140 patients with periodontal disease, by a normal distribution.[9,10] The data appear in Table 13.7. The mean blood P is 3.11 mg% and the standard deviation 0.53 mg%. Using these two values and the total (140), the appropriate normal curve can be fitted.

TABLE 13.6
Observed and Expected Frequencies of Various Manifestations of Carabelli's Cusp Assuming Equilibrium and the Validity of Kraus' Hypothesis in Blacks[8]

Phenotypes	Observed (O)	Expected (T)
CC	93	64.9
Cc	81	137.0
cc	100	72.0
Total	274	273.9

TABLE 13.7
Blood Inorganic Phosphorus Values (mg%) of 140 Patients with Periodontal Disease[10] and Fitted Normal Curve

Blood Phosphorus	Number of Patients		$(O - T)^2/T$
	Observed (O)	Normal Curve (T)	
1.70–2.09	3 ⎱ 15	3.9 ⎱ 17.5	
2.10–2.49	12 ⎰	13.6 ⎰	0.36
2.50–2.89	35	30.7	0.60
2.90–3.29	41	41.5	0.01
3.30–3.69	33	31.6	0.06
3.70–4.09	11 ⎱	14.4 ⎱	
4.10–4.49	3 ⎰ 16	3.7 ⎰ 18.7	0.39
4.50–4.89	2	0.6	
Total	140	140.0	$\chi^2 = 1.42$

The theoretical values are obtained from tables of areas of the standard normal curve and also appear in Table 13.7. The frequencies for the first two-class intervals have been combined as have those of the last three intervals, in order to obtain sufficiently large theoretical frequencies in the corresponding intervals, i.e., the "rule of 5." As indicated on page 293 this pooling destroys some of the sensitivity of the test. This restriction may be too severe, as suggested by Cochran.[16] The contributions to χ^2 appear in the last column as $(O - T)^2/T$ and the sum, $\Sigma[(O - T)^2/T] = \chi^2$. The value of χ^2 in this case is 1.42 with (categories – 3) = 5 – 3 = 2 degrees of freedom. In deducing the normal curve, there are three restrictions on the theoretical frequencies (or discrepancies) because of the use of the observed total, observed mean, and observed standard deviation. At df = 2, a χ^2 of 5.99 corresponds to P = 5%. Since the calculated value is less than 5.99, it is statistically not significant. The null hypothesis, that the distribution of blood phosphorus values in patients with periodontal disease follows a normal curve, is therefore not rejected.

Poisson

The Addis counts (red blood cells per aliquot of urine) of 100 children living in Newburgh, N.Y., a community with artificially fluoridated potable water, were obtained by Ast.[11] The urine was diluted 1:10,000 and the count made in a unit volume of the dilution. The data appear in Table 13.8 as the observed number of children with various counts. Since only a very small number of these red blood cells occur in each aliquot of the dilution, the occurrence of an erythrocyte is a rare event. A random distribution of rare events in space (or in time) can be shown to follow the Poisson distribution,

TABLE 13.8
Red Blood Cell Counts in Urine in 100 Children in Newburgh[11] and
Fitted Poisson Distribution

Red Blood Cells Per Aliquot Diluted Urine	Number of Children		$(O - T)^2/T$
	Observed (O)	Poisson (T)	
0	44	35.7	1.93
1	34	36.8	0.21
2	7	18.9	7.49
3	7 ⎫	6.5 ⎫	
4	7 ⎬	1.7 ⎬	
5	0 ⎬ 15	0.3 ⎬ 8.6	4.76
6	1 ⎭	0.1 ⎭	
Total	100	100.0	$\chi^2 = 14.39$

$y = \dfrac{\mu^x}{x!} e^{-\mu}$, where μ is the average number of red blood cells per aliquot. The Poisson distribution is actually a special case of the bi-
nomial when p' is very small and the exponent of the binomial is
very large.

μ is estimated as the observed average count (1.03). By using
tables of e^{-x} with $x = 1.03$, the values of the theoretical frequencies
according to the Poisson, were calculated and appear in the T column
in Table 13.8.

To obtain a sufficiently large theoretical frequency, the frequencies for the classes 3 through 6 red blood cells were combined and
χ^2 calculated as $\Sigma[(O - T)^2/T] = 14.39$. There are two restrictions
on the degrees of freedom (mean and the total) so that df = (categories – 2) = (4 – 2) = 2. For df = 2, $\chi^2 = 9.21$, so that the observed
distribution of children according to their Addis counts differs significantly from the fitted Poisson distribution. The null hypothesis
of random differences among the children (according to the Poisson)
is rejected.

CHI-SQUARE TESTS OF ASSOCIATION (CONTINGENCY) AND HOMOGENEITY

The fourfold table constructed from n independent items or individuals is the summary form of data gathered to demonstrate an association or lack of association between two variables, each with a
dichotomous scale. In some studies, each of the variables under consideration may have more than two categories. In these cases, the
table of n independent observations used to illustrate the degree of

association between two variables, is more extensive than the four-fold table. For example, a 4 × 2-fold table would be needed to accommodate two variables, one with a dichotomous (two) scale of classification and the other with four categories. In the typical association or contingency table, simultaneous measurements of n individuals are made with respect to two qualitative scales. In this case, neither series of marginal totals is fixed. The χ^2 test of significance of the association performed on such a table is often referred to as a χ^2 test of association or contingency.

In a typical experimental situation, one of the variables is controlled or fixed in the sense that the number of items in each category is specified by the investigator in the original design of the experiment. The most familiar type of variable that is fixed in advance is the variable "treatment." The χ^2 test of significance of the differences among the relative frequencies of the various "treatments" is often referred to as the χ^2 test of homogeneity. Actually, this is also a test of association. The arithmetic involved is the same for both types of χ^2 tests. The distinction is, in fact, equivalent to that between correlation in the case of the contingency table and regression in the case of the experimental set-up.

Chi-Square Test of Homogeneity

In the following study, four treatments are compared with respect to their clinical effectiveness. Of patients who were to have a mandibular molar extracted, 447 received inferior alveolar conductive anesthesia with four different concentrations of procaine hydrochloride with epinephrine 1:50,000.[12] The different strength solutions were given at random in a university dental clinic, the clinician not knowing which solution was being used. Standard criteria of results had been set up, so that the resultant anesthesias were classified as satisfactory or unsatisfactory, depending on the depth and duration of anesthesia sufficient for extraction of the offending molar. Results are summarized in Table 13.9.

From this study, we should like to know whether there is any relation between the concentration of procaine used and the clinical effectiveness of the resultant anesthesia. The best way of studying this question is to compare the percentage of satisfactory (or unsatisfactory) cases. Examining the right-hand column of Table 13.9, we see that the differences among the different concentrations are not great, except with 1% procaine, where the percentage of satisfactory cases is lower.

If we were to use the normal curve technique to compare the

TABLE 13.9

The Clinical Effectiveness of Different Concentrations of Procaine
HCl (Epinephrine 1:50,000) for Mandibular Molar Extraction[12]

	Observed			
Procaine Solution	Number of Satisfactory Cases	Number of Unsatisfactory Cases	Total Cases	Percent Satisfactory
1.0%	81	25	$106 = n_1$	$76.4 = p_1$
1.5%	94	10	$104 = n_2$	$90.4 = p_2$
2.0%	101	14	$115 = n_3$	$87.8 = p_3$
4.0%	113	9	$122 = n_4$	$92.6 = p_4$
Total	389	58	447	87.0%

percentages two at a time, many comparisons would be needed. In
fact, if every treatment were compared with every other treatment,
six comparisons would be necessary. By the use of χ^2, however, one
application can answer the question of significance. The null hypothesis is $p_1' = p_2' = p_3' = p_4'$. We shall test this null hypothesis at
the 5% level.

If there were no relation between concentration of procaine and
the percentage of satisfactory cases (the null hypothesis), then the
four different concentrations would produce the same results, i.e.,
87.0% satisfactory cases. Accordingly, 87.0% of the $n_1 = 106 (= 92.2)$
cases receiving the injection of 1% procaine should achieve satisfactory results, 87.0% of the $n_2 = 104 (= 90.5)$ cases receiving 1.5%
procaine should be satisfactory, etc. For the unsatisfactory cases,
13.0% of the 106 (= 13.8) cases receiving 1% procaine should be unsatisfactory, 13.0% of the 104 (= 13.5) cases receiving 1.5% procaine
should be unsatisfactory, etc. In this manner, a table of theoretical
frequencies, T, of no difference or no relation between concentration

TABLE 13.10

Theoretical Results of 447 Inferior Alveolar Injections, Assuming No Difference in the Results with Four Different Anesthetic
Concentrations

Procaine Solution	Number of Satisfactory Cases	Number of Unsatisfactory Cases	Total Cases	Percent Satisfactory
1.0%	92.2	13.8	106.6	87.0
1.5%	90.5	13.5	104.0	87.0
2.0%	100.1	14.9	115.0	87.0
4.0%	106.2	15.8	122.0	87.0
Total	389.0	58.0	447.0	87.0

TABLE 13.11
Calculation of Differences

Procaine Solution	$(O - T)$ Satisfactory Cases	Unsatisfactory Cases	Total
1.0%	81 – 92.2 = –11.2	25 – 13.8 = +11.2	0
1.5%	94 – 90.5 = +3.5	10 – 13.5 = –3.5	0
2.0%	101 – 100.1 = +0.9	14 – 14.9 = –0.9	0
4.0%	113 – 106.2 = +6.8	9 – 15.8 = –6.8	0
Total	0	0	

of anesthetic used and the ensuing results can be constructed (Table 13.10).

The computation of χ^2 proceeds as in Tables 13.11 and 13.12. It is obvious from the $(O - T)$ table (13.11) that three discrepancies serve to determine all eight. If the three $(O - T)$ values for 1.0%, 1.5%, and 2.0% in the "satisfactory" column are known to be –11.2, +3.5, and +0.9, then the discrepancy for 4.0% procaine must be +6.8, so that the sum will be zero. They must total zero since the observed and theoretical total number of satisfactory cases is the same, 389. Knowing these three discrepancies or values, the four values for the unsatisfactory cases are readily obtained since the discrepancies also total zero horizontally. Thus, we can readily see that there are 3 degrees of freedom in this table. The degrees of freedom for association tables can also be calculated from the formula,

$$df = (rows - 1)(columns - 1)$$
$$df = (4 - 1)(2 - 1) = (3)(1) = 3.$$

TABLE 13.12
Contributions to χ^2

Procaine Solution	$\dfrac{(O - T)^2}{T}$ Satisfactory Cases	Unsatisfactory Cases
1.0%	$(-11.2)^2/$ 92.2 = 1.36	$(+11.2)^2/13.8 =$ 9.09
1.5%	$(+ 3.5)^2/$ 90.5 = 0.14	$(- 3.5)^2/13.5 =$ 0.91
2.0%	$(+ 0.9)^2/100.1 = 0.01$	$(- 0.9)^2/14.9 =$ 0.05
4.0%	$(+ 6.8)^2/106.2 = 0.44$	$(- 6.8)^2/15.8 =$ 2.93
Total	1.95	12.98

$$\chi^2 = 1.95 + 12.98 = 14.93$$

From the table of the χ^2 distribution (Table 13.1), we find that at 3 degrees of freedom, a value of χ^2 of 7.82 is equaled or exceeded by chance less than 5% of the time if the null hypothesis is true. The value we have found in the procaine problem, $\chi^2 = 14.93$, is therefore equaled or exceeded less than 5% of the time by chance factors alone (P < 1%). We can state, therefore, that the differences in the percentages of satisfactory cases could not have readily occurred by chance, and that the null hypothesis that the concentration of procaine is not reflected in the clinical results, is untenable.

Seeking Where Significance Lies

The alternative hypothesis, that the concentration of procaine does affect the clinical results, can be embraced. This, however, does not answer an important question. If the concentration of procaine is important, what is the optimal concentration for the best clinical results for the procedures tested? We have just seen that the different procaine concentrations differ significantly among themselves in their clinical effectiveness. This does not necessarily mean that every concentration differs significantly from every other concentration. All the concentrations might differ considerably from each other, although none of the individual differences are significant. On the other hand, one concentration may be differentiated from all the others. These data suggest that the percentage of satisfactory cases with 1.5%, 2.0%, and 4.0% concentration of procaine have about the same percentages of satisfactory cases, but a concentration of 1.0% procaine has a much lower percentage than any of the others. This is indeed reasonable as judged by previous clinical experience. However, a test of these two new null hypotheses suggested by the data cannot be made by the usual significance tests. These tests assume that the null hypotheses were set up before the data were obtained. One way of testing these two new null hypotheses would be to conduct another experiment, which is rather impractical. Another way is to compute χ^2 as if these two null hypotheses had been decided on beforehand, but to adopt a much more stringent critical level in their interpretation.

With this precaution in mind, the arithmetic could proceed as follows. The first three concentrations, 1.5%, 2.0%, and 4.0% are compared with each other (Table 13.13). χ^2 is computed in the usual way and is found to be 1.57, with df = $(3 - 1)(2 - 1) = 2$. As expected, χ^2 is quite small, so that apparently, 1.5%, 2.0%, and 4.0% procaine (epinephrine 1:50,000) may be equally effective for the

TABLE 13.13
Observed Clinical Effectiveness of 1.5%, 2.0%, and 4.0% Procaine
for Mandibular Molar Extractions

Procaine Solution	Number of Satisfactory Cases	Number of Unsatisfactory Cases	Total Cases	Percent Satisfactory
1.5%	94	10	104	90.4%
2.0%	101	14	115	87.8%
4.0%	113	9	122	92.6%
Total	308	33	341	90.3%

procedures tested. The small size of χ^2 is not surprising here since
the three treatments being compared were chosen to be quite similar.
The pooled data for the three higher procaine concentrations are
then compared with the data derived from the 1% procaine. The
resulting fourfold table appears as Table 13.14. χ^2 is calculated as
13.71 with df = 1. This value is quite large, as anticipated, and is
well beyond the conventional .01 level of 3.84 (which, for reasons
previously mentioned, is not applicable here). A test equivalent to
the Scheffé test for *a posteriori* comparisons of means is available.[13]
The observed χ^2 with 1 df (13.71) must exceed the original critical
value of χ^2 with 3 df at the 5% level (7.82). It does exceed this value,
so that clearly 1% procaine may be considered less effective than the
three higher concentrations.

In this problem, the total χ^2 of 14.93 with df = 3 (which measured differences between four concentrations) has essentially been
divided into two parts. The first part is a χ^2 of 1.57 with 2 degrees of
freedom (which measures differences among three concentrations).
The second part is a χ^2 of 13.71 with 1 degree of freedom (which
measures the difference between three concentrations and 1.0%
procaine). The sum of the χ^2 values of the two parts (13.71 + 1.57
= 15.28) with 2 + 1 degrees of freedom is close to the overall χ^2 of

TABLE 13.14
Observed Clinical Effectiveness of 1.0% Procaine and Three Higher
Concentrations

Procaine Solution	Number of Cases Satisfactory	Number of Unsatisfactory Cases	Total Cases	Percent Satisfactory
1.0%	81	25	106	76.4
1.5%, 2%, 4%	308	33	341	90.3
Total	389	58	447	87.0

14.93 with 3 degrees of freedom. For further discussion of subdividing χ^2, see texts by Everitt[13] and by Fleiss.[14]

If the investigator had decided during the designing stage of the study to compare the three higher concentrations with each other, and to compare the lowest concentration with the three higher concentrations taken together, then the two χ^2 values of 1.57 with df = 2 and 13.71 with df = 1 could have been referred to the conventional tables of the χ^2 distribution. However, the level of significance should have been adjusted. An approximate adjustment would be to make each test at the level of $\alpha/2$, say 2.50%, so that the overall level is 5%. See page 110.

χ^2 Test of Association (Contingency)

The χ^2 technique can also be used to analyze more complicated correlation tables which appear in oral biological literature. For example, 5,690 men were classified according to their smoking habits and the presence of calculus deposits.[15] Instead of classifying them merely according to the presence or absence of the smoking habit, the investigator divided the subjects into three smoking groups: those who did not smoke, those who smoked less than 10 grains of tobacco daily, and those who smoked more than 10 grains of tobacco daily. Similarly, calculus formation was classified as no calculus, supragingival calculus, and subgingival calculus. The observations can be tabulated in a 3 × 3 fold table (Table 13.15).

In order to analyze these data, we can take as the null hypothesis the statement that smoking is not related to calculus formation. If this hypothesis were true, then the 568 men who do not smoke should not differ in their calculus accumulation from the men with other smoking habits. They should be distributed in the three classes of calculus formation in the same proportions as each of the other

TABLE 13.15
Observed Distribution of 5,690 Men By Smoking Habits and Calculus Formation[15]

	Nonsmokers	Smokers < 10 Grains/Day	Smokers > 10 Grains/Day	Total
No calculus	284 (50.0%)	606 (33.7%)	1,028 (30.9%)	1,918 (33.7%)
Supragingival calculus	236 (41.5%)	983 (54.7%)	1,871 (56.3%)	3,090 (54.3%)
Subgingival calculus	48 (8.5%)	209 (11.6%)	425 (12.8%)	682 (12.0%)
Total	568 (100.0%)	1,798 (100.0%)	3,324 (100.0%)	5,690 (100.0%)

two types of smokers. To put it another way, the individuals in each smoking status group should be distributed with respect to calculus formation in the same proportions as are given by the group as a whole.

The 568 men who do not smoke are to be distributed, theoretically, among the three classes of calculus formation according to the respective proportions, $1,918/5,690 = 0.3371; 3,090/5,690 = 0.5431$; and $682/5,690 = 0.1199$. Multiplying each proportion by the total number of men in each smoking group gives us the expected or theoretical number of men in each cell. Thus, the expected number of men who do not smoke and have no calculus is obtained as $(1,918/5,690) \times 568 = 191.46$.* As another example of the calculation, the expected number of men who smoke less than 10 grains of tobacco per day and have supragingival calculus can be calculated as $(3,090/5,690) \times 1,798 = 976.42$. In this manner, all of the T values for the 9 cells can be calculated, based on the assumption of the independence of the two variables, smoking and calculus formation.

The calculation of χ^2 for this problem can be facilitated by the construction of a calculation table, and the various steps can be listed within the table. (See Table 13.16 on page 304.) χ^2 is found to be 79.71. The number of degrees of freedom is (rows − 1)(columns − 1) $= (3 − 1)(3 − 1) = (2)(2) = 4$. From Table 13.1, we find that at df = 4, a χ^2 value of 13.28 is equaled or exceeded by chance alone 1% of the time. The value for χ^2 which we have found in this problem, $\chi^2 = 79.71$, is therefore equaled or exceeded by chance alone much less than 1% of the time, and is statistically significant. The null hypothesis that no relationship exists between smoking and calculus formation can, therefore, be rejected. The alternative hypothesis that there is an association between smoking and calculus deposition is, therefore, embraced.

The nature of this association can be ascertained, to some extent, by examining the (O − T) values in the various cells. It can be ascertained better by examining the percentage of the various smoker groups who fall into the various calculus formation categories (Table 13.15). It can be seen that nonsmoking runs more freely with no calculus, and heavy smoking (> 10 grains) runs more freely with calculus formation. In addition, subgingival calculus seems to be affected less by no smoking or heavy smoking than the two other categories of no calculus and supragingival calculus.

---

*In Table 13.16, all theoretical frequencies were calculated to two decimals to make the marginal totals of the theoretical table the same as those of the observed table.

TABLE 13.16
Calculation of χ^2

		Non-Smokers	Smokers < 10 Grains/ Day	Smokers > 10 Grains/ Day	Total
No calculus	O	284	606	1,028	1,918
	T	191.46	606.07	1,120.46	1,918.00
	(O - T)	+92.54	-0.07	-92.46	0
	(O - T)^2/T	44.73	—	7.63	52.36
Supragingival calculus	O	236	983	1,871	3,090
	T	308.46	976.42	1,805.12	3,090.00
	(O - T)	-72.46	+6.58	+65.88	0
	(O - T)^2/T	17.02	0.04	2.40	19.46
Subgingival calculus	O	48	209	425	682
	T	68.08	215.51	398.41	682.00
	(O - T)	-20.08	-6.51	+26.59	0
	(O - T)^2/T	5.92	0.21	1.77	7.89
Total	O	568	1,798	3,324	5,690
	T	568.00	1,798.00	2,324.00	5,690.00
	(O - T)	0	0	0	0
	(O - T)^2/T	67.67	0.24	11.80	79.71 = χ^2

Limitations on the Use of χ^2

Chapters 11 and 12 pointed out that because of certain theoretical considerations, sufficiently large samples are required before the normal curve approximation to the binomial may be used or before the significance test for the fourfold table may be performed by the normal curve. These same considerations also hold true for the use of χ^2 in more extensive tables. It is necessary for all the theoretical frequencies (T) to be 5 or more in order to obtain probabilities of exceeding χ^2 from the conventional Tables of the χ^2 Distribution.

Because this rule requires theoretical frequencies of at least 5, it is often necessary in the case of more extensive tables to regroup the data or to combine existing groups. In this way, the resulting T values will satisfy this requirement. Then the probabilities for χ^2 for the appropriate degrees of freedom can be obtained from the conventional tables.

If not all T values are at least 5, χ^2 can be computed, but the conventional tables do not give the correct probabilities, so considerable caution must be used. In fact, if the P found in the table were in the vicinity of the chosen critical values, the result might be called "of borderline significance." If P is greatly in excess or much less than the critical value, then, of course, the decision to be made is clear. Various studies have been made of the allowable departure from the "rule of five."[16]

MORE EXTENSIVE CORRELATED SAMPLES WITH DICHOTOMOUS SCALES

Somewhat less frequently, an oral biological study involving more than two treatments is so designed that the same individuals are used for each treatment, the outcome of the treatment being recorded on a dichotomous scale.

In a clinical study to determine whether the frequency of anesthesia changed with time, tetracaine 2% was applied to oral mucous membranes. The data were recorded as presence (plus) or absence (minus) of anesthesia at 3, 5, and 10 minutes after the initial application.[17] Results of this study on 29 normal subjects appear in Table 13.17. It may be expected that a correlation exists between the responses at the various times, since the behavior of oral mucous membranes of the same individual at different times is expected to be similar. Consequently, it is necessary to have a test similar to the McNemar test to compare the proportion of pluses for these correlated samples. The appropriate extension of the McNemar test is the Cochran Q test.[18] This test will be illustrated by using the analysis of variance approach.

Table 13.18 presents the data of Table 13.17 reaaranged so that the pluses are replaced by 1's and the minuses by 0's. An analysis of variance can be performed on this two-way layout as follows (obtaining Table 13.19):

$$\text{Between Times SS} = \left[\text{Sum of } \frac{(\text{Column sum})^2}{29} \right] - \text{CT} = \frac{128}{87},$$

$$\text{Between Individuals SS} = \left[\frac{\text{Sum of (Row sum)}^2}{3} \right] - \text{CT} = \frac{1{,}068}{87},$$

$$\text{Total SS} = \text{Sum of } x^2 - \text{CT} = \frac{1{,}880}{87},$$

and

$$\text{Residual SS} = \text{Total SS}$$
$$- (\text{Between Times SS} + \text{Between Individuals SS}) = \frac{684}{87}.$$

TABLE 13.17

Twenty-Nine Individuals Classified According to Presence or Absence of Anesthesia at Three Time Periods After Topical Application of 2% Tetracaine

Individual	Time in Minutes			Number (+)
	3	5	10	
1	−	+	+	2
2	+	+	+	3
3	−	−	−	0
4	−	−	−	0
5	−	+	−	1
6	+	+	−	2
7	+	+	+	3
8	+	+	−	2
9	+	+	+	3
10	−	−	−	0
11	−	+	+	2
12	−	−	+	1
13	+	+	+	3
14	+	+	+	3
15	−	−	+	1
16	−	−	+	1
17	−	+	−	1
18	−	−	−	0
19	−	−	−	0
20	−	−	−	0
21	−	+	+	2
22	+	+	+	3
23	−	−	−	0
24	−	+	+	2
25	−	−	−	0
26	−	−	−	0
27	−	+	+	2
28	−	−	+	1
29	−	+	+	2
Number (+)	8	16	16	40

Cochran's test criterion, Q, here called χ_Q^2, is

$$\chi_Q^2 = \frac{\text{Between Times SS}}{(\text{Between Times + Residual) Mean Square}}.$$

$$\chi_Q^2 = \frac{(128/87)}{(128/87 + 684/87) \div (2 + 56)} = 9.14.$$

TABLE 13.18
Twenty-Nine Individuals Classified According to Response to Topical Application of 2% Tetracaine at Three Time Periods (Rearrangement of Table 12.17)

	Minutes			Row Sum	Number of
	3	5	10	(+)	Individuals
	1	1	1	3	6
	1	1	0	2	2
	1	0	1	2	0
	0	1	1	2	6
	1	0	0	1	0
	0	1	0	1	2
	0	0	1	1	4
	0	0	0	0	9
Column Sum (No +)	8	16	16		29

Σx^2 = Sum of (1^2)'s = Sum of $(+)$'s = 40.

Σ (Column sum)^2 = $(8)^2 + (16)^2 + (16)^2 = 576$.

Σ (Row sum)^2 = $(3)^2(6) + (2)^2(2) + (2)^2(0) + \ldots + (0)^2(9) = 92$.

$$\text{Correction Term (CT)} = \frac{(8 + 16 + 16)^2}{(29)(3)} = \frac{(40)^2}{87}.$$

Cochran showed that this criterion, χ_Q^2, is asymptotically distributed as χ^2 with degrees of freedom equal to (number of treatments -1), in this case 2. The χ_Q^2 of 9.14 with two degrees of freedom is just about at the 1% level of significance (actually $\chi_{1\%}^2 = 9.21$).

If the three time periods in the problem under discussion pertained to independent samples, as in a one-way layout for example, different sets of subjects, the data would be presented as in Table 13.20. To compare the proportions of pluses among the three time periods, the χ^2 test with two degrees of freedom, as discussed earlier in this

TABLE 13.19
Analysis of Variance for Table 11.18

Source of Variation	Degrees of Freedom	Sum of Squares
Between Times	2	128/87
Between Individuals	28	1,068/87
Residual	56	684/87
Total	86	1,880/87

TABLE 13.20

Responses of 29 Individuals at Three Time Periods Classified as if the Three Samples were Independent

Time Period	Response		
Minutes	+	−	Total
3	8	21	29
5	16	13	29
10	16	13	29
Total	40	47	87

$$\chi^2 = 5.92$$

chapter, would be performed. χ^2 can be calculated from the standard formula:

$$\chi^2 = \sum \left[\frac{(O - T)^2}{T} \right] = 5.92, \text{ with df = 2.}$$

The probability of equaling or exceeding this value of χ^2 is slightly more than 5%. The Cochran criterion, χ_Q^2 of 9.14, is larger and corresponds to a probability of just about 1%. Both the χ^2 test for independent samples and the χ_Q^2 test exert proper control over the Type I (α) error, i.e., significance would not be asserted erroneously with more than a stated frequency. However, the use of χ^2 assuming independent samples would increase the probability of the Type II (β) error, i.e., erroneously asserting nonsignificance, thereby decreasing the power of the test.

REFERENCES

1. Pearson, K.: On the criterion that a given system of deviations from the probable in the case of a correlated system of variables is such that it can be reasonably supposed to have arisen from random sampling, Phil Mag 1:157, 1900.

2. Fisher, R. A.: The conditions under which χ^2 measures the discrepancy between observation and hypothesis, Jour Royal Stat Assn, 87:442, 1924.

3. Stern, C.: Principles of Human Genetics, 2nd ed., San Francisco (Calif.), Freeman, 1960, pp. 143–144.

4. Gasic, G.: Unpublished data, Univ of Santiago, Chile.

5. Haldane, J. B. S.: A probable new sex-linked dominant in man, J Hered 25:58, 1937.

6. Gorlin, R. H.: Unpublished data, Univ. of Minnesota.

7. Kraus, B. S.: Occurrence of the Carabelli trait in southwest ethnic groups, Amer J Phys Anthrop 17:117-123, 1959.

8. Goodman, H. O.: Genetic parameters of dentofacial development, J Dent Res 44:174-184, 1965.

9. Tenenbaum, B., and Karshan, M.: Blood studies in periodontoclasia I, J Amer Dent Ass 32:1272, 1945.

10. Karshan, M., Tenenbaum, B., Karlan, F., and Leonard, H.: Blood studies in periodontoclasia II, J Dent Res 25:247, 1946.

11. Ast, D. B.: Data modified from Schlesinger, E. R., Overton, D. C., and Chase, H. C.: Study of children drinking fluoridated and nonfluoridated water, JAMA 160:21-24, 1956.

12. Neuwirth, I., and Chilton, N. W.: The clinical effectiveness of different concentrations of procaine for mandibular extraction, Oral Surg 4:383, 1951.

13. Everitt, B. S.: The Analysis of Contingency Tables, New York, Wiley, 1977.

14. Fleiss, J. L.: Statistical Methods for Rates and Proportions, 2nd ed., New York, Wiley, 1981.

15. Pindborg, J. J.: Tobacco and gingivitis: II. Correlation between consumption of tobacco, ulceromembranous gingivitis and calculus, J Dent Res 28:461, 1949.

16. Cochran, W. G.: Some methods for strengthening the common χ^2 tests, Biometrics, 10:417, 1954.

17. Chilton, N. W., Sternberg, S., and Fertig, J. W.: Studies in the design and analysis of dental experiments. 6. Non-parametric tests (Independent samples with ordinal scales), J Dent Res 42:54, 1963.

18. Cochran, W. G.: The comparison of percentages in matched samples, Biometrika 37:256, 1950.

14

Estimation of Sample Size (Proportions)

In Chapter 6, methods were described for estimating the size of samples for problems involving means in which a true mean or a difference in true means is to be estimated with a specified precision, or in which tests of significance on one or two means are to be made with a suitable power for specified alternatives. It is the purpose of this chapter to describe comparable techniques for estimating sample sizes in problems involving relative frequencies or proportions. As in Chapter 6, before attempting to estimate sample sizes, the investigator needs a certain amount of preliminary data and information as to what contemplated result is considered important or what precision is relevant.[1]

The estimations of sample size discussed in this chapter are concerned with the simple problems of comparing the proportions of two independent or two correlated samples, and of comparing a sample proportion with a universe proportion. Since these are problems involving a single comparison, they may be referred to as "one degree of freedom" problems. They are problems that can be solved approximately by the normal curve test, or by the χ^2 test with one degree of freedom. The exact solution involves the binomial, or Fisher's Exact test for the fourfold table. Problems involving more than one degree of freedom, such as many χ^2 problems, are much more complicated and are not amenable to the solutions offered here, except insofar as they can be broken up into one degree of freedom problems.

CONFIDENCE INTERVALS

One Sample Problem

We are going to observe a single sample of n patients who are considered a random sample of some infinite universe. On this sample we are going to record the number with a definite torus palatinus and hence compute the relative frequency, p. We want this relative frequency to be within a certain distance of the true relative frequency, p', say $D = |p - p'|$. We are willing to have D exceeded only a proportion α of the time. What should n be so that the $(1 - \alpha)$ confidence interval will be $p \pm D$? Assuming n is large enough to use the normal curve instead of the binomial, evidently D should not be less than $z_\alpha(SE_p)$ where z_α is the value of $|z|$ exceeded $\alpha\%$ of the time (two tails) and $SE_p = \dfrac{p'q'}{n}$. To solve this problem, we must plug in some suitable preliminary value of p', based on a small pilot study, past experience with comparable groups, etc. This is analogous to needing some information on σ before being able to solve problems involving a specified precision of a mean $D = |\bar{x} - \mu|$.

Assume that in some group of patients somewhat comparable to the group to be studied, a relative frequency of approximately 20% was observed. Then,

$$\text{est. } SE_p = \sqrt{\frac{(20\%)(80\%)}{n}}.$$

Say the desired precision $D = |p - p'|$ is 6%, meaning that we want our p to be within a distance of 6% one way or the other of the true value p', with a probability of $(1 - \alpha)$ of, say, 95%, of not exceeding D.*

$$6\% = 1.96 \sqrt{\frac{(20\%)(80\%)}{n}}, \quad n = \frac{(1.96)^2(p'q')}{D^2} = 171.$$

This is, of course, a very large number, but relative frequencies are notoriously subject to chance variation and reducing the SE_p to 3%, as in this case, requires a large n. Very often, one cannot think of a

---

*Note that 6% is the difference between two relative frequencies and not the difference expressed as a percentage, say $|p - p'|/p'$.

preliminary value of p' other than 50%. Using 50%, this gives the maximum sample size, in this case, $n = \dfrac{(1.96)^2(50)(50)}{36} = 267$. Of course, n will be smaller if D is increased.

Obviously, after the sample of n is taken, the confidence interval will be calculated *de novo* using $\sqrt{pq/n}$ as the est. SE_p. Since the preliminary value of p' may be shaky, it is preposterous to insist that n be exactly 171. There is also an element of considerable vagueness as to the specified precision, D, and indeed, as to $(1 - \alpha)$. All that is really wanted is a fairly crude estimate of n, e.g., that it is more like 200 than like 50. The calculation is to serve as a guide to the investigator, and not as a straitjacket for his planning.

Two Independent Samples

With some preliminary information or ideas about p_1', p_2' we would know that the relative frequencies of tori in two groups, say blacks and Caucasians, will be in the vicinity of, say, 30%. We are interested in estimating the difference $(p_1' - p_2')$ with a precision of, say, 10% i.e., $D = |(p_1 - p_2) - (p_1' - p_2')| = 10\%$. Computing the

$$\text{est. } SE(p_1 - p_2) = \sqrt{\frac{1}{n}(p_1'q_1' + p_2'q_2')} \text{ with } p_1' = 30\%, p_2' = 40\%,$$

we have

$$10\% = 1.96 \sqrt{\frac{(30\%)(70\%) + (40\%)(60\%)}{n}}.$$

Solving,

$$n = \frac{(1.96)^2(p_1'q_1' + p_2'q_2')}{D^2} = 173 \text{ in each group.}$$

Again, large sample sizes are called for, but 10% implies a $SE(p_1 - p_2)$ of about 5% which is a rather small standard error for the difference in two relative frequencies. If $D = 15\%$, instead of 10%, the required n is only $(10/15)^2 = 44\%$ as large, or 77 in each group.

SIGNIFICANCE TESTS

One Sample Problem

One of the experimental designs occasionally encountered in dental research involves the comparison of a proportion, p (usually expressed as a percentage), obtained from the study of a sample group, with a generally accepted proportion (universe proportion, p'). For example, the percentage of children caries-free at a certain age, living since birth in an area with 1.0 ppm of fluoride in the drinking water, might be compared with the universe percentage of children of the same age caries-free, from nonfluoride areas.[2] Thus, studies of the dental status of many New Jersey children, age 9 at last birthday, disclosed that 29% were caries-free (p'). Examinations of 25 children, age 9, from fluoride areas might show that 10, or 40% (p), were caries-free.

The difference between the percentage of children caries-free from fluoride and nonfluoride areas would then be tested for statistical significance. The following procedure is usually employed. Percentages in repeated samples of 25 children from fluoride-free areas are distributed in a normal curve centered at p' (= 29%), with a standard deviation given by the formula:

$$SE_p = \sqrt{\frac{p'q'}{n}} ,$$

where p' is the universe percentage of children caries-free, q' (= 100% - p') is the universe percentage of children with caries, and n is the size of the sample studied. Thus:

$$SE_p = \sqrt{\frac{(29\%)(71\%)}{25}} = \sqrt{82.4} = 9.1\%.$$

The comparison of the sample from the fluoride area with the universe proportion is made in terms of

$$z = \frac{p - p'}{SE_p} = \frac{40\% - 29\%}{9.1\%} = 1.21.$$

From standard tables of the normal curve, Table 3.1, we find that the probability of equaling or exceeding a difference in percentages corresponding to z = 1.21 is 23% because of chance factors alone. The difference between the percentages of children caries-free in the fluoride and nonfluoride areas is then statistically not significant. The null hypothesis being tested — that there is no difference between the percentages of children age 9, caries-free, from these two areas — therefore cannot be rejected.

While the difference in the percentage of children caries-free is not significant, nevertheless, the investigator may feel that it is suggestive. He may feel that if he were to examine a larger group of 9-year-olds from fluoride areas, the difference would become statistically significant. The question of prime importance, then is: How many children should be examined?

If a larger group of children are examined, the percentage of caries-free individuals will not necessarily be 40%. The true percentage for fluoride areas is expected to be covered by the approximate 95% confidence range.

$$40\% \pm 1.96 \text{ est. SE}_p = 40\% \pm 1.96 \sqrt{\frac{(40\%)(60\%)}{25}}$$

$$\text{or } 20.8\% \text{ to } 59.2\%.*$$

The use of this confidence range may serve as a guide to what true percentage of children caries-free in fluoride areas (and thus, what true difference in percentages) might be important or feasible to expect. Once the true percentage to be focused on has been chosen, the size of the sample necessary in a larger, more definitive study can be estimated by the following method.

Let us suppose that the true percentage chosen is 50%, so that the true difference between the fluoride and the fluoride-free areas is $D = (p_1' - p_0') = (50\% - 29\%) = 21\%$ in favor of the fluoride areas. The investigator must decide next what level of significance he should use, e.g., 1% or 5% (probability of error of the first kind, α), and how large a chance he wants to take of having the difference be not statistically significant when, in fact, the true difference is 21%, an error of the second kind. He may want to take this chance 1% or 5% of the time (β), so that the power of the test ($1 - \beta$) would be 99% or 95%, respectively. Let us take the 1% level of significance with 99% power. The question can then be: "If the true difference between the percentages of 9 year olds, caries-free, from fluoride areas and non-fluoride areas is really 21% in favor of the fluoride areas, how many

---

*More precisely, if the binomial is used instead of the normal curve, from 21.1% to 61.3%.[3]

cases should be studied so that the probability is 99% that the obtained difference in the percentages $(p - p')$ will be statistically significant at the 1% level?" The question as stated calls for a one-tailed test.

In the normal curve of percentages centered at $p_0' = 29\%$, the upper 1% of the area of the curve is found to the right of

$$29\% + 2.33 \sqrt{\frac{(29\%)(71\%)}{n}}.$$

In the normal curve of percentages centered at $p_1' = 50\%$, the lower 1% of the area is found to the left of

$$50\% - 2.33 \sqrt{\frac{(50\%)(50\%)}{n}}.$$

The difference between 50% and 29% thus must equal the sum of

$$2.33 \sqrt{\frac{(29\%)(71\%)}{n}} \text{ and } 2.33 \sqrt{\frac{(50\%)(50\%)}{n}}$$

(Figure 14.1). Solving for n,

$$2.33 \sqrt{\frac{(29\%)(71\%)}{n}} + 2.33 \sqrt{\frac{(50\%)(50\%)}{n}} = 21\%.$$

$$\frac{2.33}{\sqrt{n}} [\sqrt{(29\%)(71\%)} + \sqrt{(50\%)(50\%)}] = 21\%$$

$$\sqrt{n} = \frac{2.33}{21\%} (45.38\% + 50.00\%) = 10.58.$$

$n = 112$ children in the sample from flouride areas. The pilot data are not used.

If the investigator desired to use the 1% level of significance with a power of 95%, the equation to be solved would be:

$$2.33 \sqrt{\frac{(39\%)(71\%)}{n}} + 1.64 \sqrt{\frac{(50\%)(50\%)}{n}} = 21\%,$$

so that n would be 80 children in the sample.

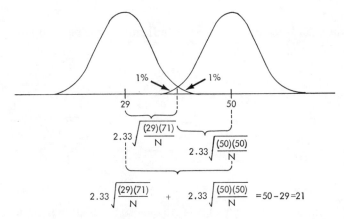

FIG. 14.1 Estimation of Sample Size (Proportions): True Difference = 21%; α = 1%; β = 1%; One-Tailed Test.

In general, for the one-tailed test, $\sqrt{n} = [z_\alpha \sqrt{p_0' q_0'} - z_\beta \sqrt{p_1' q_1'}] \div D$, where z_α is the value of z (positive) cutting $\alpha\%$ in the *upper tail* of the normal curve centered at p_0' and z_β is the value of z (negative) below which we find $\beta\%$ of the curve centered at p_1'.

In a two-tailed test with α = 1%, β = 1%, only 1/2 α, here .005, is put into the upper tail of the curve centered at 29%. Then

$$\sqrt{n} = \frac{[2.58\sqrt{(29\%)(71\%)} + 2.33\sqrt{(50\%)(50\%)}]}{21\%} = 11.12, n = 124.*$$

Again, just as in Chapter 6, note that in a confidence interval problem, the part involving the second curve centered at the alternative value is eliminated.

The solution to the one sample problem also affords the solution to the problem of two correlated samples (see the McNemar test, p. 280). In this test, the problem is transformed into a one-sample problem by considering only the untied pairs. Then the comparison is made between the proportion of untied pairs of one type and p' = 50.0%. Of course, to get a meaningful solution, one must have some idea of the proportion of samples that will be untied.

---

*Actually, two samples of 124 will have considerably more than 99% power, for a difference of 21% below 29%. This is because the curve centered at 29% – 21% = 8%, has a smaller SE_p than the one centered at 50%. It is only when the reference value p_0' is 50% that the power would be the same for plus or minus D.

TABLE 14.1
Preliminary Study of Effects of Medicaments on Sterility of Root Canal Contents

Drug	Sterile	Not Sterile	Total	% Sterile
Formocresol	9	6	$15 = n_1$	$60.0 = p_1$
Penicillin	5	10	$15 = n_2$	$33.3 = p_2$
Total	14	16	30	$46.7 = p_0$

Two Sample Problem

Although occasionally we may find a situation in which a sample proportion is to be compared to a universe proportion, such situations are rather infrequent. The more common case is that in which proportions obtained from two separate samples are compared, i.e., the four-fold table problem. For example, the proportion of cases in which infected root canals become sterile after medication with a standard root canal antiseptic, such as formocresol, may be compared with the corresponding proportion for penicillin.[4] Thirty comparable cases were treated, half with one drug and half with the other, and the results tabulated in a fourfold table (Table 14.1).

The difference in the percentages becoming sterile $(p_1 - p_2)$ was 26.7%. While this difference appears large, it is statistically not significant, as may be seen by comparison with the standard error of the difference.

$$SE_{p_1 - p_2} = \sqrt{SE_{p_1}^2 + SE_{p_2}^2} = \sqrt{\frac{2(46.7\%)(53.3\%)}{15}}$$

$$= \sqrt{2(165.94)} = \sqrt{331.88} = 18.2\%.$$

In the normal curve of differences in percentages centered at 0%, we find

$$z = \frac{(p_1 - p_2) - 0}{SE_{p_1 - p_2}} = \frac{26.7\%}{18.2\%} = 1.47.*$$

*For small samples, especially if z is significant, it is often advisable to make a "correction for continuity" (see page 270). In this case $p_1 - p_2 = 20.0\%$, and $z = \dfrac{20.0\%}{18.2\%} = 1.10$.

While this difference of 26.7% in successful results is statistically not significant, it certainly appears suggestive, so that the investigator might like to know how many cases in each group would be needed for significance to be asserted. The 95% confidence range is approximately from 26.7% – 2(18.2%) to 26.7% + 2(18.2%), or from less than 0 to 63.7% in favor of the formocresol medication. Suppose we want to know how many cases are necessary for significance to be asserted at the 5% level with a power of 95%, when the true difference between the percentages of successful cases is, say 30% in favor of the formocresol medication (a one-tailed test); $D = (p_1' - p_2') = 30\%$. Let us take the true value for the formocresol group to be 60%, the value found in the preliminary study. It then follows that the true value for the penicillin medication is assumed to be 30%, giving $(p_1' - p_2') = 30\%$. The average for the two medications is 45%. The following procedure will afford an estimate of the number of cases to be studied in each group under the above conditions.

Using $\alpha = \beta = 5\%$, in the normal curve of differences in percentages centered at 0%, the upper 5% of the curve is found to the right of

$$0\% + 1.64 \sqrt{\frac{(45\%)(100\% - 45\%)}{n_1} + \frac{(45\%)(100\% - 45\%)}{n_2}}.$$

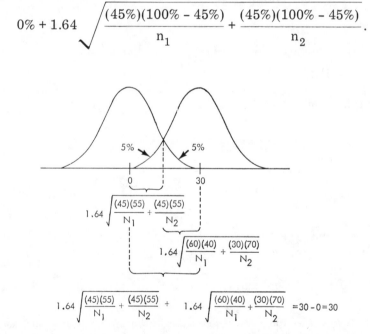

$$1.64 \sqrt{\frac{(45)(55)}{N_1} + \frac{(45)(55)}{N_2}} + 1.64 \sqrt{\frac{(60)(40)}{N_1} + \frac{(30)(70)}{N_2}} = 30 - 0 = 30$$

FIG. 14.2 Estimation of Sample Size (Proportions): True Difference = 30%; $\alpha = 5\%$, $\beta = 5\%$; One-Sided Significance Test.

In the normal curve of differences in proportions centered at the assumed true difference of 30%, the lower 5% of the area is found to the left of

$$30\% - 1.64 \sqrt{\frac{(60\%)(100\% - 60\%)}{n_1} + \frac{(30\%)(100\% - 30\%)}{n_2}}.$$

The total distance between 30% and 0% must equal the sum of

$$1.64 \sqrt{\frac{(45\%)(55\%)}{n_1} + \frac{(45\%)(55\%)}{n_2}}$$

$$\text{and } 1.64 \sqrt{\frac{(60\%)(40\%)}{n_1} + \frac{(30\%)(70\%)}{n_2}}.$$

See Figure 14.2. Since we are taking the sample size of each group to be equal ($n_1 = n_2 = n$)

$$30\% = 1.64 \sqrt{\frac{(2)(45\%)(55\%)}{n}}$$

$$+1.64 \sqrt{\frac{(60\%)(40\%)}{n} + \frac{(30\%)(70\%)}{n}}.$$

Simplifying, and solving for n,

$$\sqrt{n} = \frac{1.64}{30\%} [\sqrt{(2)(45\%)(55\%)} + \sqrt{(60\%)(40\%) + (30\%)(70\%)}]$$

$$\sqrt{n} = \frac{1.64}{30\%} (70.36\% + 67.08\%) = \frac{(1.64)(137.44)}{30} = 7.48.$$

so that n is about 56 cases in each group.* Of course, the investigator need not take *exactly* 56, which serves only as a guide in planning the study.

In the more usual question, one is interested in a difference,

---

*If the original formocresol percentage were based on a large enough series of observations so as to be considered the true or universe percentage (p'), then $p'q'/n$ is close to zero and we are back in the one sample case. The same significance and power would be obtained with only about one-half of the indicated number of cases in only one group, i.e., the penicillin group (in this instance, 28 cases).

$D = |p_1' - p_2'|$ regardless of the sign. In such a case, $\alpha/2$ is put into each tail of the curve centered at 0. The solution then becomes, for $\alpha = 5\%$ and $\beta = 5\%$,

$$\sqrt{n} = [1.96\sqrt{2(45\%)(55\%)} + 1.64\sqrt{(60\%)(40\%) + (30\%)(70\%)}] \div 30\%$$
$$= 8.26, n = 68.$$

Again, because the standard deviations of the sampling distributions are not constant under the alternatives of $(p_1' - p_2') = +30\%$ and of $(p_1' - p_2') = -30\%$, the indicated sample sizes do not give the same power for both alternatives.

The methods just described for estimating sample sizes, given the anticipated true difference, the respective true percentages on which the true difference is based, and the desired significance level and power of the test, have been utilized in the construction of Table 14.2, (one-tailed test) and Table 14.3 (two-tailed test), for $\alpha = 1\%$ with a power of the test of 99%, i.e. $(1 - \beta)$. Tables 14.3 and 14.3a are analogous tables for $\alpha = 5\%$ with a power of 95%. Tables 14.4 and 14.4a present this information for $\alpha = 5\%$ with a power of 80%, which are criteria used quite frequently in dental and oral clinical trials. For computational convenience, the values in these tables were calculated by the arc sine transformation of percentages.[5]

These tables show immediately, for any given choice of the true percentage in one group and the anticipated true difference between percentages, the sample size necessary in each group corresponding to the desired significance level and power of the test, for either a one-tailed or a two-tailed test. Thus, if the true percentage of infected root canals becoming sterile after routine medication is assumed to be 45%, and a new drug is assumed to increase the percentage becoming sterile by 30%, Table 14.2 shows us (for the one-tailed test) in the cell corresponding to 45% (vertical scale) and 30% (horizontal scale), the number of cases for each group, for $\alpha = 1\%$ with a power of 99%, namely, 111. In a similar manner, should the number of cases in each group be desired, using the criteria of $\alpha = 5\%$ with a power of 80%, for a two-tailed test, Table 14.4a would be the table of reference. Thus, if the true percentage of infected root canals becoming sterile after routine medication is assumed to be 35%, and a new drug is expected to increase the percentage becoming sterile by 40%, the number of cases for each group is found by referring to the cell corresponding to 35% (vertical scale) and 40% (horizontal scale), namely, 23. In the event that the percentage for one universe is actually known (p') so that a sample is necessary only in the other group, the necessary size in the latter group is approximately one-half the number indicated in the tables.

TABLE 14.2
Estimated Sample Sizes Necessary In Each of Two Groups Corresponding to Various Assumed True Percentages In Order to Ensure Significance at the 1% Level With a 99% Power of the Test (One-Tailed Significance Test)

Smaller True %	Anticipated True Increase in %									
	5%	10%	15%	20%	25%	30%	35%	40%	45%	50%
5%	1,169	365	191	122	86	65	51	42	35	29
10%	1,876	538	266	163	112	82	63	50	41	34
15%	2,489	683	327	195	131	95	72	56	45	37
20%	3,011	804	377	221	147	105	78	61	48	39
25%	3,446	903	417	241	158	111	82	63	50	39
30%	3,794	980	447	256	165	115	84	64	50	39
35%	4,054	1,035	466	264	169	117	84	63	48	37
40%	4,228	1,068	476	267	169	115	82	61	45	34
45%	4,315	1,079	476	264	165	111	78	56	41	29
50%	4,315	1,068	466	256	158	105	72	50	35	
55%	4,228	1,035	447	241	147	95	63	42		
60%	4,054	980	417	221	131	82	51			
65%	3,794	903	377	195	112	65				
70%	3,446	804	327	163	86					
75%	3,011	683	266	122						
80%	2,489	538	191							
85%	1,876	365								
90%	1,169									

TABLE 14.2a
Estimated Sample Sizes Necessary In Each of Two Groups Corresponding to Various Assumed True Percentages In Order to Ensure Significance at the 1% Level With a 99% Power of the Test (Two-Tailed Significance Test)

Smaller True %	Anticipated True Increase in %									
	5%	10%	15%	20%	25%	30%	35%	40%	45%	50%
5%	1,297	405	211	135	96	72	57	46	38	32
10%	2,083	597	295	181	124	91	70	56	46	38
15%	2,763	758	363	217	146	105	80	63	50	41
20%	3,343	893	419	246	163	116	87	67	53	43
25%	3,826	1,003	463	268	175	124	91	70	55	44
30%	4,212	1,088	496	284	184	128	94	71	55	43
35%	4,501	1,149	518	293	188	129	94	70	53	41
40%	4,694	1,185	529	296	188	128	91	67	50	38
45%	4,790	1,198	529	293	184	124	87	63	46	32
50%	4,790	1,185	518	284	175	116	80	56	38	
55%	4,694	1,149	496	268	163	105	70	46		
60%	4,501	1,088	463	246	146	91	57			
65%	4,212	1,003	419	217	124	72				
70%	3,825	893	363	181	96					
75%	3,343	758	295	135						
80%	2,763	597	211							
85%	2,083	405								
90%	1,297									

TABLE 14.3

Estimated Sample Sizes Necessary In Each of Two Groups Corresponding to Various Assumed True Percentages In Order to Ensure Significance at the 5% Level With a 95% Power of the Test (One-Tailed Significance Test)

		Anticipated True Increase in %									
		5%	10%	15%	20%	25%	30%	35%	40%	45%	50%
	5%	584	183	95	61	43	33	26	21	17	15
	10%	938	269	133	81	56	41	32	25	21	17
	15%	1,244	341	163	98	66	47	36	28	23	19
	20%	1,506	402	189	111	73	52	39	30	24	19
	25%	1,723	452	208	121	79	56	41	32	25	20
	30%	1,897	490	224	128	83	58	42	32	25	19
Smaller True %	35%	2,027	517	233	132	85	58	42	32	24	19
	40%	2,114	534	238	133	85	58	41	30	23	17
	45%	2,157	539	238	132	83	56	39	28	21	15
	50%	2,157	534	233	128	79	52	36	25	17	
	55%	2,114	517	224	121	73	47	32	21		
	60%	2,027	490	208	111	66	41	26			
	65%	1,897	452	189	98	56	33				
	70%	1,723	402	163	81	43					
	75%	1,506	341	133	61						
	80%	1,244	269	95							
	85%	938	183								
	90%	584									

TABLE 14.3a

Estimated Sample Sizes Necessary In Each of Two Groups Corresponding to Various Assumed True Percentages In Order to Ensure Significance at the 5% Level With a 95% Power of the Test (Two-Tailed Significance Test)

		Anticipated True Increase in %									
		5%	10%	15%	20%	25%	30%	35%	40%	45%	50%
	5%	584	219	115	73	52	39	31	25	21	17
	10%	938	323	159	98	67	49	38	30	25	20
	15%	1,244	410	196	117	79	57	43	34	27	22
	20%	1,506	483	226	133	88	63	47	36	29	23
	25%	1,723	542	250	145	95	67	49	38	30	24
	30%	1,897	588	268	153	99	69	51	38	30	23
Smaller True %	35%	2,027	621	280	159	101	70	51	38	29	22
	40%	2,114	641	286	160	101	69	49	36	27	20
	45%	2,157	648	286	159	99	67	47	34	25	17
	50%	2,157	641	280	153	95	63	43	30	21	
	55%	2,114	621	268	145	85	57	38	25		
	60%	2,027	588	250	133	79	49	31			
	65%	1,897	542	226	117	67	39				
	70%	1,723	483	196	98	52					
	75%	1,506	410	159	73						
	80%	1,244	323	115							
	85%	938	219								
	90%	584									

TABLE 14.4
Estimated Sample Sizes Necessary In Each of Two Groups Corresponding to Various Assumed True Percentages In Order to Ensure Significance at the 5% Level With an 80% Power of the Test (One-Tailed Significance Test)

		Anticipated True Increase in %									
		5%	*10%*	*15%*	*20%*	*25%*	*30%*	*35%*	*40%*	*45%*	*50%*
Smaller True %	5%	334	104	55	35	25	19	15	12	10	8
	10%	536	154	76	46	32	23	18	14	12	10
	15%	711	195	93	56	38	27	21	16	13	11
	20%	860	230	108	63	42	30	22	17	14	11
	25%	984	258	119	69	45	32	24	18	14	11
	30%	1,084	280	128	73	47	33	24	18	14	11
	35%	1,158	296	133	75	48	33	24	18	14	11
	40%	1,208	305	136	76	48	33	24	17	13	10
	45%	1,232	308	136	75	47	32	22	16	12	8
	50%	1,232	305	133	73	45	30	21	14	10	
	55%	1,208	296	128	69	42	27	18	12		
	60%	1,158	280	119	63	38	23	15			
	65%	1,084	258	108	56	32	19				
	70%	984	230	93	46	25					
	75%	860	195	76	35						
	80%	711	154	55							
	85%	536	104								
	90%	334									

TABLE 14.4a
Estimated Sample Sizes Necessary In Each of Two Groups Corresponding to Various Assumed True Percentages In Order to Ensure Significance at the 5% Level With an 80% Power of the Test (Two-Tailed Significance Test)

		Anticipated True Increase in %									
		5%	*10%*	*15%*	*20%*	*25%*	*30%*	*35%*	*40%*	*45%*	*50%*
Smaller True %	5%	424	132	69	44	31	24	19	15	13	11
	10%	680	195	96	59	40	30	23	18	15	12
	15%	982	248	119	71	48	34	26	20	12	13
	20%	1,092	292	137	80	53	38	28	22	17	14
	25%	1,250	328	151	88	57	40	30	23	18	14
	30%	1,376	355	162	93	60	42	31	23	18	14
	35%	1,470	375	169	96	61	42	31	23	17	13
	40%	1,533	387	173	97	61	42	30	22	12	12
	45%	1,565	391	173	96	60	40	28	20	15	11
	50%	1,565	387	169	93	57	38	26	18	13	
	55%	1,533	375	162	88	53	34	23	15		
	60%	1,470	355	151	80	48	30	19			
	65%	1,376	328	137	71	40	24				
	70%	1,250	292	119	59	31					
	75%	1,092	248	96	54						
	80%	982	195	69							
	85%	680	132								
	90%	424									

If other levels of significance and/or powers are desired, the reader can resort to appropriate substitution for the critical values in the equations developed in this chapter, or he can refer to other tables which are also available, which give sample sizes for different values of D, α, and β.[6-8] Many of the tables try to improve on the normal curve approximation by introducing continuity corrections. These requirements may not be of too great an importance, however, since there are so many qualitatively assessed factors: α, β, D, and a provisional p'. After all, what is needed is an *idea* of n, *not* whether it is 112 or 113!

REFERENCES

1. Chilton, N. W., and Fertig, J. W.: The estimation of sample size in experiments. 2. Using comparison of proportions, J Dent Res 32:606–612, 1953.

2. Wisan, J. M.: Dental caries and fluorine-water, Trenton (N.J.), N.J. Dept of Health, Pub Health News 27:139, 1944.

3. Mainland, D.: Elementary Medical Statistics, 2nd ed., Philadelphia, Saunders, 1963, pp. 358–361.

4. Ostrander, F. D., Crowley, M. C., and Dowson, J.: A clinical study of the treatment of root canal and periapical infections with penicillin, J Dent Res 26:403, 1947.

5. Statistical Research Group, Columbia Univ: Selected Techniques of Statistical Analysis, Chap. 16, New York, McGraw-Hill, 1947.

6. Feigl, P.: A graphical aid for determining sample size when comparing two independent proportions, Technical Report No. 6, Department of Biostatistics, School of Public Health and Community Medicine, Seattle, Washington, 1977.

7. Natrella, M. G.: Experimental Statistics, Washington, DC, National Bureau of Standards, Handbook 91, 1963.

8. Fleiss, J. L.: Statistical Methods for Rates and Proportions, 2nd ed., New York, Wiley, 1981.

15
Ranking Tests

The data analyzed in Chapters 3 through 10 were primarily bona fide measurements, such as mg% salivary calcium. The results of many oral biological studies are expressed in this form. Other studies, however, give rise to qualitative or nominal scales, such an Angle's Classification of Malocclusion. Many of these nominal scales are, in fact, dichotomous (plus or minus, react or nonreact). The analysis of such qualitatively scaled data was discussed in Chapters 11, 12, 13, and 14. Still other studies yield data expressed in terms of scores or indices (such as P-M-A Index)*, which, while being numerical and simulating measurements, are not really conventional measurements. They may be considered as an ordering mechanism, thus giving rise to an ordinal scale. Although ordinally scaled data simulate measurement data, the methods of analysis are often different. It is the purpose of this chapter to present some of these methods.

The usual method of analyzing measurements makes some assumption about the underlying form of the distribution that involves certain parameters, such as the normal curve with its mean and standard deviation. The data are then analyzed by estimating the parameters and comparing the estimates. These various techniques in the field of measurements have been referred to as *parametric methods* and include such well-known tests as the t-test, analysis of variance, etc. Parametric methods exist for many types of experimental de-

---

*The statistical methods described in this chapter apply equally as well to other indices. For a discussion of these indices, the reader is referred to Chilton, N.W., ed., International Conference on Agents Used in the Prevention/Treatment of Periodontal Diseases. Jour Perio Research, supplement 14, 1974.

signs, such as independent samples, correlated samples, and Latin squares.

The parametric methods are not suitable for analyzing data classified according to a nominal scale, nor are they particularly appropriate for data of the ordinal variety, e.g., many types of scores. Appropriate methods for dealing with data of these types are often referred to as *nonparametric* or, better, *distribution-free methods*. These methods are independent of the explicit form of, and the values of the parameters in, the underlying distribution.

Some nonparametric methods for nominally scaled data have already been discussed in Chapters 11 through 14, e.g., binomial, χ^2 goodness of fit test, normal curve or χ^2 test for the fourfold table. Many of the nonparametric tests for *ordinal scales are ranking tests*. A number of these ranking tests will be discussed in the present chapter. The nonparametric methods, suitable for nominal or ordinal scales, may also be used with measurements from a distribution whose form is unknown, or difficult to manipulate.

Data in an ordinal scale may be indicated as scores or some qualitative variable, such as mild, moderate, or marked response. Such data have the inherent property of a grading, so that one measurement is not only different from, but also has a definite order relation with, the others, i.e., "greater than" or "less than," "more marked," or "less marked." Another property of such data is that equal differences between measurements may not have the same meaning all along the scale. For example, it does not necessarily follow that P-M-A indices of 4 and 9 differ to the same extent in meaning as P-M-A indices of 16 and 21. The underlying distributions of such data may be of forms that in general are unknown.

The tests to be described here are valid for data that are truly ordinal in nature. They are also applicable to weak measurements, such as some scores that may often be interpreted better when transformed to an ordinal scale. They may also be used with measurements from a distribution whose form is unknown so that the appropriate parametric test is not available, or whose form is known but difficult to manipulate so that the appropriate parametric test is not feasible. On occasion, economy of time justifies the use of these tests even when the appropriate assumptions as to distribution form are satisfied and the parametric test is well known (e.g., the use of ranks in the case of two independent samples of measurements where the assumptions of normality and equality of variance are satisfied so that the conventional t-test could be performed).

In this chapter, we shall present analogues of parametric tests for two samples and more than two samples, correlated as well as independent, where the appropriate parametric tests would be the t-test or the analysis of variance and F-test. The tests that will be presented are, as in the parametric case, most sensitive to differences in location (i.e., centering constants) and are based on ranks assigned to the original data.

TWO INDEPENDENT SAMPLES

As part of a larger clinical study of the effect of dentifrices on gingival inflammation, Chilton and Di Dio[1] measured existing gingival inflammation of 19 dental students in terms of their P-M-A scores (Table 15.1). The students were first randomly assigned to two groups, A with 10 individuals and B with 9. These groups were the subjects of a further experiment not discussed at this time. The initial P-M-A scores of these two independent groups of students will be used for illustrative purposes. The standard parametric test of

TABLE 15.1
P-M-A Scores of 19 Dental Students Divided Randomly Into Two Groups

Group A	Group B
17	6
2	2
2	17
13	9
6	6
10	7
3	7
0	9
12	29
3	
Total 68	92
N_A 10	N_B 9

$$\Sigma x = \text{Total of all scores} = 160,$$

$$\Sigma x^2 = 2{,}230,$$

$$\frac{(\text{Group A total})^2}{N_A} + \frac{(\text{Group B total})^2}{N_B} = \frac{(68)^2}{10} + \frac{(92)^2}{9} = 1{,}402.73,$$

$$\text{Correction term (CT)} = \frac{(160)^2}{19} = 1{,}347.38.$$

TABLE 15.2
Analysis of Variance of Measurements of Table 15.1

Source of Variation	Degrees of Freedom	Sum of Squares (SS)	Mean Square (MS)
Between Groups	1	55.35	55.35
Within Groups	17	827.27	48.66
Total	18	882.62	

statistical significance of the difference in means is the t-test, or the equivalent F-test for two independent samples. The sums of squares (SS) for the one-way analysis of variance are calculated as follows:

Between Groups SS = Sum of $[(\text{Group Sum})^2/\text{No. Indiv. in Group}]$ - CT,

Total SS = Sum of x^2 - CT,

Within Groups SS = Total SS - Between Groups SS (Table 15.2).

$$F_{1,17} = \frac{\text{Between Groups MS}}{\text{Within Groups MS}} = \frac{55.35}{48.66} = 1.14;$$

not significant at the 5% level.

In the case of two samples, $F_{1,17}$ is the square of t with 17 degrees of freedom.

The preceding parametric analysis would be appropriate if the data were actual measurements and satisfied the necessary criteria. However, this analysis may not be appropriate for the P-M-A units, which are scores and whose distribution, furthermore, may be fairly skew. Moreover, the necessary assumption of equal variability may often not be tenable. For these reasons, one might feel more comfortable using a distribution-free or nonparametric technique in this case.

If the division of the 19 individuals into two groups were truly random, then the high scores and the low scores should be about equally divided between the two groups. Contrariwise, the high scores should tend to fall predominantly in one group and the low scores in the other. The *Wilcoxon Rank Sum test*[2] may be applied to analyze the data to investigate the randomness of the division of the scores. The scores are ordered without regard to group, and ranks assigned to them. The distribution of the ranks between the two groups is then examined. Thus the lowest score, 0, occurs in Group A and is given a rank of 1. The score of 2 occurs twice in Group A and once in Group B, using up ranks 2, 3, and 4. When ties such as this occur, the average rank is given to each member of the tie. In this case, the average rank is 3. The next ordered score is 3, which occurs twice in Group A, so that the average of ranks 5 and 6, or 5.5, is assigned to each of these subjects. Table 15.3 was constructed in this manner.

The ranks are now summed for one of the groups, say, the smaller one, Group B, giving a rank sum, T_B, of 101.5. To evaluate the significance of T_B, it is necessary to have the sampling distribution under the null hypothesis (i.e., equally likely assignment of ranks).

TABLE 15.3
Ranked P-M-A Scores of Two Groups of Dental Students

Group A		Group B	
Scores	Ranks (Low to high)	Ranks (Low to high)	Scores
0	1.0		
2	3.0		
2	3.0		
		3.0	2
3	5.5		
3	5.5		
6	8.0		
		8.0	6
		8.0	6
		10.5	7
		10.5	7
		12.5	9
		12.5	9
10	14.0		
12	15.0		
13	16.0		
17	17.5		
		17.5	17
		19.0	29

Sum = T_A = 88.5,   *Sum* = T_B = 101.5,

Σx = Sum of all ranks = $T_A + T_B = (N_A + N_B)(N_A + N_B + 1)/2 = 190.0$,

Σx^2 = Sum of squared ranks

$= [(1)^2 + (3)^2 + (3)^2 + (3)^2 + (5)^2 + (5)^2 + (8)^2 + \ldots + (19)^2]$

$= 2,464.00.$

Exact Test

The distribution of T_B can be evaluated by forming all possible divisions of the ranks from 1 to $(N_A + N_B)$ into two groups of size N_A and N_B, respectively [i.e., all possible ways in which N_B ranks can be picked out of $(N_A + N_B)$ ranks]. The total number of divisions is given by $(N_A + N_B)!/(N_A!)(N_B!)$. In our example, this is 92,378. Each of these ways is equally likely under the null hypothesis and leads to a value of T_B, not all values of which are distinct, however. The distribution is symmetrical about its mean, Mean $T_B = N_B(N_B + N_A + 1)/2 = 9(9 + 10 + 1)/2 = 90$. An observed value of T_B would be referred to this distribution to assess its significance (i.e., to see how far out it lies in either tail of the distribution). In the present example, T_B exceeds the mean. The probability of a value of T_B of 101.5 or more is 0.19, or $2(0.19) = 0.38$ for a two-tailed test. Limited tables of the distribution of T are readily available,[3] and more extensive tables can also be found.[4]

Approximate Test

The normal curve approximation may be used even for samples as small as 9 and 10, because of the symmetry of the distribution. The mean and the standard deviation of the distribution of T_B are given by

$$\text{Mean } T_B = \frac{N_B(N_B + N_A + 1)}{2} = \frac{9(9 + 10 + 1)}{2} = 90;$$

$$\text{SE}_{TB} = \sigma_{TB} = \sqrt{\frac{N_A N_B (N_A + N_B + 1)}{12}}$$

$$= \sqrt{\frac{(9)(10)(9 + 10 + 1)}{12}} = \sqrt{150}.$$

To see whether T_B of 101.5 is significantly different from its mean of 90, the normal deviate is computed as

$$z = \frac{(T_B - \text{mean } T_B)}{\sigma_{TB}} = \frac{(101.5 - 90)}{\sqrt{150}} = 0.939.$$

The probability of exceeding this value is 0.35, for a two-tailed test.

It is often simpler arithmetically to compute χ^2 with one degree of freedom, instead of the normal deviate. In this example,

$$\chi^2 = \frac{(T_B - \text{mean } T_B)^2}{\sigma_{TB}^2} = \frac{(101.5 - 90)^2}{150} = 0.882,$$

where χ^2 is the square of the normal deviate and corresponds to the same probability, 0.35.

The normal curve approximation to the exact distribution can be improved by using a continuity correction in which T_B is brought $\frac{1}{2}$ unit closer to the mean. Then,

$$\text{Corr. } \chi^2 = \frac{(101 - 90)^2}{150} = 0.807; P = .37.$$

This probability is close to that obtained with the exact test (0.38).

Little work has been done on the distribution of T in the event of ties, but from what has been done, it appears that the effect of a moderate number of ties is negligible. The presence of ties decreases the variance of T, so that the use of the exact or the approximate distribution of T is conservative, i.e., the probability (tail areas) under the null hypothesis is actually less than that given in the tables.

Several comments are worthwhile at this point. If the scores were ranked from high to low instead of from low to high, the value of $(T_B - \text{mean } T_B)$ would be the same except for sign. If the ranks for Group A were summed instead of those for Group B, the distribution of T_A would have to be used. The mean of this distribution would have to be calculated by interchanging the role of A and B in the formulas already given. The variance of T_A, σ_{TA}^2, is the same as σ_{TB}^2. The same normal deviate or χ^2 would be obtained when making the significance test since $(T_A - \text{mean } T_A) = - (T_B - \text{mean } T_B)$.*

---

*A test equivalent to the Wilcoxon Rank Sum Test is the Mann-Whitney U test,[5] in which a statistic, U, is calculated, where

$$U = (N_A)(N_B) + \frac{N_B(N_B + 1)}{2} - T_B = (10)(9) + \frac{(9)(10)}{2} - 101.5 = 33.5$$

$$\text{Mean } U = \frac{(N_A)(N_B)}{2} = 45.0$$

$$\sigma_U^2 = \sigma_{TB}^2 = 150.$$

Thus, $\chi^2 = (U - \text{mean } U)^2/\sigma_U^2 = 0.882$.

Some investigators use the "T-test", while others use the "U-test," but they are equivalent.

TABLE 15.4
Analysis of Variance of Ranks of Table 15.3

Source of Variation	Degrees of Freedom	Sum of Squares
Between Groups	1	27.92
Within Groups	17	536.08
Total	18	564.00

Analysis of Variance Approach

The value of χ^2 obtained with the approximate test can easily be computed from a one-way analysis of variance performed on the ranks referring to the ranks as x. Thus, referring to the ranks from the second and third columns of Table 15.3 on page 331.

$$\text{Between Groups SS} = \frac{(T_A)^2}{N_A} + \frac{(T_B)^2}{N_B} - \frac{(T_A + T_B)^2}{N_A + N_B}$$

$$= \frac{(88.5)^2}{10} + \frac{(101.5)^2}{9} - \frac{(190)^2}{19} = 27.92;$$

$$\text{Total SS} = \Sigma x^2 - \frac{(T_A + T_B)^2}{N_A + N_B} = 2,464 - \frac{(190)^2}{19} = 564.00;$$

$$\text{Within Groups SS} = \text{Total SS} - \text{Between Groups SS}$$

$$= 536.08 \text{ (Table 15.4).}$$

$$\chi^2 = \frac{\text{Between Groups SS}}{\text{Total Mean Square}} = \frac{27.92}{564.00 \div 18}$$

$$= 0.891 \text{ with one degree of freedom.}$$

This value does not agree exactly with the value computed previously (0.882). The reason for this is that, in the analysis of variance approach, due account has been taken of the ties in computing the Total SS. If the original scores of Table 15.1 contained no ties, then the corresponding ranks would be all the integers from 1 to 19. In that case,

$$\text{Total SS} = \frac{(N_A + N_B)[(N_A + N_B)^2 - 1]}{12} = \frac{19(360)}{12} = 510.00,$$

and

$$\chi^2 \text{ not corrected for ties} = \frac{\text{Between Groups SS}}{\text{Total MS}} = \frac{27.92}{570.00 \div 18}$$

$$= 0.882.$$

A continuity correction can also be included in the analysis of variance method of calculation. The values of T_A and T_B are brought into closer accord with each other by deducting $\frac{1}{2}$ from the larger and adding $\frac{1}{2}$ to the smaller and recomputing Between groups SS:

$$\text{Between Groups SS} = \frac{(101.5 - 0.5)^2}{9} + \frac{(88.5 + 0.5)^2}{10} - \frac{(190)^2}{19}$$

$$= 25.54,$$

$$\chi^2 = \frac{\text{Between Groups SS}}{\text{Total MS}} = \frac{25.54}{465.00 \div 18}$$

$$= 0.815$$

The difference between this value and the previous value of χ^2 corrected for continuity (0.807; see page 333) is due to the latter's not having been corrected for ties.

This method of calculating the ratio of mean squares from the analysis of variance table differs from the method used in an analysis of variance with actual measurements. In that case, we would calculate

$$F = \frac{\text{Between Groups MS}}{\text{Within Groups MS}}.$$

This would be referred to the F tables with appropriate degrees of freedom. In the usual analysis of variance model, the measurement data have to meet certain requirements (equal variance or homoscedasticity, normality, etc.). We are not concerned with these assumptions in our particular use of the analysis of variance table with ranks. The analysis of variance table is presented merely because it represents a particularly simple way of calculating χ^2 and, in addition, immediately points the way for an extention to the case with more than two samples.

MORE THAN TWO INDEPENDENT SAMPLES

Studying the effect of three different types of diets on the production of periodontal disease in rats, Baer and White[6] utilized a scoring method[7] for measuring the amount of periodontal breakdown. For illustrative purposes, the data for 30 female rats, 10 in each dietary group, were chosen from the overall study. Of course, the numbers in the groups do not have to be equal.

The standard parametric test for the statistical significance of the differences between the mean periodontal scores of the three dietary groups is the F-test, computed by means of the analysis of variance on the scores of Table 15.5. Using the computations presented in Table 15.5, Table 15.6 is obtained.

A distribution-free test may be more appropriate in this case, because of the nature of the data (i.e., scores rather than actual measurements), and because the assumptions underlying the analysis of variance may not be satisfied. The *Kruskal-Wallis test*,[8] an extension of the Wilcoxon Rank Sum test,[9] is an example of this.

The 30 scores of Table 15.5 are ranked in order of magnitude, maintaining the distinction of dietary grouping (Table 15.7). Thus,

TABLE 15.5
Periodontal Scores of 30 Female Rats on Three Different Diets

Diet A	Diet B	Diet C
13	4	10
13	7	10
21	9	10
21	9	20
19	16	17
18	13	17
21	15	16
21	10	21
18	9	19
21	10	17
Total 186	102	157

$$\Sigma x = \text{Total of all scores} = 445,$$
$$\Sigma x^2 = 7,335.00,$$
$$\frac{(\text{Total A})^2}{10} + \frac{(\text{Total B})^2}{10} + \frac{(\text{Total C})^2}{10} = \frac{(186)^2 + (102)^2 + (157)^2}{10} = 6,964.9,$$
$$\text{Correction Term (CT)} = \frac{(445)^2}{30} = 6,600.8.$$

TABLE 15.6
Analysis of Variance of Measurements of Table 15.5

Source of Variation	Degrees of Freedom	Sum of Squares	Mean Square
Between Groups	2	364.1	182.0
Within Groups	27	370.1	13.4
Total	29	734.2	

$$F_{2,27} = \frac{\text{Between Groups MS}}{\text{Within Groups MS}} = \frac{182.0}{13.4} = 13.0; \text{significant.}$$

the lowest periodontal score of 4 occurs in Group B and is given a rank of 1. A score of 7 is next, also in Group B, and is ranked 2. The next score of 9, occurring three times in Group B, corresponds to ranks 3, 4, and 5. Each of the three tied scores is assigned the average rank, 4. A score of 10 occurs twice in Group B and three times in Group C, using up ranks 6, 7, 8, 9, and 10. Each of the tied scores is given the average rank, 8. Similarly, ranks were assigned to the other scores (Table 15.7).

If the diets had no effect on the periodontal scores, then the high scores and the low scores should be about equally divided among the

TABLE 15.7
Periodontal Scores of 30 Female Rats on Three Different Diets Ranked in Order of Increasing Scores

Diet C	Diet B	Diet C
12.0	1.0	8.0
12.0	2.0	8.0
20.5	4.0	8.0
20.5	4.0	15.5
22.5	4.0	18.0
27.5	8.0	18.0
27.5	8.0	18.0
27.5	12.0	22.5
27.5	14.0	24.0
27.5	15.5	27.5
Sum = T_A = 225.0	T_B = 72.5	T_C = 167.5

Σx = Sum of all ranks = $T_A + T_B + T_C$ = 465.0,

Σx^2 = Sum of squared ranks

$= [(12)^2 + (12)^2 + (20.5)^2 + \ldots + (27.5)^2] = 9,420.00,$

$$\text{Correction Term (CT)} = \frac{(465.0)^2}{30} = 7,207.50.$$

TABLE 15.8
Analysis of Variance of Ranks of Table 15.7

Source of Variation	Degrees of Freedom	Sum of Squares
Between Diets	2	1,186.25
Within Diets	24	1,026.25
Total	29	2,212.50

three dietary groups (the null hypothesis). Consequently, the ranks from 1 to 30 would be so distributed as to give about the same sums for the three diets. The Kruskal-Wallis test examines the variation among these diet sums. The test will be illustrated by using the analysis of variance approach:

$$\text{Between Diets SS} = \frac{(T_A)^2}{N_A} + \frac{(T_B)^2}{N_B} + \frac{(Tc)^2}{N_C} - \frac{(T_A + T_B + Tc)^2}{N_A + N_B + N_C}$$

$$= \frac{(225)^2 + (72.5)^2 + (167.5)^2}{10} - \frac{(465)^2}{30}$$

$$= 8,393.75 - 7,207.50 = 1,186.25;$$

$$\text{Total SS} = \Sigma x^2 - \frac{(T_A + T_B + T_c)^2}{N_A + N_B + N_C} = 9,420.00 - 7,207.50$$

$$= 2,212.50;$$

$$\text{Within Diets SS} = \text{Total SS} - \text{Between Diets SS}$$

$$= 1,026.25 \text{ (Table 15.8).}$$

$$\chi^2 = \frac{\text{Between Diets SS}}{\text{Total MS}} = \frac{1,186.25}{2,212.50 \div 29} = 15.55.$$

Kruskal and Wallis showed that the ratio above (H in their terminology) is asymptotically distributed as χ^2, with degrees of freedom equal to (number of groups - 1), in this case, 2. A χ^2 of 15.55 is significant well beyond the 1% level.

The computation of χ^2 by means of the above analysis of variance has taken account of the ties. If the original scores of Table 15.5 contained no ties, then the corresponding ranks would be all the integers from 1 to 30. In that case,

$$\text{Total SS} = \frac{30[(30)^2 - 1]}{12} = 2,247.50,$$

and

$$\chi^2 = \frac{1{,}186.25}{2{,}247.50 \div 29} = 15.31.$$

This value of χ^2 takes no account of the ties. The formula usually given for calculating χ^2 following the method described by Kruskal and Wallis corresponds to the above value, uncorrected for ties.* Methods are available to control the probability level when making multiple comparisons.[19]

The exact distribution of χ^2 can be evaluated by forming all possible divisions of the $N_A + N_B + N_C$ ranks into three groups of N_A, N_B, and N_C, respectively. In the present example, there would be $30!/(10!)^3$ divisions. Each division is equally likely under the null hypothesis and leads to a value of χ^2 not all values of which are distinct. An observed value of χ^2 would be referred to this distribution to assess its significance. Only limited tables are available, however.[9]

CORRELATED OR PAIRED SAMPLES

Correlation between samples occurs when, for example, the same individuals are used under different conditions or for different treatments or when the individuals in the two samples are paired for some other reason, e.g., twins. In the parametric case, such data are analyzed by the analysis of variance technique for the two-way classification, or, alternatively, in the case of two samples, by the t-test for two samples. This answers the question, "Do the treatment means differ significantly from each other?" When the data in an ordinal scale have been replaced by ranks, the analysis provides a method of answering a much broader question, i.e., "Can the different samples of ranks all come from the same universe?" Thus, the question pertains not only to possible differences in location of the distributions, but also to possible differences in dispersion, skewness, etc. Ob-

---

$$*H = \frac{12}{(N_A + N_B + N_C)(N_A + N_B + N_C + 1)} \left[\frac{T_A^{\,2}}{N_A} + \frac{T_B^{\,2}}{N_B} + \frac{T_C^{\,2}}{N_C} \right]$$

$$-3(N_A + N_B + N_C + 1) = \frac{12}{(30)(31)} \left[\frac{(225)^2 + (72.5)^2 + (167.5)^2}{10} \right]$$

$$- 3(30 + 1) = 15.31.$$

viously, if the distributions are similar in all respects except for centering constants, the question pertains solely to location parameters.

Two Correlated Samples

The first rank order test to be discussed in this chapter is the analogue of the t-test applied to the sample of differences obtained from two correlated samples. The question of deciding whether the mean of the differences is significantly different from zero is now changed to the equivalent question in terms of the median. Because of its simplicity, it is the natural introductory topic in the study of rank-order statistics for more than two correlated samples.

Studying the effect of a new dentifrice on gingival inflammation, Chilton and Di Dio[1] scored the gingivae of 10 dental students prior

TABLE 15.9

P-M-A Scores of 10 Dental Students at a Preliminary Examination and After an 8-Week Experimental Period

Individual	P-M-A Scores Prelim. Period	Exper. Period	Prelim. – Exper. Difference (d)	Sum
1	14	8	+ 6	22
2	2	1	+ 1	3
3	3	7	– 4	10
4	12	0	+12	12
5	7	6	+ 1	13
6	10	3	+ 7	13
7	0	0	0	0
8	1	0	+ 1	1
9	6	3	+ 3	9
10	3	2	+ 1	5
Total	58	30	+28	88

Σx = Total of all scores = $58 + 30 = 88$,

$\Sigma x^2 = [(14)^2 + (2)^2 + \ldots + (8)^2 + (1)^2 + \ldots + (2)^2] = 720.0$.

$$\frac{\text{Sum of (Period sum)}^2}{\text{Number Individuals}} = \frac{[(58)^2 + (30)^2]}{10} = 426.4,$$

$$\frac{\text{Sum of (Individual sum)}^2}{\text{Number Periods}} = \frac{[(22)^2 + (3)^2 + \ldots + (5)^2]}{2} = 591.0,$$

$$\text{Correction Term (CT)} = \frac{(88)^2}{20} = 387.2.$$

to the use of the dentifrice, and again after 8 weeks of dentifrice usage, in terms of the P-M-A index. The data appear in Table 15.9. For each individual, there is a pair of observations — P-M-A index before treatment, and P-M-A index after treatment. If the necessary assumptions were tenable, these data could be analyzed by a two-way analysis of variance to test the effect of treatment (Table 15.10) as follows:

$$\text{Between Periods SS} = \frac{\text{Sum of (Period sum)}^2}{\text{No. Individuals}} - CT = 39.2,$$

$$\text{Between Individuals SS} = \frac{\text{Sum of (Individual sum)}^2}{\text{No. Periods}} - CT = 203.8,$$

$$\text{Total SS} = \text{Sum of } x^2 - CT = 332.8,$$

$$\text{Residual SS} = \text{Total SS}$$

$$- (\text{Between Periods SS} + \text{Between Individuals SS}) = 89.8.$$

$$F_{1,9} = \frac{\text{Between Periods MS}}{\text{Residual MS}} = \frac{39.20}{9.98} = 3.93;$$

not significant at 5% level.

Equivalent results are obtained by performing a t-test on the difference (d) between the two periods. The calculations proceed as follows:

$$SE_{\bar{d}} = \sqrt{\frac{\Sigma d^2 - (\Sigma d)^2/N}{N(N-1)}} = \sqrt{\frac{258 - (28)^2/10}{(10)(9)}} = \sqrt{1.9956} = 1.41;$$

$$t = \frac{\bar{d}}{SE_{\bar{d}}} = \frac{2.80}{1.41} = 1.98, \text{ with 9 degrees of freedom;}$$

$$t_9^2 = (1.98)^2 = 3.93 = F_{1,9}.$$

TABLE 15.10
Analysis of Variance of Measurements of Table 15.9

Source of Variation	Degrees of Freedom	Sum of Squares	Mean Square
Between Periods	1	39.2	39.20
Between Individuals	9	203.8	22.64
Residual	9	89.8	9.98
Total	19	332.8	

Sign Test

The parametric test is not very satisfactory because of the nature of the data, i.e., scores rather than true interval measurements. Since the data are ordinal, the scores for each individual may be replaced by their ranks. Rank 1 is assigned to the lower score, and rank 2 to the higher score. The null hypothesis to be tested is that treatment has no effect on P-M-A scores. If the hypothesis were true, then, for each individual, the P-M-A scores should be about the same for the two periods. Equivalently, if the hypothesis were true, the ranking (1, 2) or (2, 1) should occur with equal frequency.

For the first individual in Table 15.9, the P-M-A score is lower in the experimental period and is assigned rank 1, the score in the preliminary period is assigned rank 2. The same situation occurs for the second individual. For the third, the ranks are 1 for the lower score

TABLE 15.11
Ranks of P-M-A Scores of 10 Dental Students at a Preliminary Examination and After an 8-Week Experimental Period

| Individual | Ranks of P-M-A Scores | | Prelim. – Exper. Difference (d) |
	Prelim. Period	Exper. Period	
1	2.0	1.0	+1
2	2.0	1.0	+1
3	1.0	2.0	−1
4	2.0	1.0	+1
5	2.0	1.0	+1
6	2.0	1.0	+1
7	1.5	1.5	0
8	2.0	1.0	+1
9	2.0	1.0	+1
10	2.0	1.0	+1
Total	18.5	11.5	+7

Σx = Total of all ranks = 30,

$\Sigma x^2 = [(2.0)^2 + (1.0)^2 + \ldots + (1.5)^2 + \ldots + (2.0)^2 + (1.0)^2] = 49.50,$

$$\frac{\text{Sum of (Period sum)}^2}{\text{Number Individuals}} = \frac{[(18.5)^2 + (11.5)^2]}{10} = 47.45,$$

$$\frac{\text{Sum of (Individual sum)}^2}{\text{Number Periods}} = \frac{[(3)^2 + (3)^2 + \ldots + (3)^2]}{2} = 45.00,$$

$$\text{Correction Term (CT)} = \frac{(30)^2}{20} = 45.00.$$

of the preliminary period and 2 for the higher experimental period score. For individual 7, the P-M-A scores are tied, so the average of 1 and 2 or a rank of 1.5 is given to each period. The complete ranking for these data is shown in Table 15.11.

It is clear that if an individual has ranks (1, 2) in that order — i.e., his preliminary score is lower than his experimental score — then the difference in ranks, "before" - "after," equals - 1. If an individual has ranks (2, 1), then the difference equals +1. If an individual has tied scores, the difference between his ranks is 0. If the null hypothesis is true, we would expect the number of +1 differences to be close to the number of -1 differences. Consequently, the statistical analysis concerns itself only with the number of +1 differences among the total number of nonzero differences in the ranked scores. If the rankings (1, 2) and (2, 1) are equally likely, as under the null hypothesis, the total number of +1 differences would be expected to be close to half the total number of individuals with untied scores, which are referred to as "untied pairs." The test is equivalent to comparing the division of the untied pairs into the two types -1 and +1, with a 50:50 division. The test is known as the *Sign test*,[10] and is associated with the binomial distribution $\left(\dfrac{1}{2} + \dfrac{1}{2}\right)^N$, where N is the number of untied pairs. The test calls for the use of the binomial distribution in exactly the same form as on page 281, where the McNemar test for paired nominal dichotomous data was described. In fact, the McNemar test may be considered a special case of the Sign test.

From Table 15.11, it can be seen that there are nine untied pairs, eight of which are (2, 1), giving eight +1 differences; the remaining pair is (1, 2), giving one -1 difference. From the binomial $\dfrac{1}{2} + \dfrac{1}{2}\,^9$, the probability of obtaining a departure from the 50:50 division as large as that obtained or larger (two-tailed) is found to be 0.039. Tables of this binomial are readily available.[3]

Because of the symmetry of the binomial $\dfrac{1}{2} + \dfrac{1}{2}\,^N$, the normal curve approximation or the equivalent χ^2 approximation with one degree of freedom can be used even for an N as small as 9. Thus

$$\chi^2 = \frac{[(\text{Number of } +1\text{'s}) - (\text{Number of } - 1\text{'s})]^2}{(\text{Number of } + 1\text{'s}) + (\text{Number of } - 1\text{'s})}$$

$$= \frac{(7)^2}{9} = 5.44, \text{ with 1 degree of freedom}; P = 0.020.$$

Correcting for continuity,[10]

$$\text{Corr.}\ \chi^2 = \frac{(|8-1|-1)^2}{9} = 4.00; P = 0.045.$$

Wilcoxon's Matched-Pairs Signed-Ranks Test

In the Sign test, only information relative to the sign or direction of the differences between the scores for members of each pair is utilized. A more powerful test can be performed if the ranked size of these differences, as well as their directions, can be put to use, as in the *Wilcoxon Matched-Pairs Signed-Ranks test.*[12]

The data for the differences (d) in the before and after P-M-A scores in Table 15.9 are ranked in order of increasing magnitude, without regard to sign. Zero differences are not used. We find that individuals numbered 2, 5, 8 and 10 are all tied with a difference of 1. These four individuals all receive ranks of 2.5, since $(1 + 2 + 3 + 4)/4 = 2.5$. Individual number 9, with a difference of 3 P-M-A units, receives a rank of 5; individual 3 receives a rank of 6, etc. After these ranks have been assigned, the sign for each specific difference is put back on the ranks, as shown in Table 15.12.

The sum of the negative ranks is $T^- = 6$, and of the positive rank is $T^+ = 39$. The sum of all the ranks without regard to sign is

TABLE 15.12
Signed Ranks (x) of Differences of Table 15.9

		Signed Rank of $|d|$	
Individual	d	x^-	x^+
1	+ 6		7
2	+ 1		2.5
3	- 4	-6	
4	+12		9
5	+ 1		2.5
6	+ 7		8
7	0		
8	+ 1		2.5
9	+ 3		5
10	+ 1		2.5
Total	+28	$T^- = 6$	$T^+ = 39$
$\Sigma|x| = 45 = N(N+1)/2$*			

*N is now the number of individuals whose d is not zero.

$N(N + 1)/2 = 90/2 = 45$. The smallest T^- is 0 when all the ranks have a plus sign, and the largest T^- value is $N(N + 1)/2 = 45$ when all the ranks have a minus sign. For $N = 9$, there are $2^9 = 512$ possible ways of assigning signs to the ranks 1, 2, 3, ... 9, and hence 512 values of T^- (not all distinct). On the assumption of a symmetrical distribution of d, these 512 possible values of T^- are equally likely under the null hypothesis that the median (as well as the mean) of d is zero.

$$\text{Mean } T^- = N(N + 1)/4 = (9)(10)/4 = 22.5$$

$$SE_T^{\,2} = \sigma_T^{\,2} = N(N + 1)(2N + 1)/24 = (9)(10)(19)/24 = 285/4.$$

The *Exact test* is based on the distribution of T^- as actually enumerated by forming all possible values of T^-, in this case 512. The distribution of T^- is symmetrical about the mean. The observed value of T^- is referred to this distribution to assess its significance (i.e., to see how far out it lies in either tail of the distribution). In the present example, T^- is less than the mean. The probability of a value of T^- of 6 or less is .027, or .054 for a two-tailed test. Limited tables of the distribution of T^- are available,[3] and more extensive tables can also be found.[4] Obviously, one could focus attention on T^+ instead of T^-. The distributions of T^+ and T^- are the same, except that as T^- increases, T^+ decreases since $T^+ = N(N + 1)/2 - T^-$.

Because of the symmetry of the distribution, the normal curve approximation can be used, even for samples as small as 9. To determine whether T^- of 6 is significantly different from its mean of 22.5, we calculate

$$\chi^2 = z^2 = \frac{(6 - 22.5)^2}{71.25} = \frac{1,089}{285} = 3.82, df = 1.$$

The probability of exceeding this value is .051. The approximation can be improved by using a continuity correction in which T^- is brought ½ unit closer to the mean. Then,

$$\chi^2 = z^2 = \frac{(6.5 - 22.5)^2}{71.25} = 3.59, df = 1, P = .059.$$

Whereas the reputedly more powerful Wilcoxon Matched-Pairs Signed-Ranks test did not show significance at the 5% level, the less powerful Sign test did. This should remind one that the concept of power in significance testing is a long-run proposition, derived from a consideration of all possible samples under a given alternative hypothesis, and not from a single sample.

MORE THAN TWO CORRELATED SAMPLES

Howell et al.[13] studied the effect of oxalate in the drinking water on dental caries of rats, using litter-mate controls. The caries extent was measured in several ways, one of which was a total-extent score. The data for the animals on the various diets appear in Table 15.13. Diet A was a basic caries diet + distilled drinking water; Diet B was the basic caries diet + 0.020% potassium oxalate in drinking water; and Diet C was the basic caries diet + 0.220% potassium oxalate in the drinking water.

If the necessary assumptions were satisfied, these data could be analyzed by a two-way analysis of variance, as given in Table 15.14.

$$F_{2,10} = \frac{\text{Between Diets MS}}{\text{Residual MS}} = \frac{396.17}{106.63} = 3.72; \text{ not significant at the 5\% level.}$$

TABLE 15.13
Dental Caries Extent of Rats with Different Diets, by Litter

Litter Number	Diet A	B	C	Total
C-30	45	43	32	120
C-31	18	22	30	70
C-33	35	21	45	101
C-37	30	13	30	73
C-38	60	23	67	150
C-41	40	27	34	101
Total	228	149	238	615

$$\Sigma x = \text{Total of all scores} = 228 + 149 + 238 = 615,$$
$$\Sigma x^2 = [(45)^2 + (43)^2 + (32)^2 + \ldots + (34)^2] = 5,457.75,$$
$$\frac{\text{Sum of (Diet sum)}^2}{\text{Number Litters}} = \frac{[(228)^2 + (149)^2 + (238)^2]}{6} = 2,893.58,$$
$$\frac{\text{Sum of (Litter sum)}^2}{\text{Number Diets}} = \frac{[(120)^2 + (70)^2 + \ldots + (101)^2]}{3} = 3,599.08,$$
$$\text{Correction Term (CT)} = \frac{(615)^2}{18} = 2,101.25.$$

TABLE 15.14
Analysis of Variance of Measurements of Table 15.13

Source of Variation	Degrees of Freedom	Sum of Squares	Mean Square
Between Diets	2	792.33	396.17
Between Litters	5	1,497.83	299.57
Residual	10	1,066.35	106.63
Total	17	3,356.50	

Since the data are scores rather than bona fide measurements, a non-parametric test may be preferable, such as Friedman's method of ranks.[14] This is an extension of the analysis of ranks (Sign test) for more than two samples. The scores in each litter are ranked as 1, 2, or 3. In the case of ties, the average rank is assigned to each member of the tie. The ranks assigned to the data in this manner appear in Table 15.15. A two-way analysis of variance is performed on the ranks in Table 15.15, and is given in Table 15.16.

TABLE 15.15
Ranks (Within Litters) of Dental Caries Extent of Rats on Different Diets

Litter Number	Diet			Total
	A	B	C	
C-30	3.0	2.0	1.0	6
C-31	1.0	2.0	3.0	6
C-33	2.0	1.0	3.0	6
C-37	2.5	1.0	2.5	6
C-38	2.0	1.0	3.0	6
C-41	3.0	1.0	2.0	6
Total	13.5	8.0	14.5	36

Σx = Total of all ranks = 36,

$\Sigma x^2 = [(3.0)^2 + (2.0)^2 + (1.0)^2 + \ldots + (2.5)^2 + (1.0)^2 + (2.5)^2 + \ldots + (2.0)^2$
$= 83.50,$

$$\frac{\text{Sum of (Diet sum)}^2}{\text{Number Litters}} = \frac{(13.5)^2 + (8.0)^2 + (14.5)^2}{6} = 76.08,$$

$$\frac{\text{Sum of (Litter sum)}^2}{\text{Number Diets}} = \frac{6(6)^2}{3} = 72.00,$$

$$\text{Correction Term (CT)} = \frac{(36)^2}{18} = 72.00$$

TABLE 15.16
Analysis of Variance of Ranks of Table 15.15

Source of Variation	Degrees of Freedom	Sum of Squares
Between Diets	2	4.08
Between Litters	5	0.00
Residual	10	7.42
Total	17	11.50

$$\chi^2 = \frac{\text{Between Diets SS}}{(\text{Between Diets SS} + \text{Residual SS})/12} = \frac{4.08}{11.50/12} = 4.26.$$

Except for the fact that the ties were taken into account in the Total SS in the above analysis of variance, χ^2 is the same as Friedman's test criterion, χ_r^2. On the assumption that all ranks were integers, the Total SS would be 12.00, and χ^2 would be 4.08, agreeing exactly with Friedman's criterion, χ_r^2.

Friedman showed that χ_r^2 is asymptotically distributed as χ^2, with degrees of freedom equal to (number of treatments - 1), in this case, 2. The same asymptotic distribution applies to χ_r^2 corrected for ties (4.26), which is the χ^2 found above. A value of 4.26 for χ^2 with 2 degrees of freedom is not significant at the 5% level. The exact distribution of χ^2 is obtained by permuting the ranks 1, 2, and 3 in all possible ways for each of the 6 litters. The total number of permutations necessary to consider is very large — $(3!)^5$. Under the null hypothesis, each of these permutations is equally likely. Each of these permutations would produce a χ^2 value, many of which, of course, would be the same. A limited table of exact probabilities is available.[15]

RIDIT ANALYSIS

It is not uncommon for the outcome variable in some clinical dental studies to be an ordered categorical scale. An example would be the measurement of pain relief on an ordered scale ranging from none to very good.

The statistical technique known as *ridit analysis* may be considered an appropriate method of analysis for data of this type. It was originally proposed by Bross[16] for both the description of differences between groups on an ordered categorical scale, and the testing of the significance of those differences. The word "ridit" is based on an acronym for "relative to an identified distribution." Virtually the only assumption made in ridit analysis is that the discrete categories

TABLE 15.17
Overall Degree of Pain Relief by Treatment (Proportions in Parenthesis)

Category of Pain Relief	Ibuprofen		Placebo	Aspirin
	Low Dose	High Dose		
None	0 (0.000)	1 (0.012)	0 (0.000)	1 (0.011)
Poor	6 (0.064)	3 (0.035)	18 (0.186)	4 (0.045)
Fair	10 (0.106)	5 (0.058)	10 (0.103)	11 (0.125)
Good	17 (0.181)	25 (0.291)	37 (0.381)	25 (0.284)
Very good	61 (0.649)	52 (0.605)	32 (0.330)	47 (0.534)
Total	94 (1.000)	86 (1.001)	97 (1.000)	88 (0.999)

represent intervals of an underlying but unobservable, continuous distribution.

To illustrate, a consecutive series of 365 patients presented for extraction in a university oral surgery clinic and returned within one week of surgery for evaluation of overall pain relief.[17] Each patient received one of the following four drugs immediately after extraction, in a random, double-blind, fashion: placebo, ibuprofen* (low dose: 200 mg), ibuprofen* (high dose: 400 mg), or aspirin 325 mg, packaged 16 to a bottle. The patients were instructed to take two tablets of their assigned medication if they experienced postoperative pain, and to take additional doses at minimal intervals of four hours, up to a total of eight tablets a day. If, after taking eight tablets, the patient was still in pain, he had the option of taking another analgesic of his choice. The data on pain relief generated from this study appear in Table 15.17. The value of chi square is statistically significant at less than the .001 level ($\chi^2 = 38.10$; df = 12), but it is obvious that no account has been taken of the ordering of the response variable, pain relief. In addition, it is not clear how to summarize the results in an informative way. These deficiencies can be remedied by the use of ridit analysis.

Ridit analysis begins with the identification of a population to serve as a standard or reference group. In the postextraction analgesic study, the aspirin group will serve as reference since aspirin is the current standard analgesic for postoperative pain in ambulatory patients. For the reference group, the proportion is estimated of all patients whose value on the underlying continuum falls at or below the midpoint of each interval, i.e., each interval's *ridit*. The required arithmetic is illustrated in Table 15.18 for the responses by the aspirin group.

*Motrin (Upjohn Co.)

TABLE 15.18
Calculation of Ridits with Aspirin Group as Standard

Category	(1)	(2)	(3)	(4) = ridit
None	0.011	0.0055	0.000	0.0055
Poor	0.045	0.0225	0.011	0.0335
Fair	0.125	0.0625	0.056	0.1185
Good	0.284	0.1420	0.181	0.3230
Very good	0.534	0.2670	0.465	0.7320

1. In general, column 1 contains the proportionate distribution over the several categories for the reference group. In Table 15.18, the distribution is over the five categories of pain relief for the 88 patients on aspirin, taken from Table 15.17.
2. The entries in column 2 are simply half the corresponding entries in column 1.
3. The entries in column 3 are the accumulated entries in column 1, but displaced one category downward.
4. The entries in column 4, finally, are the sums of the corresponding entries in columns 2 and 3.

The final values are the ridits associated with the various categories. The ridit for a category, then, is nothing but the proportion of all subjects from the reference group falling in the lower ranking categories, plus half the proportion falling in the given category.

Uses of Ridit Analysis

The mean ridit for a particular group may be calculated if the distribution of this group over the same categories is available. The resulting mean value can be interpreted as a probability. The mean ridit for one of the four medication groups is the probability that a randomly selected patient from the particular group will obtain better pain relief than a randomly selected patient from the standard aspirin group. The mean ridits for each of the four groups are given in Table 15.19.

TABLE 15.19
Mean Ridits for Four Treatment Groups

	Ibuprofen		Placebo	Aspirin
	Low Dose	High Dose		
Sample size	94	86	97	88
Mean ridit	.548	.545	.383	.500
Critical ratio	1.12	1.30	2.75	—

Mathematically, the mean ridit for the reference group must always be .500. This is in accordance with the fact that, if two patients are randomly selected from the same population, the first patient will be at least as well off half the time, and will be at least as poorly off also half the time. Let us suppose that, in addition to the standard group, there are k groups being studied; in this case, k = 3. Then, let n_s denote the number of patients in the reference group, n_i the number of patients in group i, and $\bar{r}_i$ the mean ridit in group i, where i = 1, ... k. We can define

$$\bar{r} = \frac{\sum_{i=1}^{k} n_i \bar{r}_i}{\sum_{i=1}^{k} n_i} \, ,$$

as the weighted average of the k mean ridits. The hypothesis of equal mean ridits in all k + 1 groups (including the standard or reference group) may be tested by referring the value of

$$\chi^2 = 12 \sum_{i=1}^{k} n_i (\bar{r}_i - .5)^2 - \frac{12 \sum_{i=1}^{k} n_i^2}{n_s + \sum_{i=1}^{k} n_i} (\bar{r} - .5)^2$$

to tables of chi square with k degrees of freedom.[18] In the postextraction analgesic study, $\bar{r} = 0.489$ and $\chi^2 = 20.32$, with df = 3; P < .001. Statistically significant differences therefore exist among the four treatment groups.

Pairwise Comparisons

Since statistically significant differences have been found among the four treatment groups, pairwise contrasts comparing one treatment group with another, are in order in clinical studies such as this one.

There are, in general, $c = k(k + 1)/2$ possible pairwise comparisons among the $k + 1$ groups, so that there are $c = 6$ in this ibuprofen trial. Because there are multiple comparisons involved, the Bonferroni criterion[19] (see page 110) will be used to assess statistical significance. If the desired level of significance, α, is .05, then $\alpha/c = .0083$, and the corresponding critical normal curve value is 2.64. This is the value used for determining the statistical significance for each pairwise comparison.

An excellent approximation to the standard error of the mean ridit of a group (other than the standard group) is [18]

$$SE_{\bar{r}_i} = \frac{\sqrt{n_s + n_i}}{2\sqrt{3n_s n_i}}.$$

The critical ratio for comparing the mean ridit associated with any group and the reference group is

$$z_i = \frac{\bar{r}_i - .5}{SE_{\bar{r}_i}} = \frac{2(r_i - .5)\sqrt{3n_s n_i}}{\sqrt{n_s + n_i}}.$$

The critical ratios for comparing both of the ibuprofen groups and placebo with aspirin are presented in the last row of Table 15.19. Since the critical ratio for placebo exceeds the Bonferroni criterion value of 2.64 and the other two do not, the inference may be drawn that pain relief with the placebo medication is significantly poorer than pain relief with aspirin, but that neither ibuprofen group (high or low dose) is different from aspirin.

In order to compare two mean ridits, $\bar{r}_i$ and $\bar{r}_j$, they should both be close to .5, say between .35 and .65. Then one of these two mean ridits would be subtracted from the other and .5 added, in order to obtain an estimate of the probability that a typical patient from one group experiences greater pain relief than a typical patient from the other group. To illustrate, we can compare high dose ibuprofen ($\bar{r}_2 = .549$) with placebo ($\bar{r}_3 = .383$). Then, $(.545 - .383) + .500 = 0.662$ is a simple estimate of the probability of greater pain relief with high dose ibuprofen than with placebo. This value is close but not identical to that obtained by taking one of the two groups being compared as the new reference group, recalculating the ridits, and then finding the mean ridit for the other group. It is immaterial which group is taken as the standard group. This latter approach is more accurate, but requires more calculations. In the analgesic study, this approach yields .661 as the probability of greater pain relief with high dose ibuprofen than with placebo, which, of course, is just trivially different from the simpler estimate of .662 just found. When, however, $\bar{r}_i$ and $\bar{r}_j$ become further away from .500, the simpler method no longer is applicable, and the longer method must be used.

The critical ratio for comparing two groups is

$$z_{i-j} = \frac{\bar{r}_i - \bar{r}_j}{SE(\bar{r}_i - \bar{r}_j)} = \frac{2(r_i - r_j)\sqrt{3n_i n_j}}{\sqrt{n_i + n_j}}.$$

In the study under discussion, $n_2 = 86$, $n_3 = 97$ and $z_{2-3} = 3.79$. This value exceeds the Bonferroni value of 2.64, so that high dose ibuprofen may be stated to be statistically significantly superior to placebo for postextraction pain relief. In a similar manner the critical ratios for comparison of low dose ibuprofen with placebo is found to be 3.95, indicating superiority for ibuprofen, but the critical ratio obtained when the two dose levels of ibuprofen are compared is 0.07, confirming the absence of a difference between them. Summarizing these pairwise comparisons, the three active medications do not differ significantly among themselves, but each is significantly superior to placebo.

The standard errors defined in the preceding discussion may be used to set confidence limits about the probability that a typical patient in one group experiences greater pain relief than a typical patient in another group.[20]

The key descriptive feature of ridit analysis is the estimation of the probability that a randomly selected patient from one group is "better off" than a randomly selected patient from another group. If this probability is .5, the inference is drawn that members of one group tend to be neither better off nor worse off than members of the other group. If the probability is greater than .5, the inference is drawn that members of the first group tend to be better off than members of the second. The closer the probability is to 1, the more superior is the outcome in the first group than in the second. If the probability is less than .5, the conclusion is the opposite.

Ridit analysis is similar in many ways to ranking tests described earlier in this chapter.[21] For example, the Kruskal-Wallis test is a suitable alternative to the chi-square analysis of Table 15.17. This test also refers the test statistic (which is H in their terminology, see page 339) to the chi square table with df = number of groups − 1. The H value for the analysis of Table 15.17 is 19.69, which is only slightly different than the χ^2 of 20.32. When the sample sizes are small (when the smallest sample size is less than 15 or so, for example), the Kruskal-Wallis test, corrected for ties, should be used for significance testing, but the mean ridits may still be used for descriptive purposes. (See Fleiss[22] for further discussion of the role of ridit analysis in clinical research.)

Comments on the Use of Nonparametric Methods

Parametric rather than nonparametric methods are often used with pseudomeasurements. The two approaches usually yield about the same criteria of significance.[23] In the event of marked statistical significance, however, the test statistic for the nonparametric analysis has an upper bound because of the discontinuity of the distribution. There often seems to be little reason to insist on nonparametric analysis just because one does not see interval measurements. In addition, the scores are often averages of many constituent scores so that one profits from the Central Limit Theorem. Of course, when there is order but no numbers are assignable, there is no question that nonparametric methods should be used.[24]

Since nonparametric methods do not explicitly estimate parameters of a distribution, it is difficult to speak of confidence intervals, but methods have been devised in some cases, such as for the median and quartile.

Other problems that have been solved by the use of distribution-free methods are: rank correlation; comparing cumulative distributions (*Kolmogorov-Smirnov test*); and some higher order designs, such as incomplete three-way layouts. Distribution-free methods have not been elaborated for many other types of higher order designs, however.

REFERENCES

1. Chilton, N. W., Sternberg, S., and Fertig, J. W.: Studies in the design and analysis of dental experiments. 6. Nonparametric tests (Independent samples with ordinal scales), J Dent Res 42:54, 1963.

2. Wilcoxon, F.: Individual comparisons by ranking methods, Biometrics 1:80, 1945.

3. Dixon, W. J., and Massey, F. J., Jr.: Introduction to Statistical Analysis, 3rd ed., New York, McGraw-Hill, 1969.

4. Wilcoxon, F., Katti, S. K., and Wilcox, R. A.: Critical Values and Probability Levels for the Wilcoxon Rank Sum Test and the Wilcoxon Signed Rank Test, New York, American Cyanamid Company, and Florida State Univ.

5. Siegel, S.: Nonparametric Statistics, New York, McGraw-Hill, 1956.

6. Baer, P. N., and White, C. L.: Studies on periodontal disease in the mouse. 4. The effect of a high protein, low carbohydrate diet, J Periodont 32:328, 1961.

7. Baer, P. N., and Lieberman, J. E.: Observation on some genetic characteristics of the periodontium in three strains of inbred mice, Oral Surg 12:820, 1959.

8. Kruskal, W. H., and Wallis, W. A.: Use of ranks in one-criterion variance analysis, J Amer Stat Assn 7:583, 1952.

9. Seigel, S.: Op. cit., Ref. 5, p. 282.

10. Dixon, W. J., and Massey, F. J., Jr.: Op. cit., Ref. 3, p. 335.

11. Fertig, J. W., Chilton, N. W., and Sternberg, S.: Studies in the design and analysis of dental experiments. 5. Nonparametric tests (correlated samples with dichotomous scales), J Dent Res 41:1021, 1962.

12. Siegel, S.: Op. cit., Ref. 5, p. 75.

13. Howell, S. R., Schlack, C. A., Taylor, B. L., and Berzinskas, V. J.: The role of oxalates on the incidence and extent of dental caries in the cotton rat, J Dent Res 27:136, 1948.

14. Friedman, M.: The use of ranks to avoid assumption of normality implicit in the analysis of variance, J Amer Stat Assn (32:675, 1937.

15. Siegel, S.: Op. cit., Ref. 5, p. 280.

16. Bross, I. D. J.: How to use ridit analysis, Biometrics 14:18-38, 1958.

17. Chilton, N. W., and Mohnac, A.: Unpublished data, Temple Univ. School of Dentistry.

18. Selvin, S.: A further note on the interpretation of ridit analysis, Amer J Epidem 105:16, 1977.

19. Miller, R. G.: Simultaneous Statistical Inference, 2nd ed., New York, Springer-Verlag, 1981.

20. Fleiss, J. L., Chilton, N. W., and Wallenstein, S.: Ridit analysis in Dental Clinical Studies, J Dent Res 58:2080-2084, 1979.

21. Kantor, S., Winkelstein, W., and Ibrahim, A.: A note on the interpretation of the ridit as quantile rank, Amer J Epidem 87:609-615, 1968.

22. Fleiss, J. L.: Statistical Methods for Rates and Proportions, 2nd ed., New York, Wiley, 1981, pp. 151-156.

23. D'Agostino, R. B., Heeren, T., and Meeks, S. L.: Robustness of the Two Independent Sample t-Test on Sealed Ordinal Data, Pharmacol Ther Dent 7:1, forthcoming, Boston University, Department of Mathematics.

24. Wallenstein, S., Fleiss, J. L., and Chilton, N. W.: The Logistic Analysis of Categorical Data from Dental and Oral Experiments, Pharmacol Ther Dent 6:65, 1981.

16
Sequential Analysis

In the usual type of experimental study, particularly of a clinical nature, the number of subjects to be included in the various treatment groups under comparison is often determined by the availability of these subjects, or funds, or of the substance being studied. More "exactly," however, the size of the groups used should depend on the anticipated difference in treatment effects, or on the size of the treatment difference considered important by the investigator. The size of the groups should also depend on the magnitude of probability of error in rejecting or accepting i.e., not rejecting the working null hypothesis (errors of the first and second kind) the investigator is willing to tolerate. Methods for determining the sample size of experiments, under various conditions, have been presented in Chapters 6 and 14.

In many experiments, the investigator would like to check the results before the preassigned total number of subjects has been studied. Thus he could perform significance tests part way through the study, and make a decision about the feasibility of continuing the experiment or, if the results did not look promising or because a difference was already apparent, discontinuing it. Unfortunately, however, this procedure changes his agreed-on probabilities of errors of the first and second kind. A desire to check the results periodically and still control the probabilities of error leads logically to a sequential type of design. Finney has stated:

> The use of a time sequence of pairs suggests a sequential design. If the results for any subject are obtainable fairly rapidly, any large difference in effectiveness of A and B is likely to betray itself from tests on only a few pairs: to continue until a preassigned number has been tested not

only seems uneconomic experimentation but also offends against the ethical principle that a remedy shall not be used after it has been proved inferior. On the other hand, if the difference between A and B is small, a preassigned number of subjects may fail to point decisively to either as the better, and to stop the experiment at that total could be almost equivalent to wasting all the work already done. In practice, most clinical experimenters no doubt decide whether to continue or to end an experiment from study of the results already obtained, and what is wanted is an objective rule of conduct.[1]

During the second World War, the need for determining as rapidly as possible which of two products was better gave impetus to the development of the theory and application of sequential analysis by Wald and his co-workers.[2,3] Since that time, there have been many applications of these methods in medical experimentation. Armitage has written a text on the subject,[4] and articles have appeared on oral biological applications.[5-8]

SEQUENTIAL SIGN TEST

The simplest type of problem for the application of sequential analysis is probably the binomial one in which a sample proportion is compared with a standard or universe proportion.

The binomial problem does not actually arise frequently in its direct form in oral biological research, because a suitable standard proportion is not usually available against which to compare an experimental proportion. However, data are sometimes analyzed in such a way that they conform to this binomial pattern. A good illustration is the Sign test performed on paired observations. These observations may be numerical measurements, or may be measurements according to an ordinal (ranking) scale, or even according to a dichotomous scale.

Sign Test with Measurements on an Ordinal Scale

The observations which are paired need not be bona fide numerical measurements, but may be scores according to an ordinal scale rather than numerical measurements. Even with such a scale, it is not actually necessary to note each response for the two members of the pair; it is sufficient merely to obtain a decision which is larger or smaller, better or worse, etc. for the two members of the pair. The

Sign test when applied to this type of problem may also be called a *Preference test*.

As an example of the type of problem where the Sequential Sign test would have been possible, a double-blind clinical study was conducted, in a dental school clinic, to determine the relative effectiveness of a new relaxing drug as compared to a placebo in reducing tension in extremely apprehensive patients undergoing dental procedures.[9,10] Of the total subjects in the study, 20 received both medications in a random assignment. Each patient's reactions were classified according to a four-point relaxation score scale (++, +, − and − −). The results of the study were listed in Table 16.1. The first patient, TC, was scored as ++ with the new drug and − with the placebo, and was classified as preferring the new drug. The second patient was scored as + with the new drug and ++ with the placebo, and was therefore classified as preferring the placebo. The third patient was scored as + with both the new drug and the placebo, and so was classified as giving no preference; he gave no information

TABLE 16.1

Relaxation Scores with Two Medications for 20 Apprehensive Dental Patients[9,10]

Patient	Age	Sex	Relaxation Score		Preference		
			Drug	Placebo	Drug	Placebo	Tied
TC	11	M	++	−	√		
CY	24	F	+	++		√	
LK	62	F	+	+			√
RH	40	F	++	+	√		
AI	11	F	++	+	√		
MW	60	F	+	++		√	
RS	16	M	+	++		√	
TA	49	F	+	+			√
NH	11	F	++	++			√
DO	25	F	++	+	√		
RM	28	M	+	+			√
JR	20	F	+	−	√		
BJ	13	F	−	++		√	
RN	30	F	+	−	√		
IT	27	F	++	+	√		
AM	28	M	++	++			√
DS	12	F	+	+			√
BZ	55	M	++	+	√		
CS	30	F	+	−	√		
TL	26	M	++	++			√
				Total	9	4	7

which medication was "better." As in the Sign test with actual measurements, the ties are not utilized. Here, because of the type of measurement scale used, there may be an appreciable number of ties. In similar manner, the scores and preferences of the remaining 17 patients are listed.

The sample size (20) was chosen for convenience. The number of individuals expressing a preference is 13, of whom 9 prefer the new drug and 4 the placebo. If there were no difference between the relaxation effectiveness of the two drugs (the null hypothesis), then half of the preferences would be for the new drug, and half for the placebo. The test can be performed by comparing the observed proportion of preferences for the new drug (9 out of 13) with $\frac{1}{2}$, its value under the null hypothesis, by means of the binomial expansion or its normal curve approximation. We are interested only in determining whether the new drug is more effective than the placebo, not whether the placebo is better than the new drug; therefore, a one-sided test is appropriate.

The calculation of the normal curve, z, for the Sign test (see Chapter 15) with its correction for continuity yields,

$$z = \frac{(|\,9 - 4\,| - 1)}{\sqrt{9 + 4}} = 1.11.$$

For a one-sided test, this corresponds to $P > 5\%$ so that the number of patients preferring the new drug is not significantly larger than the number preferring the placebo, i.e., the proportion preferring the new drug (among those stating a preference) is not significant greater than $\frac{1}{2}$. While the analysis is correct, the verdict of nonsignificance attained with a sample size (20), fixed without reference to a suitable alternative hypothesis, may not be very pointed. Specifications should be set up in advance and the sample size determined accordingly.

Fixed Sample Size Approach

If 80% of the patients who stated a preference chose the new drug (the alternative hypothesis $p = p_1 = .80$), this would be of clinical importance to the investigator and would merit rejecting the null hypothesis ($p = p_0 = .50$). The level of significance is chosen as $\alpha = .05$ and the power of the test is chosen as .90, so that β, the probability of an error of the second kind, is .10. According to these specifications, the number of untied preferences needed to reach a decision may be calculated as described in Chapter 14. Thus, for a one-sided test with $\alpha = .05$ (in one tail) and $\beta = .90$,

$$(p_1 - p_0) = 1.64 \sqrt{\frac{p_o q_0}{n}} + 1.28 \sqrt{\frac{p_1 q_1}{n}}.$$

Substituting, and solving for n,

$$\sqrt{n} = \frac{1.64 \sqrt{(50\%)(50\%)} + 1.28 \sqrt{(80\%)(20\%)}}{30} = 4.44$$

$$n = 20.$$

This is the number of individuals with untied preferences required. If it is known that about 2/3 of the individuals express a preference, the number of individuals required in order to yield 20 with a preference, can be estimated as $20 \div 2/3 = 30$.

Sequential Approach

In spite of the paucity of data, the problem under discussion here will be utilized to illustrate sequential analysis. According to the specifications already mentioned, we can determine the formulae for the parallel lines which constitute the boundaries for the sequential plan. The calculation proceeds as follows:

$$a = \log \frac{(1 - \beta)}{\alpha} = \log \frac{0.90}{0.05} = \log 18 = 1.25527$$

$$b = \log \frac{(1 - \alpha)}{\beta} = \log \frac{0.95}{0.10} = \log 9.5 = 0.97772$$

$$c = \log \frac{q_o}{q_1} = \log \frac{0.5}{0.2} = \log 2.5 = 0.39794$$

$$d = \log \frac{p_1 q_0}{p_0 q_1} = \log \frac{(0.80)(0.50)}{(0.50)(0.20)} = \log 4 = 0.60206$$

$$y_1 = \frac{a}{d} + \frac{c}{d} n = 2.0849 + 0.66096n$$

$$y_0 = -\frac{b}{d} + \frac{c}{d} n = -1.6240 + 0.66096n.$$

These two lines are plotted in Figure 16.1. The abscissa refers to the number of individuals with untied responses, i.e., showing a

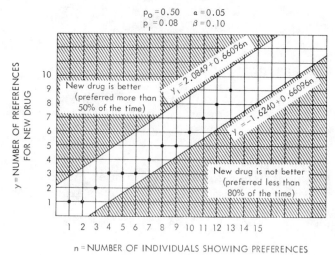

$$P_O = 0.50 \quad a = 0.05$$
$$p_1 = 0.08 \quad \beta = 0.10$$

FIG. 16.1 One-Sided Sequential Plan for Sign Test with Ordinal Data.

preference, and the ordinate, y, refers to the number of these individuals preferring the new drug. The points for the individuals with untied responses are plotted as follows: The first patient showed a preference for the new drug, so he is recorded one unit to the right on the abscissa and one unit up on the ordinate. The second patient preferred the placebo, so he is recorded one unit to the right on the abscissa. The third patient showed no preference for either the new drug or the placebo (i.e., tied) and is, therefore, not recorded on the sequential chart. The fourth and fifth patients each exhibited a preference for the new drug, and are each recorded one unit to the right on the abscissa and one unit up on the ordinate. The next two patients preferred the placebo, and are each recorded one unit to the right on the abscissa. The next two patients show no preferences, and are not recorded on the graph. This procedure is continued for the rest of the patients' responses in the study.

It is noted that all of the 13 plotted points, representing those patients who manifest a preference, fall within the boundaries of the sequential plan. Since the points do not cross the upper boundary, it cannot be stated that the new drug is preferred to the placebo more than 50% of the time. Since the points do not cross the lower boundary, the conclusion cannot be drawn that the new drug was preferred to the placebo less than 80% of the time. The only statement possible is that no decision can be made about the difference between the two medications. If enough individual preferences were available, one of the lines would eventually have to be crossed, no matter what the true difference between the drugs may be.

The failure to make a decision appears at first glance to contradict the results of the original significance test ($z = 1.11$; $P > 5\%$). However, when the data in Table 16.1 were collected, there was no prior specification as to an alternative to 50% nor as to a value for β. Thus, to accept the null hypothesis that $p = .50$, it was not necessary at the same time to reject a particular alternative hypothesis. In the sequential procedure, and also in the fixed sample size method, the particular alternative hypothesis and β for that alternative are specified and the acceptance of the null hypothesis must at the same time imply the rejection of that specific alternative. Reviewing the data of this example sequentially, we fail to make a decision since we do not have enough information to rule out either the null hypothesis that $p = .50$, or the alternative hypothesis that $p = .80$. The confidence interval for p is still wide enough to include both .50 and .80. In fact, the 95% confidence interval as determined from tables of the binomial is 38.6% to 90.9%.[11]

A batch of data obtained without basing the sample size on a consideration of suitable alternatives may well yield a decision of nonsignificance when the standard type of analysis is performed. A sequential review of these same data need not result in a decision, however. The data may still be wandering in the channel where no decision can be made, unless the alternative hypothesis chosen is sufficiently different from the null hypothesis. Obviously a decision by the sequential procedure can be forced for any available batch of data by an appropriate choice of one or more of the quantities a, β, and the specified alternative.

In a sequential design the sample size is not fixed but is variable. However, it is possible to estimate the average sample size (ASN) necessary to arrive at a decision, i.e., to cross one of the two lines in sequential analysis. When the null hypothesis is true and half of the preferences are theoretically for the placebo,

$$ n = \left[\frac{b}{d} - a \left(\frac{a}{d} + \frac{b}{d} \right) \right] \div \left(\frac{c}{d} - p_0 \right). $$

Substituting,

$$ n = \frac{1.6240 - .05(2.0849 + 1.6240)}{(0.66096 - 0.50000)} = 9, $$

where n is the number of untied pairs. Thus, if the null hypothesis is true, then, on the average, we will need 9 preferences to arrive at a decision; 95% of the time, this decision will be one of nonsignificance (crossing the lower line). If 2/3 of the patients express a preference, the total number of patients required, on the average, is equal to 9 ÷ 2/3, or 14 individuals.

If the alternative hypothesis corresponding to 80% of the preferences for the new drug is true,

$$n = \left[\frac{a}{d} - \beta \left(\frac{a}{d} + \frac{b}{d} \right) \right] \div \left(p_1 - \frac{c}{d} \right).$$

Substituting,

$$n = \frac{2.0849 - 0.10(2.0849 + 1.6240)}{(0.80000 - 0.66096)} = 12.$$

If the specified alternative hypothesis is true, we will need, on the average, 12 preferences to reach a decision. Since $\beta = .10$, this means that 90% of the time the decision will be that the new drug is preferred to the placebo. If 2/3 of the patients express a preference, this means that the number of patients required will be 18 if the alternative hypothesis is true.

If the true situation is somewhere in between the null hypothesis $(p = p_0 = 1/2)$ and the postulated alternative hypothesis $(p = p_1 = .80)$, the average amount of testing will be maximized. The average sample size required by the sequential method is less than that required as a fixed sample (30). In fact, this is one of the advantages of sequential analysis. Another advantage of sequential analysis is that if a new drug is truly preferred more than 80% (the specified alternative) of the time, or if the placebo is truly preferred more frequently than the new drug, a decision will be reached with even less testing.

Sign Test with Numerical Measurements

With a series of paired measurements, interest may be focused on the magnitude of the differences or merely on their direction. The pairing arises, for example, when two different methods have been applied to specimens of the same material, or when the patient serves as his own control, the "before-and-after" problem.

For example, Wessinger performed pH determinations on the saliva of 50 patients, using a quinhydrone electrode and a glass electrode.[12] The data appear in Table 16.2 together with the differ-

TABLE 16.2
Comparison of pH Determinations with Quinhydrone Electrode and with Glass Electrode on Saliva of 50 Patients[12]

Patient Number	pH Glass Electrode (x_1)	pH Quinhydrone Electrode (x_2)	$x_2 - x_1$ (d)
1	6.77	6.70	-0.07
2	6.90	6.81	-0.09
3	7.05	6.93	-0.12
4	6.95	6.84	-0.11
5	7.03	6.93	-0.10
6	7.12	7.20	+0.08
7	7.20	7.27	+0.07
8	6.97	6.88	-0.09
9	6.99	6.93	-0.06
10	6.79	6.70	-0.09
11	6.85	6.79	-0.06
12	6.95	6.87	-0.08
13	6.61	6.52	-0.09
14	6.70	6.74	+0.04
15	7.09	7.01	-0.08
16	6.84	6.77	-0.07
17	6.73	6.64	-0.09
18	6.93	6.82	-0.11
19	6.84	6.71	-0.13
20	6.57	6.48	-0.09
21	6.87	6.77	-0.10
22	6.81	6.75	-0.06
23	6.49	6.41	-0.08
24	6.38	6.29	-0.09
25	7.09	6.97	-0.12
26	6.76	6.71	-0.05
27	6.84	6.77	-0.07
28	6.92	6.90	-0.02
29	7.12	7.15	+0.03
30	6.73	6.64	-0.09
31	6.81	6.75	-0.06
32	6.94	6.90	-0.04
33	6.88	6.81	-0.07
34	6.77	6.65	-0.12
35	7.25	7.18	-0.07
36	6.16	6.15	-0.01
37	6.88	6.78	-0.10
38	6.63	6.51	-0.12
39	6.71	6.65	-0.06
40	6.95	6.83	-0.12
41	6.31	6.25	-0.06
42	6.47	6.44	-0.03
43	6.60	6.63	+0.03
44	6.85	6.73	-0.12
45	6.60	6.50	-0.10
46	6.52	6.42	-0.10

TABLE 16.2 *(Continued)*

Patient Number	pH Glass Electrode (x_1)	pH Quinhydrone Electrode (x_2)	$x_2 - x_1$ (d)
47	6.83	6.74	−0.09
48	6.23	6.15	−0.08
49	7.10	7.22	+0.12
50	6.71	6.64	−0.07
Total	340.09	336.83	−3.26

ence (quinhydrone − glass). The usual test that focuses attention on the actual size of the difference between the two methods is the t-test, in which the average difference is compared with zero (the null hypothesis). The two-sided version of the t-test is used since a negative or a positive average difference elicits the same interest.

$$t = \frac{(\bar{d} - 0)}{\sqrt{\dfrac{\Sigma d^2 - (\Sigma d)^2/N}{N(N-1)}}} = \frac{-0.065}{0.008} = -8.0, \text{ with 49 degrees of freedom.}$$

P is much less than 1% so that the statistical significance of the average difference is overwhelming. Statistical significance could have been shown with fewer than 50 patients if one had known where to stop collecting data. If some particular alternative, together with values of a and β, had been specified in advance, it would have been possible to determine the necessary sample size to discriminate between the null hypothesis and the alternative. In that event, a sequential t-test would also be possible, as will be described later in this chapter.

If interest were focused merely on whether one method produced a higher pH reading than the other, then a Sign test (Chapter 15) could be performed. In Table 16.2, six of the differences between the pH readings with the two electrodes (quinhydrone − glass) are positive and 44 are negative. Again, a two-sided test is appropriate since departure from the null hypothesis in either direction is of interest. Using the χ^2 test, with the correction for continuity:

$$\chi^2 = \frac{(|6 - 44| - 1)^2}{44 + 6} = \frac{1,369}{50} = 27.4, \text{ with df} = 1.$$

With measurements recorded to the accuracy of those in Table 16.2, ties are not very likely to occur, but if they do occur, such individuals are not utilized in the Sign test. As with the parametric t-test, the significance is overwhelming. The verdict of significance could have been arrived at much sooner if it had been known when to stop.

The investigator's motivation in choosing 50 patients is not known, but presumably this was a convenient sample size. An appropriate sample size could have been determined in advance if, in addition to the significance level (a), an alternative to the null hypothesis and the power of the test $(1 - \beta)$ for that alternative had been specified. Suppose that the investigator specifies in advance, for example, that if the true proportion (p) of plus signs (or minus signs) exceeds 0.70, then it is appropriate to state that the quinhydrone electrode gives higher (or lower) values. This calls for a two-sided test against the null hypothesis of 0.50.

H_0: Null Hypothesis	H: Alternative Hypotheses
$p = p_0 = .50$	$H_1: p = p_1 = .70$
	$H_2: p = p_2 = .30$

Furthermore, suppose that the investigator selects a significance level a of .02, a_1 (= .01) in the upper tail of the normal curve, and a_2 (= .01) in the lower tail because the test is two-sided — and a power of .90 (β = .10). With these specifications, the investigator could determine the necessary sample size for a fixed sample plan, or he could determine a sequential plan.

If the analysis is performed sequentially, there will be a gain on two scores: smaller samples will be needed, on the average, to effect the same discrimination, and if p is actually much greater than .70(p_1), or much less than .30(p_2), a decision may be reached quickly.

The data in Table 16.2 will be reviewed by the sequential method merely for illustrative purposes. Obviously, when a batch of data has already been collected, as in the comparison of electrodes, the correct analysis has already been described on page 73 ff.

For a two-sided sequential test, it is necessary to have two sets of parallel lines to form the boundaries of the sequential plan. The upper pair of parallel lines corresponding to the alternative hypothesis H_1 is given by the following formulae:

$$a = \log \frac{(1 - \beta)}{a_1} = \log \frac{0.90}{0.001} = \log 90 = 1.95424$$

$$b = \log \frac{(1 - a_1)}{\beta} = \log \frac{0.99}{0.10} = \log 9.9 = 0.99564$$

$$c = \log \frac{q_0}{q_1} = \log \frac{0.50}{0.30} = \log (5/3) = 0.22185$$

$$d = \log \frac{p_1 q_0}{p_0 q_1} = \log \frac{(0.70)(0.50)}{(0.50)(0.30)} = \log (7/3) = 0.36798$$

$$y_1 = \frac{a}{d} + \frac{c}{d} n = 5.3107 + 0.60289n$$

$$y_0 = -\frac{b}{d} + \frac{c}{d} n = -2.7057 + 0.60289n.$$

The lower pair of parallel boundaries corresponding to the alternative hypothesis H_2 follows simply by symmetry, since $p_2 = (1 - p_1)$,

$$y_0' = \frac{b}{d} + \left(1 - \frac{c}{d} \right) n = 2.7057 + 0.39711n$$

$$y_1' = -\frac{a}{d} + \left(1 - \frac{c}{d} \right) n = -5.3107 + 0.39711n.$$

These two pairs of parallel lines are drawn on graph paper, as in Figure 16.2.

The signs of the differences between the pH reading with the two types of electrodes (quinhydrone – glass) appear in Table 16.2. Thus, the first patient has a lower reading with the quinhydrone electrode, so he is recorded one unit to the right on the abscissa. Recordings are made similarly for the next four patients. The sixth patient, however, has a higher reading with the quinhydrone electrode, so his point is graphed one unit up on the ordinate and one to the right on the abscissa. At the nineteenth patient, the lower line (y_1') is crossed and the experiment is terminated with the decision of statistical significance, namely, that the quinhydrone electrode yields lower salivary pH readings than the glass electrode more than half the time.* A decision is reached long before the fiftieth individual. As in

---

*The line y_0 has actually been crossed at the fifth patient, indicating that the quinhydrone electrode does not yield higher pH reading than the glass electrode (or at least not higher by an important amount). From this point on, it is only necessary to decide whether the quinhydrone electrode actually yields lower reading than the glass electrode (cross line y_1') or whether there is no important difference (cross line y_0'). The line for y_0' may actually be crossed before reaching the shaded area.

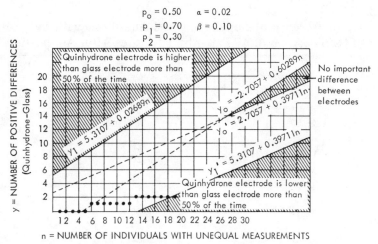

FIG. 16.2 Two-Sided Sequential Plan for Sign Test with Numerical Measurements.

the case of the usual Sign test, with a fixed sample size, the individuals showing ties would not be utilized.

Sign Test with Measurements on a Dichotomous Scale

When both measurements for the paired observations are scaled dichotomously, e.g., yes-no, react-not react, plus-minus, etc., the data correspond to two correlated samples according to a dichotomous scale, i.e., a double dichotomy in which the samples are not independent. The standard method of analysis (McNemar test see Chapter 12) utilizes the disagreements or changes in the two observations of the pairs. Again the data from the tied pairs, of which there may be a considerable number, are not utilized. If the changes in one direction are called plus and those in the other direction minus, then the data offer merely another illustration of the Sign test.

Kutscher studied the effectiveness of two topical anesthetic drugs, a standard one in long usage (B) and a newer one (A).[13] Both drugs were applied simultaneously to the oral mucous membrane of 47 patients in the apical area of the maxillary canines. The side to which a particular drug was applied was determined by tossing a coin. After four minutes, each area was tested with a probe for topical anesthesia, and the results recorded as + or –. The data were collected sequentially. Four possible types of paired responses were

TABLE 16.3
Presence or Absence of Topical Mucosal Anesthesia with Two Drugs,
in Both Canine Areas of 47 Patients, 4 Minutes After Application[13]

Patient Number	Drug A	B	Patient Number	Drug A	B
1	-	-	25	+	+
2	-	-	26	-	+
3	-	+	27	+	+
4	+	-	28	+	+
5	-	-	29	+	-
6	-	-	30	+	+
7	-	-	31	-	-
8	-	-	32	-	+
9	+	-	33	+	+
10	+	-	34	+	-
11	+	-	35	-	-
12	-	-	36	-	-
13	-	-	37	+	-
14	+	+	38	+	-
15	+	+	39	-	-
16	+	+	40	-	-
17	+	+	41	+	+
18	+	+	42	+	+
19	+	+	43	+	-
20	+	-	44	+	-
21	-	-	45	+	+
22	-	-	46	-	-
23	+	-	47	+	-
24	+	+			

observed (1) ++; (2) --; (3) +-; and (4) -+. Forty-seven individuals, of whom 19 had untied responses (+-, or -+), were necessary to reach a decision. The data appear in Table 16.3.

According to the null hypothesis, the proportion of individuals reacting with Drug A (p_A) is the same as that with Drug B (p_B), so that ($p_A - p_B$) = 0. This can be translated into a null hypothesis that half the individuals with untied responses react with A and not with B, and that the other half react with B and not with A. If the proportion reacting with A is larger than that with B, i.e., ($p_A - p_B$) > 0, this implies that more than half the individuals with untied responses will react to A and not to B. Thus, it is obvious that a comparison of the proportion of untied individuals who react to A and not to B with one half, is at the same time a comparison of p_A, the proportion reacting with Drug A, and p_B, the proportion reacting with

Drug B. If, then, we stipulate a certain value alternative to one-half as representing the proportion of untied individuals who react to Drug A and not to Drug B, this alternative refers to some difference $(p_A - p_B)$, although the difference implied cannot be determined unless the correlation between A and B results is taken into account.

In this study, we are interested only in whether the new drug, A, is better than the older standard drug, B. A one-sided sequential plan using $p_0 = 0.50$ as the null hypothesis and $p_1 = 0.75$ as the alternative was constructed, with $a = .05$ and $\beta = .10$. Utilizing the formulae previously described, the boundaries for the one-sided sequential plan are given by:

$$y_1 = 2.6309 + 0.63093n$$
$$y_0 = -2.0492 + 0.63093n.$$

These lines are shown in Figure 16.3 and the points plotted as described previously. At the 16th individual showing untied responses (the 47th individual in the experiment), the upper line is crossed, giving a verdict that Drug A produces topical anesthesia significantly more frequently than Drug B.

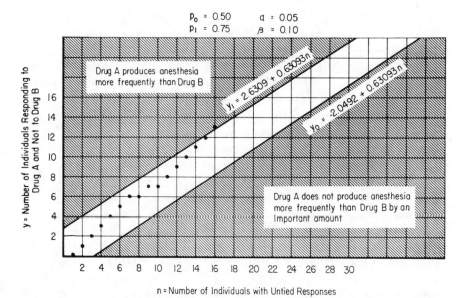

FIG. 16.3 One-Sided Sequential Plan for Sign Test with Dichotomous Data.

If the data yielding these 16 untied pairs, which led to the decision of statistical significance, are now reviewed *erroneously* by the standard test procedure (McNemar Test), one obtains

$$z = \frac{[|\ 13 - 3\ | - 1]}{\sqrt{13 + 3}} = \frac{9}{\sqrt{16}} = 2.25.$$

For a one-sided test this corresponds to P approximately 1%. Rejection of the null hypothesis by the sequential method would usually lead to even more emphatic rejection by the use of the conventional method. This latter procedure is not justified, however, after the data have been collected and analyzed sequentially.

The fact that the conventional test exhibits greater statistical significance than that obtained by the sequential test does not represent a disadvantage of the sequential procedure. After all, how would one have known exactly where to stop the experiment to perform this test? If the investigator were to stop repeatedly to examine the data and make this conventional test, he would be losing control over the errors of the first and second kind.

DOUBLE DICHOTOMY

In the more usual double dichotomy problem, the samples are not correlated but are independent, e.g., one group of individuals treated with A is compared with an independent group treated with B. The two sample proportions of reactors are to be compared. A convenient way to deal with this problem sequentially is to have the individuals paired at random and the data for each pair examined and recorded.* Sometimes the individuals favor one treatment, sometimes the other, and sometimes they are equal or tied in response. The data are now in the same form as for correlated pairs discussed under the Sign test with measurements on a dichotomous scale. The null hypothesis that the two proportions of reactors are equal is equivalent to the null hypothesis that one-half the untied pairs will favor one treatment over the other. The alternative hypothesis specifying a certain difference in the proportions, because of the independence of the members of the pair, can be translated into an alternative hypothesis specifying the proportion of untied pairs favoring one of the treatments. Thus, the trick of forming random

---

*This problem can also be dealt with sequentially by pairing groups of individuals.[8]

pairs has translated this double dichotomy problem into a form that resembles the Sign test and hence into a binomial problem.

An experiment was designed to determine the relative effectiveness of 5% lidocaine in two different ointment bases as a topical anesthetic.[5] Previous experience had indicated that 5% lidocaine in a mineral oil-polyethylene base ointment would produce discernible topical anesthesia of oral mucous membranes about 70% of the time. The investigators thought that an increase of 15% (from 70% to 85%) in the performance of the lidocaine in gelatin, pectin, carboxymethyl cellulose in mineral oil-polyethylene base ointment (Orabase) compared to lidocaine in Plastibase, would be of practical importance. With these baseline data, a sequential scheme was developed.

The two preparations were applied to the oral mucous membranes of the right side of the mouth of patients under treatment at the School of Dental and Oral Surgery, Columbia University, in a random fashion, so that half the subjects received preparation A (Orabase vehicle), and the other half preparation B (Plastibase vehicle). For each pair of subjects, the decision was made by a coin toss which one would receive A and which one would receive B. The sequence of drug application appears in Table 16.4. The preparations were applied in a double-blind manner — i.e., neither the subject nor the investigator knew the composition of the preparations applied.

The effectiveness of topical anesthesia was determined at various time intervals, but only the observations at 12 minutes after application are presented here, because this was chosen at the beginning of the experiment as the time of critical comparison. The presence or

TABLE 16.4
Order of Application of Two Topical Anesthetic Preparations to Individuals in Each Pair[5]

Pair	Preparation Used		Pair	Preparation Used	
	1st Member	2d Member		1st Member	2d Member
1	A	B	11	B	A
2	B	A	12	A	B
3	B	A	13	A	B
4	B	A	14	A	B
5	A	B	15	A	B
6	A	B	16	A	B
7	B	A	17	A	B
8	B	A	18	A	B
9	A	B	19	B	A
10	A	B	20	A	B

absence of anesthesia was determined for each patient, and then a comparison was made between the two members of each pair. Thus there are four possibilities for the outcome of a pair:

A	B	Probability	
1. Produced anesthesia	Did not produce anesthesia	$p_A q_B$	untied pairs
2. Did not produce anesthesia	Produced anesthesia	$q_A p_B$	
3. Did not produce anesthesia	Did not produce anesthesia	$q_A q_B$	tied pairs
4. Produced anesthesia	Produced anesthesia	$p_A p_B$	

Only alternatives 1 and 2, the "untied pairs," give information about the relative value of the preparations, i.e., A is better than B, or A is not better than B (actually, A is worse than B). The tally of the results appears in Table 16.5.

In preparing the sequential plan for this experiment, the following considerations entered: (1) past experience indicated that 5% lidocaine in a Plastibase vehicle (preparation B) produced topical

TABLE 16.5
The Relative Effectiveness of Two Topical Anesthetic Preparations (A and B) for Each Pair of Patients 12 Minutes After Application[5]

Pair	A Effective B Ineffective	B Effective A Ineffective	A and B Both Ineffective	A and B Both Effective
1		✓		
2	✓			
3	✓			
4	✓			
5	✓			
6				✓
7				✓
8	✓			
9			✓	
10	✓			
11	✓			
12		✓		
13				✓
14	✓			
15	✓			
16	✓			
17	✓			
18			✓	
19				✓
20	✓			

anesthesia of the oral mucous membranes in about 70% of the cases, i.e., $p_B = .70$; (2) the investigators felt that an increase in the percentage of patients having topical anesthesia with the new preparation A of 15% was important, i.e., $p_A = 0.70 + 0.15 = 0.85$; (3) the investigators then chose appropriate probabilities of errors of the first kind (a) and of the second kind (β). They took $a = .05$ and $\beta = .20$.

Utilizing the criteria above, the one-sided sequential plan was calculated as follows: Let θ = proportion of untied pairs favorable to preparation A under the alternative hypothesis; then

$$\theta = \frac{p_A \, q_B}{(p_A \, q_B + p_B \, q_A)}$$

where

$$p_B = 0.70 \text{ and } q_B = (1 - 0.70) = 3.30,$$
$$p_A = 0.85 \text{ and } q_A = (1 - 0.85) = 0.15.$$

Thus

$$\theta = \frac{(0.85)(0.30)}{[(0.85)(0.30) + (0.70)(0.15)]} = .7083.$$

Actually, the same θ includes other combinations of p_B and p_A differing by more than 15% (for p_B less than 70%) and by less than 15% (for p_B greater than 70%). Under the null hypothesis that $p_A = p_B$, $\theta = 1/2$. (If A is actually less effective than B, so that $p_A < p_B$, then, of course, $\theta < 1/2$).

The parallel lines constituting the boundaries of the one-sided sequential plan are calculated from the formulas already given for the Sign Test, replacing p_1 by θ and p_0 by 1/2. Thus,

$$a = \log \frac{(1 - \beta)}{a} = \log \frac{0.80}{0.05} - \log 16 = 1.20412$$

$$b = \log \frac{(1 - a)}{\beta} = \log \frac{0.95}{0.20} = \log 4.75 = 0.067669$$

$$c = \log \frac{1}{2(1 - \theta)} = \log \frac{1}{2(0.2917)} = \log 1.7141 = 0.23403$$

$$d = \log \frac{\theta}{(1 - \theta)} = \frac{(0.7083)}{(0.2917)} = \log 2.4282 = 0.38529.$$

The equations of the line are:

$$y_1 = 3.125 + 0.6074n$$
$$y_0 = -1.756 + 0.6074n,$$

where y is the number of untied pairs favoring the new preparation A and n is the number of untied pairs.

Reject $\theta = 1/2$ and declare preparation A is better than preparation B when $y > y_1$. Reject $\theta = 0.7083$ and declare preparation A is not better than B when $y < y_0$ (not better than B by 15% if, in fact, $p_B = 70\%$).

These two lines are drawn on arithmetic graph paper (Figure 16.4). On the abscissa scale, n is plotted as the number of untied pairs, and on the ordinate scale, y is plotted as the number of these pairs favorable to the new preparation, A. From the results in Table 16.5, we note that the first pair is untied, favoring preparation B. On the sequential graph, we plot one unit to the right on the abscissa for an untied pair. The next pair is also untied but favoring preparation A, so we go one unit to the right on the abscissa scale for an untied pair, and one unit up on the ordinate scale for an untied pair favoring preparation A. The next three pairs are also untied, favoring preparation A, so in each case we go one unit to the right and one up. We continue in this manner until we record the twentieth pair, which is untied and favoring A, at which point the upper line is crossed. This then terminates the experiment. The decision is to

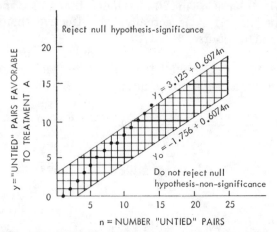

FIG. 16.4 One-Sided Sequential Plan for a Double Dichotomy Problem: $a = .05; \beta = .20; \theta = .7083$.

reject the null hypothesis, declaring that preparation A is better than preparation B under the conditions set forth at the beginning of the experiment. In other words, the observed proportion of the A cases showing effective topical anesthesia is significantly higher than the corresponding proportion of the B cases.

SEQUENTIAL t-TEST

When naturally paired samples of numerical measurements are available, the usual test of significance is to compare the average difference with zero by the t-test. The significance test can also be performed sequentially. When two independent samples of measurements are available, the difference between the two means is compared with zero by the two-sample t-test. In order to perform the test for independent samples sequentially, it is usually necessary to introduce random pairing and proceed as with the case of natural pairing.

If the standard deviation (σ_d) of the difference (d) between paired measurements were known, the fixed sample size test calls for the use of the normal curve. A sequential plan could easily be constructed using the normal curve, which would be sensitive to any specified difference in means expressed as a multiple, D, of the standard deviation, i.e., $D = (\mu_1 - \mu_2)/\sigma_d$. The cumulative sum of the d's, Σd, is then referred to the boundaries given by the plan. Occasionally, on the basis of a long, stable past experience, it is possible to calculate σ_d for use in the sequential design. However, when σ_d is not known and has to be estimated from the data, the appropriate fixed sample size test is the t-test, and the appropriate sequential test is the sequential t-test. Unfortunately, this test has not been developed as fully as that based on the normal curve, nor has it been developed as fully as sequential tests utilizing dichotomous scales illustrated earlier in this chapter. It is the purpose of this section to present the application of the sequential t-test to a clinical dental research problem.

An experiment was designed to determine whether a new local anesthetic, Carbocaine HCl 2% with 1:20,000 Neo-Cobefrin, would produce conduction anesthesia of the inferior alveolar nerve more rapidly or more slowly than the widely used Xylocaine HCl 2% with 1:100,000 epinephrine.[14] Each patient received an inferior alveolar nerve block with 1.8 cc of each solution with roughly two or three days between injections. The side of the mandible injected and the order in which the solutions were used was determined by a prear-

ranged randomized scheme. Each patient started a stop watch when
the needle was inserted and stopped it as soon as the onset of local
anesthesia at the midline of the lip was noted. A decision of nonsignificance was reached after testing 14 patients. The data appear in
Table 16.6.

TABLE 16.6
Onset Times of Inferior Alveolar Nerve Anesthesia in 14 Patients
Given Xylocaine and Carbocaine Injections (X, C)[14]

| Patient | Order of Administration | | Time of Onset of Anesthesia at Midline of Lower Lip | | Xylocaine – Carbocaine |
	Side	Solution	Min	Sec	(d) Seconds
1	L	X	1	23.0	+ 11.7
	R	C	1	11.3	
2	R	X	4	48.2	+ 81.6
	L	C	3	26.6	
3	L	X	0	27.0	– 63.0
	R	C	1	30.0	
4	R	X	3	12.8	–310.0
	L	C	8	22.8	
5	L	C	2	10.2	+ 53.0
	R	X	3	3.2	
6	R	C	5	17.1	+ 55.8
	L	X	6	12.9	
7	L	X	4	12.5	–425.5
	R	C	11	18.0	
8	R	C	3	18.9	+ 82.5
	L	X	4	41.4	
9	R	C	9	23.3	–310.4
	L	X	4	12.9	
10	R	X	5	1.5	+105.7
	L	C	3	15.8	
11	R	C	4	18.2	+ 54.1
	L	X	5	12.3	
12	L	X	2	31.1	– 90.7
	R	C	4	1.8	
13	R	C	2	6.8	+ 12.9
	L	X	2	19.7	
14	L	X	3	31.0	+ 82.4
	R	C	2	18.6	

The average time of onset of inferior alveolar nerve block with Xylocaine may be estimated from prior experience to be about four minutes. From the preliminary inspection of a few individuals who had Xylocaine injection in both jaws, to note how the difference in onset times between the sides varies from individual to individual, it was estimated that the interindividual standard deviation of the difference in onset times between the sides of the jaw is approximately two minutes. A new drug that changed the average induction time by as much as two minutes is of interest. This leads one to pick a ratio of difference in average induction time to standard deviation of $|D| = (|\mu_1 - \mu_2|)/\sigma_d = 2 \text{ min}/2 \text{ min} = 1.00$ as an alternative to the null hypothesis that $D = 0$. The test is two-sided, since interest is focused on a change in either direction. A two-sided test can be thought of as a three-decision problem: Carbocaine is faster than Xylocaine; there is no important difference in onset time; or Carbocaine is slower than Xylocaine.

In the preliminary planning for the sequential t-test, the values $a = .02$ and $\beta = .05$ were decided on. Thus, if the investigator controls the probability of an error of the first kind at $a = .02$ ($a = .01$ for each side of the two-sided test), he is taking a chance of 2 in 100 of declaring significance when, in fact, the true difference is zero. If he takes the risk of an error of the second kind as $\beta = .05$, he has a chance of 5 in 100 of declaring nonsignificance when the true difference is as specified ($|D| = 1.00$). Thus, the test has a power, $1 - \beta$, of .95. The fixed sample size necessary to effect the desired discrimination with the indicated a and β is approximately 20.

The sequential t-test to be illustrated here is that ascribed to Barnard. The advantage of using Barnard's[15] method over that described by Wald[2] for the two-sided test is that the sequential scheme can be constructed by combining two one-sided tests, thus making it more analogous to the test described previously for the Sign test and for the double dichotomy. Wald's sequential t-test, on the other hand, is two-sided automatically by construction rather than a two-sided test composed of two one-sided tests. In that sense, it is a two-decision, rather than a three-decision test. If the null hypothesis is rejected, the reason for its rejection must still be ascertained. The advantage of Wald's test is that extensive tables of boundaries have been prepared by the National Bureau of Standards.[16] The tables of boundaries for Barnard's test are in a much more sketchy form, but are available. Actually, the Wald test and the Barnard test (two-sided) do not differ materially in their boundaries.[4]

In the experiment discussed here, the difference in time of onset

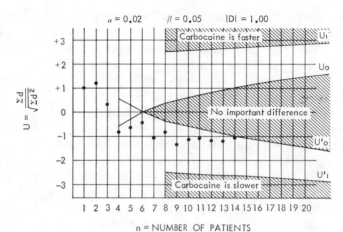

FIG. 16.5 Two-Sided Sequential Plan for t-Test.

of local anesthesia in seconds between the two solutions (d = Xylocaine – Carbocaine) is determined for each individual. The cumulative sum of the differences is then calculated, taking the sign into
account. Any zero values of d — a remote possibility — are not dis-
regarded as are ties in the Sign Test. The cumulative sum of the
squares is also calculated (Σd^2), as well as the value, $U = \Sigma d/\sqrt{\Sigma d^2}$.
It is this function of the observations that is given in Table 16.7* and
plotted in Figure 16.5. By referring to the appropriate table (Table
16.8), one obtains the boundary values of U_0 and U_1 appropriate to
the one-sided test with D = +1.00. The values for D = -1.00 are the
negatives of U_0 and U_1. The boundaries are plotted in Figure 15.5.
It is noted that the boundaries are not pairs of parallel lines as they
would be if σ_d were known and the sequential normal curve test
could be used. The boundaries U_1 and U_1', can, however, be extended rather well by extrapolated straight lines after about N = 20
in this problem.

The successive values of U from Table 16.7 are then plotted as in
Figure 16.5. It will be noted that the plot of the fourteenth individual just crosses the U_0' line, i.e., into the zone of no important difference. The experiment is terminated with the decision that no
important difference exists in the average time of onset of local
anesthesia for Carbocaine and Xylocaine under the conditions of the
experiment. That is, |D| is less than one.

---

*This value, U, is related to the usual t of the t-test as

$$t = (U\sqrt{N-1})/\sqrt{(N-U^2)}.$$

TABLE 16.7
Calculation for the Sequential t-Test

n	d	Σd	Σd^2	$\sqrt{\Sigma d^2}$	U
1	11.7	11.7	136.89	11.7	1.000
2	81.6	93.3	6,795.45	82.4	1.132
3	- 63.0	30.3	10,764.45	103.8	0.292
4	-310.0	-279.7	106,864.45	326.9	-0.856
5	53.0	-226.7	109,673.45	331.2	-0.685
6	55.8	-170.9	112,787.09	335.8	-0.509
7	-425.5	-596.4	293,837.34	542.1	-1.100
8	82.5	-513.9	300,643.59	548.3	-0.937
9	-310.4	-824.3	396,991.75	630.1	-1.308
10	105.7	-718.6	408,164.24	638.9	-1.125
11	54.1	-664.5	411,091.05	641.2	-1.036
12	- 90.7	-755.2	419,317.54	647.5	-1.166
13	12.9	-742.3	419,483.95	647.7	-1.146
14	82.4	-659.9	426,273.71	652.9	-1.011

TABLE 16.8
Boundary Values for Two-Sided Sequential t-Test[a]
$a = .02; \beta = .05.$

	One-Sided Test $a = .01; \beta = .05; D = 1.00$		One-Sided Test $a = .01; \beta = .05; D = 1.00$	
n	U_0	U_1	$U_0' = - U_0$	$U_1' = -U_1$
4	-0.55	. . .	0.55	. . .
6	0.01	. . .	-0.01	. . .
8	0.35	2.49	-0.35	-2.49
10	0.62	2.52	-0.62	-2.52
15	1.10	2.65	-1.10	-2.65
20	1.46	2.79	-1.46	-2.79
25	1.75	2.95	-1.75	-2.95
30	2.01	3.11	-2.01	-3.11
35	2.24	3.26	-2.24	-3.26
40	2.44	3.40	-2.44	-3.40
45	2.63	3.54	-2.63	-3.54
50	2.82	3.67	-2.82	-3.67

[a]Adapted from Davies.[15]

SEQUENTIAL SAMPLING VERSUS FIXED SAMPLES

Advantages of Sequential Sampling

There are two basic advantages of the sequential method. First, the average sample size necessary to assert significance is less than that calculated on the basis of a fixed sample size. Second, if the difference between the two treatments, A and B, exceeds that specified in the preparation of the plan, a decision is usually reached much sooner. In a one-sided plan, if A is worse than B instead of being better than B as specified in the alternative hypothesis, then a decision of nonsignificance is reached even more rapidly.

Disadvantages of Sequential Sampling

One of the basic disadvantages is that the nature of the study may not lend itself readily to this method, as, for example, when there is an appreciable time lag between the (intake) treatment of the subjects and the evaluation of the results, so that many subjects may still be in the process of evaluation when a decision is reached. Another problem sometimes encountered is that, because of random variation, the testing may go on much longer than the calculated average sample size. To circumvent this difficulty, the investigator can decide in advance to stop the experiment (truncation) at, for example, twice the calculated fixed sample size. If this truncation is performed far out on the sequential graph, such as at twice the fixed sample size, it does not materially change the values previously selected for a and β. In the event of truncation, the decision made corresponds to the upper line (y_1) or to the lower line (y_0), according to whether the last point plotted falls above or below a line drawn through the origin parallel to the y_1 and y_0 lines.

One further disadvantage of the sequential method is largely an administrative one. In setting up a study, it is often necessary to prepare a suitable budget and also to hire additional personnel, such as technicians, who are usually hired for a definite period of time. If the study is terminated more rapidly or continued longer than originally planned, problems often arise concerning the staff.

REFERENCES

1. Finney, D. J.: Experimental Design and Its Statistical Basis, Chicago, Univ. Chicago Press, 1955, pp. 118–119.

2. Wald, A.: Sequential Analysis, New York, Wiley, 1947.

3. Statistical Research Group, Columbia Univ., Sequential Analysis of Statistical Data: Applications, New York, Columbia Univ. Press, 1945.

4. Armitage, P.: Sequential Medical Trials, 2nd ed., New York, Wiley, 1975.

5. Chilton, N. W., Fertig, J. W., and Kutscher, A. H.: Studies in the design and analysis of dental experiments. 3. Sequential Analysis (double dichotomy), J Dent Res 30:331, 1961.

6. Fertig, J. W., Chilton, N. W., and Varma, A. A. O.: Studies in the design and analysis of dental experiments. 9. Sequential analysis (sign test), J Oral Ther 1:45, 1964.

7. Chilton, N. W., Fertig, J. W., and Varma, A. A. O.: Studies in the design and analysis of dental experiments. 10. Sequential analysis (t-test), J Oral Ther 1:175, 1963.

8. Varma, A. A. O., and Chilton, N. W.: Studies in the design and analysis of dental experiments. 11. Sequential analysis (two dichotomous populations where the data are collected in groups), J Oral Ther 2:44, 1965.

9. Sherman, H., Fiasconaro, J. E., Cain, E. A., Jr., and Fertig, J. W.: Control of dental anxiety with mephenesin, J Amer Dent Ass 58:63, 1959.

10. Chilton, N. W., and Fertig, J. W.: The clinical dental trial. II. Evaluation of a relaxing drug for operative dentistry, J Dent Res 37:444, 1958.

11. Mainland, D., Herrera, L., and Sutliffe, M. I.: Statistical Tables for Use with Binomial Samples, New York. Dept. of Medical Statistics, New York Univ. College of Medicine, 1965.

12. Wessinger, G.: Comparative measurements of salivary pH, J Dent Res 20:123, 1941.

13. Kutscher, A. H.: Unpublished data, Columbia Univ. School of Dental and Oral Surgery.

14. Chilton, N. W., and Leventhal, S.: Unpublished data, Temple Univ. School of Dentistry, 1962.

15. Davies, O. L., ed.: The Design and Analysis of Industrial Experiments, London, Oliver and Boyd, 1960.

16. National Bureau of Standards: Tables to Facilitate Sequential t-Tests, Applied Mathematics Series #7, Washington (D.C.), U.S. Dept of Commerce, 1951.

17

Experiment Design

Our preceding chapters have explained comparisons — comparison of a sample value with a hypothetical value, of two independent samples, of more than two independent samples (the one-way layout of data), of two paired or correlated samples, and of more than two correlated samples (the two-way layout of data). The data were measurement, nominal (including dichotomous) and ordinal in nature.

The methods expounded were not limited to experimental data, but were also used with naturally formed groups or observational data, i.e., nature's experiments. Many epidemiological studies are of this type. The method of analysis and the method of drawing inferences are the same with experimental and observational data, but one has to be careful with the resulting inferences if the data have not been derived from actual experiments. In the preceding chapters, no clear distinction was made between data of the experimental type and of the observational type. In this chapter, attention will be focused on experimental data in which the investigator determines the makeup of the groups and the treatments to be applied to these groups or units. While some references have already been made to the problems of comparability, randomization, and selection of treatments, this chapter will expand these concepts.

PLANNING THE EXPERIMENT

When an experiment is to be performed, the investigator should be prepared to spend a considerable amount of time in its planning. First he should define the basic objective of the research study. Then he should define clearly the various "treatments" he expects to compare; the units (patients, animals, chemical aliquots, tissues) to which he expects to apply these treatments; the methods of assigning the various treatments to these experimental subjects or units; and the types of observations, records or measurements he expects to make on each subject so treated. These factors constitute the basic concepts in the design of an experiment.

In general, the purpose of an experiment is to measure the effect of one or more procedures or treatments on experimental units by a comparison with some other treatment which may, in fact, be no treatment or an orthodox treatment. The general desideratum of a good experiment is the similar application of objective criteria to similar groups, which should be large enough so that effects having practical importance will be detected. Experiments will differ greatly as to how these requirements are satisfied.

The treatments must be completely defined, including such details as dosage and frequency of administration, and once agreed on should be adhered to throughout the experiment. The purpose of the experiment will determine just what type of controls, if any, are necessary and what precautions must be taken to ensure comparability of the various groups.

The planning phase of the experiment should also give consideration to the way in which the results are going to be reported, what tables are to be compiled, how the data are to be analyzed, and what comparisons and significance tests are to be performed. Detailed consideration of these steps will also suggest what subgroupings of the experimental subjects are appropriate, and how large the groups may need to be so that any real effects of practical importance may be detected.

The objectives of the experiment consist of a series of questions to be answered or hypotheses to be tested. Often a number of questions are put to a single experiment, but one should not be too ambitious and try to answer too many questions from the same experiment, or none may be answered satisfactorily. Variations in the form of extra questions can come in later experiments. A clear statement of the questions to be answered will also determine what measurements need to be obtained and what precautions must be taken to avoid bias in the measurements.[1]

Measurements Used

The measurements will be of various kinds, such as blood pressure, gain in weight, carious or noncarious teeth, grade of improvement; and these will determine what records are to be kept. Quantitative measurements, such as mg% of salivary calcium or gain or loss of weight, are generally preferred to such evaluations as improved or worse, cured or not cured, if they are equally relevant. The precision of the experiment is usually increased by using more refined measurements. In general, objective measurements or assessments, where the human observer is only incidental, are preferred to subjective measurements.

Reducing Experimental Error

It is to the selection of the units or subjects to which the treatments are to be applied, and the methods of assigning the treatments to these experimental units, that a great deal of attention must be devoted. It is the purpose of this chapter to expound on these and related aspects, in order to assist the investigator in determining the best type of design for the experiment he plans to perform.

Experimental subjects are variable, so that two subjects usually differ from each other even when given the same treatment. Because of this inherent variability, the effects of a given treatment will not be consistent and some uncertainty is thus introduced into the conclusions. It is this biological variability plus the lack of standardization of the various steps and measurements made in the experiment that causes the experimental error, which may mask the effects of the treatments. A well-designed experiment attempts to minimize these experimental errors.

The usual way of decreasing the experimental error is to increase the number of subjects utilized in the various treatment groups. The dependence of the precision of the comparison on the sample size has been covered in preceding chapters in terms of standard errors, t-test, F-test, fourfold table, χ^2, and so on. One way of reducing experimental error is to use more homogeneous material, so that the more obvious variations are eliminated. Thus, an experimental study of the effect of a chelating agent on supragingival calculus formation may be limited to subjects who are nonsmokers. Since smoking is believed to have an effect on calculus deposition, this restriction on the subjects included makes them more homogeneous and also reduces the experimental error. It must be remembered, however, that whatever conclusions are drawn must be limited to nonsmokers, and generalizations to other types of subjects cannot safely be made.

Pairing or Blocking Experimental Units

Another widely used method of increasing the precision of the experiment is to group the experimental subjects so as to control extraneous sources of variation, so that the subjects to which the treatments are applied are more closely comparable. In the simplest case where only two treatments are involved, pairs are formed. The subjects available are grouped into pairs in such a manner that the members of a pair are as similar as possible, and then one member from each pair is assigned to each treatment. It is important that the selection of a member of a pair for a particular treatment be made randomly and independently, as by tossing a coin or using a table of random numbers. This pairing improves an experiment by bringing together subjects who are alike for the variable under study except for the effects of treatment difference. As Finney pointed out, "Any character that can be assessed before the experiment begins may be used as the basis of the pairing. The experimenter should try to use a character closely associated with the measurement eventually to be made, but his choice will be limited by convenience and practicability."[2] Obvious examples are naturally occurring pairs, such as in twin studies or in littermate control studies, where one member of the litter serves as the experimental member of the pair and a litter mate as the control member. The experimenter may also form pairs on the basis of some presumably relevant factor, such as the P-M-A Index. The pairs may be formed by matching on a number of variables forming what is usually referred to as "matched pairs."

Crossover Designs

The use of the same individual in each of two treatments, A and B, if possible, is an obvious form of pairing in which "each individual serves as his own control." This design is often referred to as a "cross-over design." Obviously, the order of presenting the two treatments must be chosen at random for each individual. Special steps may be taken, in fact, to ensure that both possible orders, AB and BA, occur with the same frequency.[3] Crossover designs may present difficulties, however, because the effect of the first treatment may be partly exhibited while the second treatment is being given, the "carry-over" effect. This difficulty can often be avoided by allowing enough time to elapse before instituting the second treatment. Problems may still exist where there may be differential carry-over effects.[4] Detailed critiques of the crossover design in clinical studies have been published by Varma and Chilton[5] and by Brown.[6]

What appears to be a special type of crossover design is the "before and after" experiment, in which a control reading is taken before treatment is instituted and again after completion of the treatment. Unfortunately, the sequence in which the measurements are made cannot be randomized. Furthermore, the experimental errors in the two time periods may not be independent of each other. For this reason, it is frequently necessary to use a control group of subjects who receive a placebo treatment and who are studied before and after the application of this "treatment."

The discussion with regard to the formation of pairs can obviously be extended to cover the case of more than two treatments. In this case, blocks of experimental units are formed instead of pairs, the number of units in the block being equal to the number of treatments involved. If, for example, four treatments were being compared, we should have to speak of quadruplet studies, litters of size four, blocks of four subjects having the same P-M-A Index, and blocks of four subjects formed by matching on a number of variables.

If the same individual can be used for all four treatments, A, B, C, and D, we have an obvious extension of the crossover design. The order of the four treatments would be determined at random for each individual. Special steps may, in fact, be taken to ensure that each succeeding treatment appears as frequently as the first treatment. This control of order yields a four by four Latin square when only four subjects are used. Replicated Latin squares would be formed with further groups of four subjects.[7]

The extension of the before-and-after experiment would arise, for example, if we had a control reading before treatment was instituted and a series of readings at various times during the treatment, or subsequent to the completion of the treatment. Again, it might be necessary to run a comparable group of patients on a placebo treatment for comparison.

Stratification

Frequently, the number of subjects forming the block is large enough so that more than one subject from the block can be allocated to each treatment. In effect, the block is a stratum homogeneous with respect to one or more relevant variables. The subjects within the stratum are allocated at random to the various treatments. Similarly, the subjects in the other strata are divided at random among the treatments. It is not necessary that the number of subjects in the various strata be the same. It is advisable, however, that within each stratum the number of subjects allocated to the various treatments be equal; otherwise the statistical analysis may present some difficulty. The formation of pairs or blocks equal in size to the number of treatments is, in fact, merely a special case of the more general stratification.

STATISTICAL ANALYSIS AND
SIGNIFICANCE TESTS

The design of the experiment dictates the type of statistical analysis and tests to be performed. If no pairing or blocking is performed, we have the unrestricted randomized design. The appropriate analysis for such data, in the field of measurements, is the t-test for two independent samples, or the one-way analysis of variance in the general case of two or more treatments. In the case of a dichotomous scale, the corresponding methods are the fourfold table analysis for two treatments, and the χ^2 test of homogeneity for two or more treatments. In the case of an ordinal scale, the corresponding methods are the Wilcoxon rank sum test and the Kruskal-Wallis test.

When pairing or blocking has been performed, i.e., the randomized block design, the appropriate analysis with measurements is the paired t-test in the case of two treatments. In the case of two or more treatments, the appropriate analysis is the two-way analysis of variance with the associated F-test. With dichotomous scales, the comparable methods of analysis are the McNemar test and the Cochran Q test. With ordinal scales, the comparable tests are the Sign test and the Friedman two-way analysis of variance on ranks. For the special case of two paired samples with ordinal scales, the Wilcoxon signed rank test is also available. (For these tests, see Chapters 7, 12, 13, and 15.)

The analysis of a crossover design where the order of the sequence of treatments is controlled, and also a Latin square design, has been described for measurement data in standard texts.[3,8] The analysis for corresponding designs in the field of dichotomous and ordinal data has generally not been developed to any great extent.

The analysis of the before-and-after design for measurements in which a placebo control group is also utilized involves two independent samples of differences with the associated t-test. In the general case of two or more time periods, the test is derived from appropriate terms of the incomplete three-way analysis of variance. Corresponding tests generally do not seem to be available for dichotomous and ordinal scales.

The analysis of measurement data in the general case of stratification involves the two-way analysis of variance with replication in the cells. The particular F-test required depends on the type of model assumed, i.e., fixed or mixed. Various solutions to stratification problems involving dichotomous and ordinal scales have been proposed.[9-13]

CONSIDERATIONS IN A CLINICAL STUDY

Selection of subjects for a clinical study is often made on the basis of personal contacts or relationships with administrators of schools or public or private institutions, or even of industrial organizations. While such personal contacts are helpful, in fact even desirable, in order to ensure full cooperation of the various administrators of the study population, there are other very important considerations in the selection of these subjects. Since dental caries inhibition is the object of extensive clinical study, the following discussion will refer to this type of study.[14]

Selection of Subjects in a Dental Caries Study

Because dental caries is most active during childhood and adolescence, the best trial would be run in a group in which these ages were heavily represented rather than in an older population in which the carious process is no longer so active. While this may seem obvious, the first clinical trials of some agents have been run in such older age groups. The lowest age group studied should be one in which a sufficient number of permanent teeth are present at the start to give a large enough susceptible tooth population. While deciduous teeth are also attacked by caries, accurate records and final evaluation of results are extremely difficult because of the normal exfoliation of these teeth in a variable pattern. Thus, unless a study is specifically set up to evaluate the effectiveness of the caries-inhibitory agent on deciduous teeth, it would be advantageous to eliminate consideration of these teeth from the study. Similarly, while some clinical trials may be run for specific problems, the chronological ages that would provide the most suitable "dental ages" for the clinical trial would usually range from 10 or 11 to 19 years. While the study need not be confined to these age groups, the distribution of subjects should be concentrated within them.

The population selected for the clinical trial should be fairly stable. This stability should be reflected in a relatively low loss of population in the groups over the study period, as well as in the consistency of carrying out the desired method of utilization of the agents being compared. Undoubtedly, a "captive" type of population would meet these requirements to a greater extent than one consisting of individuals who are together only part of the time, i.e., an institutionalized population rather than a public school population.

Children attending school as day students can, of course, be used as the subjects under study, but the investigator must make every effort to obtain the wholehearted cooperation of the parents as well as the school administrators, teachers, and the children themselves. When this cooperation is not fully obtained, it is not inconceivable that extraneous factors may be introduced that can influence the outcome of the clinical trial. For example, some children may receive topical applications of fluoride salts by their private dentists, or may use any one of a number of dentrifices now on the market that may or may not have a caries-inhibitory effect, or may be inconsistent in their oral hygiene patterns away from the routine prescribed at school.

With institutionalized populations, these extraneous factors are amenable to control. Furthermore, such possible influencing factors as dietary intake can also be better controlled, or at least recorded. On the other hand, institutionalized populations may not be representative of children of similar ages in the population as a whole, and any conclusions drawn from the results of the clinical trial may not apply to the overall population.

Assignment of Subjects to Groups

In order to understand the formation of the experimental groups and the assignment of different treatments to them, let us consider a simple clinical trial. Comparability of the groups is usually attained by some form of random allocation of the subjects to the various groups. If all the subjects to be used in an experiment were arbitrarily divided into two groups without any apparent bias or prejudice, it could not be claimed that randomization had been performed. Rather, such a division might be called "haphazardization." If, in addition to haphazardization, a different treatment were assigned to each group in such a way that each individual knew what he was receiving and each examiner also knew, this experiment might very well be poorly conducted. Any difference in the results obtained from the two groups could be due to one of five factors, or to a combination of them: chance variation, treatment difference, bias because of haphazard selection of subjects, bias on the part of the subjects, and bias on the part of the examiners in determining the response to treatment.

This experiment can be improved by assigning the subjects to the two groups in a random manner, substituting "randomization" for "haphazardization." This is important, because significance tests are based on the concept of random sampling. In this simplest case of two groups, there would be an experimental and a control group, or a treated and an untreated group, or perhaps two treatment groups. One way to divide the subjects into two groups in a randomized manner would be to order them by lot. Suppose, for example, that it is desired to divide a group of 20 patients into two groups. Each of the 20 patients is assigned a number from 1 to 20; the numbers are placed on tickets, which are put into a hat and shuffled. The patients corresponding to the first 10 numbers pulled from the hat would be assigned to one group, and the remainder to the other.

Use of Tables of Random Numbers

Rather than perform a lottery each time patients are selected for a study, one may use tables of random numbers, readily available. Table 17.1 is composed, typically, of numbers from 00 to 99, arranged for convenience in blocks of five rows with five two-digit numbers each. The number 00 stands for 100. We start anywhere in the table, perhaps by closing our eyes and placing our pencil at random. Our pencil falls in the third block in and one block down on the table, on the first figure in the second row, 61. Reading the numbers in this block, row by row for each column, we obtain 61, 59, 62, 90, 15, 54, 63, 61, 18, 70, 13, 69, 65, 48, 11, etc. The first 10 numbers less than 20 would designate the individuals assigned to the first group. Thus, numbers 15, 18, 13, 11, etc. belong to the first group of 10 patients. Since 20 is a number much smaller than 100, we find that this is a wasteful procedure, since many of the numbers exceed 20 and cannot be used. A more convenient procedure, in this case, is to express the numbers as remainders from 20 or multiples of 20, i.e., to reduce them modulo 20. Thus, $61 - (3)(20) = 1$, so that number 1 is obtained. The next number is 59, or, reduced modulo 20, is 19. The third number is 62, which becomes 2. The next number is 90, which becomes $90 - (4)(20) = 10$. The next number in the next column in the block is 15, which does not have to be reduced. If a number is repeated, it is discarded, so that 61 and 70, which would again yield 1 and 10, are not used. Using this procedure, the first 10 random numbers are 1, 19, 2, 10, 15, 14, 3, 18, 13, and 9. The 10 patients bearing these numbers are then assigned one treatment, and the other 10 the other treatment.

In the case of more than two treatment groups, say six treatments to be assigned to 24 patients, the numbers from 1 to 96 are reduced modulo 24. The numbers 97, 98, 99 and 00 must be dis-

TABLE 17.1
Random Numbers

```
53 74 23 99 67   61 32 29 69 84   94 62 67 86 24   98 33 41 19 95   47 53 53 38 09
63 38 06 86 54   99 00 65 26 94   02 82 90 23 07   79 62 67 80 60   75 91 12 81 19
35 30 58 21 46   06 72 17 10 94   25 21 31 75 96   49 28 24 00 49   55 65 79 78 07
63 43 36 82 69   65 51 18 37 88   61 38 44 12 45   32 92 85 88 65   54 34 81 85 35
98 25 37 55 26   01 91 82 81 46   74 71 12 94 97   24 01 71 37 07   03 92 18 66 75

02 63 21 17 69   71 50 80 89 56   38 15 70 11 48   43 40 45 86 98   00 83 26 91 03
64 55 22 21 82   48 22 28 06 00   61 54 13 43 91   82 78 12 23 29   06 66 24 12 27
85 07 26 13 89   01 10 07 82 04   59 63 69 36 03   69 11 15 83 80   13 29 54 19 28
58 54 16 24 15   51 54 44 82 00   62 61 65 04 69   38 18 65 18 97   85 72 13 49 21
34 85 27 84 87   61 48 64 56 26   90 18 48 13 26   37 70 15 42 57   65 65 80 39 07

03 92 18 27 46   57 99 16 96 56   30 33 72 85 22   84 64 38 56 98   90 01 30 98 64
62 95 30 27 59   37 75 41 66 48   86 97 80 61 45   23 53 04 01 63   45 76 08 64 27
08 45 93 15 22   60 21 75 46 91   98 77 27 85 42   28 88 61 08 84   69 62 03 42 73
07 08 55 18 40   45 44 75 13 90   24 94 96 61 02   57 55 66 83 15   73 42 37 11 61
01 85 89 95 66   51 10 19 34 88   15 84 97 19 75   12 76 39 43 78   64 63 91 08 25

72 84 71 14 35   19 11 58 49 26   50 11 17 17 76   86 31 57 20 18   95 60 78 46 75
88 78 28 16 84   13 52 53 94 53   75 45 69 30 96   73 89 65 70 31   99 17 43 48 76
45 17 75 65 57   28 40 19 72 12   25 12 74 75 67   60 40 60 81 19   24 62 01 61 16
96 76 28 12 54   22 01 11 94 25   71 96 16 16 88   68 64 36 74 45   19 59 50 88 92
43 31 67 72 30   24 02 94 08 63   38 32 36 66 02   69 36 38 25 39   48 03 45 15 22

50 44 66 44 21   66 06 58 05 62   68 15 54 35 02   42 35 48 96 32   15 52 41 52 48
22 66 22 15 56   26 63 75 41 99   58 42 36 72 24   58 37 52 18 51   03 37 18 39 11
96 24 40 14 51   23 22 30 88 57   95 67 47 29 83   94 69 40 06 07   18 16 36 78 86
31 73 91 61 19   60 20 72 93 48   98 57 07 23 69   65 95 39 69 58   56 80 30 19 44
78 60 73 99 84   43 89 94 36 45   56 69 47 01 41   90 22 91 07 12   78 35 34 08 72
```

```
84 37 90 61 56   70 10 23 98 05   85 11 34 76 60   76 48 45 34 60   01 64 18 39 96
36 67 10 08 23   98 93 35 08 86   99 29 76 29 81   33 34 91 58 93   63 14 52 32 52
07 28 59 07 48   89 64 58 89 75   83 85 62 27 89   30 14 78 56 27   86 63 59 80 02
10 15 83 87 60   79 24 31 66 56   21 48 24 06 93   91 98 94 05 49   01 47 59 38 00
55 19 68 97 65   03 73 52 16 56   00 53 55 90 27   33 42 29 38 87   22 13 88 83 34

53 81 29 13 39   35 01 20 71 34   62 33 74 82 14   53 73 19 09 03   56 54 29 56 93
51 86 32 68 92   33 98 74 66 99   40 14 71 94 57   45 94 19 38 81   14 44 99 81 07
35 91 70 29 13   80 03 54 07 27   96 94 78 32 66   50 95 52 74 33   13 80 55 62 54
37 71 67 95 13   20 02 44 95 94   64 85 04 05 72   01 32 90 76 14   53 89 74 60 41
93 66 13 83 27   92 79 64 64 72   28 54 96 53 84   48 14 52 98 94   56 07 93 89 30

02 96 08 45 65   13 05 00 41 84   93 07 54 72 59   21 45 57 09 77   19 48 56 27 44
49 83 43 48 35   82 88 33 69 96   72 36 04 19 76   47 45 15 18 60   82 11 08 95 97
84 60 71 62 46   40 80 81 30 37   34 39 23 05 38   25 15 35 71 30   88 12 57 21 77
18 17 30 88 71   44 91 14 88 47   89 23 30 63 15   56 34 20 47 89   99 82 93 24 98
79 69 10 61 78   71 32 76 95 62   87 00 22 58 40   92 54 01 75 25   43 11 71 99 31

75 93 36 57 83   56 20 14 82 11   74 21 97 90 65   96 42 68 63 86   74 54 13 26 94
38 30 92 29 03   06 28 81 39 38   62 25 06 84 63   61 29 08 93 67   04 32 92 08 09
51 29 50 10 34   31 57 75 95 80   51 97 02 74 77   76 15 48 49 44   18 55 63 77 09
21 31 38 86 24   37 79 81 53 74   73 24 16 10 33   52 83 90 94 76   70 47 14 54 36
29 01 23 87 88   58 02 39 37 67   42 10 14 20 92   16 55 23 42 15   54 96 09 11 06

95 33 95 22 00   18 74 72 00 18   38 79 58 69 32   81 76 80 26 92   82 80 84 25 39
90 84 60 79 70   24 36 59 87 38   82 07 53 89 35   96 35 23 79 18   05 98 90 07 35
46 40 62 98 82   54 97 20 56 95   15 74 80 08 32   16 46 70 50 80   67 72 16 42 79
20 31 89 03 43   38 46 82 68 72   32 14 82 99 70   80 60 47 18 97   63 49 30 21 30
71 59 73 05 50   08 22 23 71 77   91 01 93 20 49   82 96 59 26 54   66 39 67 98 60
```

[From Fisher and Yates: *Statistical Tables for Biological, Agricultural and Medical Research*, Edinburgh, Oliver & Boyd Ltd., 1949, p. 105, by permission of the authors and publishers.]

carded, since they do not allow for a complete sequence and their use would lead to some degree of bias. The patients corresponding to the first four numbers in the sequence would be assigned to the first group, the patients with the next four numbers to the second group, etc. Many hand-held calculators can generate random numbers which can be used instead of resorting to existing tables.

Subjects Selected over a Period of Time

Frequently the subjects do not come into the study at the same time, so that they are selected for the study groups over a period of time. Again, illustrating with two groups, one method of selecting patients would be to have a box of black beads and white beads thoroughly mixed (in equal numbers if equal sample sizes are desired)* and to pick blindly one bead each time a patient came into the study, replacing it each time. All patients with black beads would go into the first group, and those with white beads into the second group. This procedure effects a random division of the subjects; however, the groups will not necessarily be of the same size. Furthermore, any systematic trend in the makeup of the material will not be completely controlled, since there can be runs of blacks and whites, i.e., group 2 and group 1 patients. Of course, tossing a coin for each patient would have been equally as good as selecting beads, and far simpler.

Another method often employed is systematic alternation, which, of course, is not randomization. In this scheme, the first patient goes into the first group, and the second into the second group, the third into the first group and the fourth into the second group, for a scheme A,B, A,B, A,B. While this has the advantage of yielding groups of equal size, it may introduce a bias if there is a systematic trend in some property of the material, such as weight or severity, which is related to the measurement under study. Thus, if there is a consistent downward trend of weight of animals utilized in an experiment, for example, the animals assigned to group A would always be somewhat heavier than those assigned to group B. This may influence the outcome of the experiment if weight is a relevant factor.

---

*Occasionally, one may want to put more individuals in one treatment group than in another. This may be the case when several treatments plus a control are used and individual comparisons of each treatment with the control group are to be made. In such a case, more individuals may be allocated to the control group.

A simple way of obtaining randomization and the advantages of alternation is random alternation. A coin is tossed for each pair of patients to determine the disposition of the two members of the pair. If heads comes up, the first member of the pair is assigned to group A and the second to group B. If tails comes up, the opposite assignment is used. Random alternation can also be achieved by taking random permutations of the numbers 1 and 2 from tables of random numbers, or more easily, odd and even numbers. All schemes for dividing the material into treatment groups should preferably be decided before the subjects present themselves for the study.

With more than two, say four, groups of subjects, the toss of a die could be used to determine the assignment of the patients, or a box containing beads of four different colors, or the numbers 1 to 4 from a table of random numbers. If the numbers (or beads or tosses of a die) are taken as they come, the ultimate sizes of the groups will not necessarily be equal. Greater efficiency of the experiment results when the groups are equal. Equality can be forced by using random permutations of the numbers 1 to 4. These can be constructed by discarding repeated numbers until each sequence of 1 through 4 is completed, that is, not accepting a number more than once until each cycle of four groups is completed. Various tables of random permutations are available.[15]

Treatment Assignment in a Clinical Caries Trial

In the clinical trial of a caries-inhibitory agent, the composition of the groups receiving the test or experimental agent and the control agent should be such that they are comparable with respect to those factors (known and unknown) that influence dental caries susceptibility. Among the known factors are age, sex, race, caries experience, fluoride intake, dietary practices, and, perhaps, socioeconomic status. This comparability usually cannot be accomplished by assigning one dentifrice to an intact group in one school and another dentifrice to another group in a different school. While the employment of such intact groups certainly will ease the administrative problems involved in any clinical study, one group may be quite different from the other with respect to the ponderable factors listed above, which could produce confusion in interpreting the results obtained from such a study. How different the groups may be with respect to imponderable factors is problematic.

While a random assignment of the children available to the study groups would assure comparability within chance limits, for the known as well as the unknown factors, it is usually advisable (and often simpler) to control some of the known factors by a procedure of stratification. The randomization is then performed within the various strata. This is one of the standard devices for reducing experimental error. With an institutionalized population, the children may be stratified with respect to age, and then the distribution of the dentifrices randomized within these age strata. Stratification by age also affects some stratification for other known factors, such as caries experience. The use of grades produces an approximate age stratification. In an institutionalized population, the factor of sex can easily be controlled, since the domiciles are usually separated by sex.

After the initial examinations have been performed and, if possible, even before the clinical trial has commenced, it is wise to check the comparability of the control and experimental groups with respect to the known factors, even though the dentifrices assignment has been determined by randomization. One has to be reassured that randomization has not played any tricks. Fortunately, if one has ensured comparability with respect to age by stratification procedures, the two groups are likely to be comparable with respect to many other relevant factors. If intact groups have been used, or if the selection of subjects has been by "haphazardization" rather than randomization, a check of comparability is of even greater importance. In such studies, however, the demonstration of comparability with respect to certain known factors does not reassure one to the same degree.

Reducing Bias in Observations

Many oral biological experiments involve subjective measurements. In such cases, certain precautions must be taken so that the observer does not change his scale of measurement or criteria from one treatment group to another. To ensure lack of bias on the part of the observer, various blindfold techniques are used. The aim of these techniques is to have the observer make the measurements without knowing to which group the subjects belong, so that he cannot let his personal likes or dislikes enter into the observation. There are many examples of such techniques, such as reading the x-ray plates without knowing to which of the several groups they pertain, having the treatments given by one person and the measurements made by another, or having the treatments in identical form and assigning them according to some code unknown to the person who treats and assesses.[1]

Lack of objectivity may result from a bias on the part of not only the observer but also the observed. Consequently, the subjects may also have to be blindfolded, so they do not know to which group they belong. This generally involves giving the control group a placebo. The general aim is to expose the control group to the same manipulation as the treated group except for the actual treatment involved. There may be some cases where this is not feasible, for example, when treatment involves operation and removal of a functioning part.[1] Obviously, the control group cannot be given a blank operation. Many of the issues involved in avoiding bias on the part of the observer and the subjects are admirably discussed by Bradford Hill in his papers, "The Clinical Trial."[16,17]

Blindfolding of both the observer and the observed has been called the double-blind technique. "Briefly, it is a control device to prevent bias from influencing results. On the one hand, it rules out the effects of the hopes and anxieties of the patient by giving both the drug under investigation and a placebo of identical appearance in such a way that the subject (the first "blind" man) does not know what he is receiving. On the other hand, it also rules out the influence of preconceived hopes of, and conscious communication by, the investigator or observer by keeping him (the second "blind" man) ignorant of whether he is prescribing a placebo or an active drug. At the same time, the technique provides another control, a means of comparison with magnitude of placebo effects."[18]

Coding (Labeling) of Treatment Agents

Making both treatments — that is, placebo and active drug — the same in appearance, packaging, smell, taste, and mode of administration is usually effective in masking the identity of the agent. Since it is necessary, however, to be able to identify each treatment for recording and later for analyzing the results, it is important not to disclose the secret by the labeling procedure. Here some type of coding is useful. There are many variations of coding that can be utilized, but is should always be remembered that the code employed should be as simple as possible and should not be capable of being broken easily by the observer, in order to keep bias minimized.

The agents employed in the clinical study are usually identified by either a letter or a numerical code. Needless to state, the code should be unknown to both observer and patient. The type of code used depends on the type of clinical study. For example, in a study of the clinical effectiveness of four local anesthetics in dental procedures,[19] the solutions were supplied in cartridges for injection, all identical in appearance, numbered continuously from 1 to 100, in boxes of 100. One-fourth of the numbers were randomly assigned to each solution in a manner similar to that described previously. Since each injection utilized only one anesthetic solution, it was not necessary to provide resupply of the drug. If this had been necessary, the code would have had to be broken in order to identify the solution used. Randomization of the four treatments among the 100 cartridges actually results in the random assignment of the 100 patients to the four treatments without any further steps. Furthermore, at the end of the study of 100 patients, the four treatments will be equally represented. In fact, the randomization of the cartridges could be so arranged as to obtain equality after every four patients. This method of randomization of the patients into the four groups at the treatment-assignment level is simpler from an administrative view than that described previously in terms of the patient-assignment level.

Where resupply is necessary, as with a study involving prolonged use of a dentifrice or mouthwash, a continuous coding method may not be convenient. If two treatments are used, a simple letter code like A and B may be too easy to identify, particularly if a therapeutic effect is manifested early in the study, and such identification can produce severe bias in the later assessment of patient response. To help avoid this possibility, multiple coding with letters or numbers is often helpful. Thus, if two dentifrices are to be included, numbers from, say, 1 to 12 can be used with six numbers obtained from a table of random numbers, assigned to one formula, and the remaining six numbers assigned to the other formula. While the same assignment of dentifrice formulas to numbers is used throughout the study, a different permutation of the numbers from 1 to 12 is used for each cycle of 12 patients. The number of patients in the two treatment groups will be equal after every 12 patients. When the patient needs an additional supply of the dentifrice, he is given the same number-coded package as he had been using.

Comments on Analysis of Clinical Caries Trials

In studies of the clinical effectiveness of caries-inhibitory agents, the data for each individual are usually expressed as differences between the number of DMF teeth (DMFT) or DMF surfaces (DMFS)* from the initiation of the study to the time of last examination. The DMF is a discontinuous or discrete measurement; therefore, the increment of DMF is also discrete. The distributions of the DMF increment in the various treatment groups may not closely resemble normal curves. In the usual clinical trial of caries-inhibitory agents, however, the samples are usually of sufficient size so that one would not hesitate to compute mean DMF increments and compare these means by normal curve procedures. With small samples, some investigators might prefer to use some nonparametric procedures rather than the t-test.[13]

REFERENCES

1. Fertig, J. W.: Design of medical experiments, Texas Rep Biol Med 12:758, 1955.

2. Finney, D. J.: Experimental Design and Its Statistical Basis, Chicago, Univ. of Chicago Press, 1955.

3. Cochran, W. G., and Cox, G. H.: Experimental Designs, 2nd ed., New York, Wiley, 1957.

4. Varma, A. A. O., Fertig, J. W., Chilton, N. W., and Mandel, I. D.: Restricted Latin square design in a plaque disclosant study, J Periodont Res 9:386, 1974.

5. Chilton, N. W., ed.: International conference on clinical trials of agents used in the prevention/treatment of periodontal diseases, Varma, A. A. O. and Chilton N. W.: Crossover designs involving two treatments, J Period Res 9; (Supplement 14):160, 1974.

6. Brown, W. B. Jr.: The crossover experiment for clinical trials, Biometrics 36:69, 1980.

7. Varma, A. A. O. Chilton, N. W., and Kutscher, A. H.: Studies in the design and analysis of dental experiments: Replicate Latin squares, J Dent Res 52:23, 1973.

8. Chilton, N. W.: Latin square design in clinical experimentation, J Dent Res 34:421, 1955.

9. Cochran, W. G.: Some methods for strengthening the common χ^2 test, Biometrics 10:417, 1954.

---

*Studies can be conducted in terms of "teeth" or "tooth surfaces," provided either criterion is used *exclusively* in the study (and is so stated). The results obtained by using either one as the measuring unit have usually led to the same overall conclusions. The use of tooth surfaces necessitates, however, a much more elaborate method of record keeping (always employing roentgenographic as well as clinical examination). In addition, independent studies utilizing measurements in terms of tooth surfaces may not be comparable, since the method of counting different surfaces (particularly on anterior teeth) may differ with different investigators. Such difficulties are not usually encountered when "teeth" constitute the unit of measurement.

10. Kincaid, W. M.: The combination of 2×2 contingency tables, Biometrics 18:224, 1962.

11. Mantel, N., and Haenszel, W.: Statistical aspects of the analysis of data from retrospective studies of disease, J Nat Cancer Inst 22:719, 1958.

12. Wilcoxon, F.: Some Rapid Approximate Statistical Procedures, Stamford (Conn.), Amer. Cyanamid Company, 1949.

13. Varma, A. A. O., Fertig, J. W., and Chilton, N. W.: A nonparametric approach to the comparison of various dental agents in a stratified experimental design, Pharm & Thera in Dentistry 4:1, 1979.

14. Chilton, N. W., and Fertig, J. W.: The clinical dental trial: I. A new caries-inhibitory agent, J Dent Res 37:335, 1958.

15. Cochran, W. G.: Sampling Techniques, 3rd ed., New York, Wiley, 1967.

16. Hill, A. B.: The clinical trial, Brit Med Bull 7:278, 1951.

17. Hill, A. B.: The clinical trial, New Engl J Med 247:113, 1952.

18. Modell, W., and Houde, R. W.: Factors influencing clinical evaluation of drugs, JAMA 167:2190, 1958.

19. Epstein, S., and Chilton, N. W.: The clinical effectiveness of certain local anesthetics in dental procedures, Oral Surg 12:93, 1959.

18

Sampling from Existing Populations

In the inductive reasoning utilized in statistical methodology, conclusions based on observations of individuals or of small groups lead to inferences applicable to the population as a whole. The individuals on whom the observations have been made constitute merely a sample from some population or universe. From the information obtained by studying the sample or samples, the observer desires to estimate the characteristics of the universe distribution, the parameters. The estimate of the parameter obtained from the sample is often called a "statistic."

The universe is distributed according to either a qualitative or a quantitative scale. When the scale is qualitative, a series of relative frequencies characterize the population, while with a quantitative scale of classification, generally some sort of average and some measure of variation or dispersion describe the particular universe in question. The sample distributions are used to estimate the universe distributions, so that the characteristics of the sample distribution — e.g., the means and medians as centering constants and the variances (or standard deviations) and ranges as measures of variation — are used to estimate the corresponding characteristics of the population.

The concepts of sampling employed thus far in connection with experiments of various types and the testing of hypotheses (significance tests), have been based on the idea of universes of infinite size. In fact, the universes are often hypothetical in nature. Thus, if we have a sample of germ-free Golden Syrian hamsters infected with *Streptococcus odontolyticus*, we think of this sample as coming from a universe or population of Golden Syrian hamsters similarly infected. Although this universe is hypothetical and does not actually exist, conceivably it could be made to exist. The formulas for the sampling errors employed for the various types of designs assume random sampling from populations of infinite size.

When we want to draw samples from an existing population, we find that this population is finite in size, although it will usually be much larger than the size of the sample drawn from it. As with infinite populations, the value of the characteristic, e.g., the mean, relative frequency, etc., calculated from the sample will differ somewhat from the true or universe value, either on the plus or minus side, due to the chance factors operating in the selection of the samples. That is, the estimates computed from the sample are subject to sampling errors.

NONPROBABILITY SAMPLING

Samples can be classified into two general types, probability and nonprobability samples. While nonprobability samples may provide good estimates of the parameters, they usually cannot give an idea of the size of the difference between the sample estimate and the true value or parameter. The following are examples of nonprobability samples whose accuracy cannot be assessed quantitatively. The dental investigator may find it convenient to select a particular group, such as the dental clinic with which he is associated, on which to test a new caries-inhibitory agent. This *convenience sample* may or may not represent the universe; there is no way of knowing. Such relevant factors entering into the characteristics and alterations of caries attacks as age, dietary patterns, socioeconomic status, racial and genetic patterns, cooperation of the subjects, etc. may or may not be referable to the overall population. Intact groups, as, for example, all the children in one school as a sample of all school-children in a particular community, also fall into the category of a convenience sample. *Volunteer samples* and other *self-selected samples* are special cases of a convenience sample.

In some instances, the investigator may have a good knowledge of the characteristics of the universe and, if he can maintain the proper objectivity, he may possibly obtain a good *judgment sample*. Unfortunately, much depends on the talents of the investigator, plus the fact that there is no way of assessing quantitatively how the sample estimate may differ from the true value. Judgment samples must, therefore, be viewed with caution.

In some instances, the investigator selects the sample without any evident bias, by a so-called blind or unprejudiced technique; thus, he may go into a classroom and arbitrarily pick several children in an "unbiased" manner. This constitutes a *haphazard* sample rather than a random sample. It is practically impossible to avoid some type of bias in selection of samples in this way, and, once again, there is no way of assessing how the sample estimate may differ from the true value.

PROBABILITY SAMPLING

As distinguished from nonprobability samples, randomization procedures are utilized in selecting probability samples. The advantages of probability sampling are that an unbiased estimate of the parameter can be obtained and the sampling error can be determined. Thus, a quantitative assessment can be made to show how far from the true value the estimate may be. For example, we know that the estimate will differ from the parameter by more than twice its standard error only 5% of the time (for cases where the estimates are normally distributed). This sampling fluctuation decreases as the number of cases in the sample increases, as intuition would lead us to believe. Sampling errors resulting from methods of selection of the sample are not the only errors that may occur. Other errors may arise from errors of measurement, errors in the preparation of estimates, errors due to time trend changes in the population characteristics, and errors due to nonresponse.

In a probability sample, whether an individual is selected or not depends neither on the characteristic possessed by the individual nor on the judgment of the investigator. Each individual element in the population has an assigned probability of being included in the sample, but no individual has a probability of zero. In the simplest case, all the individuals have equal probabilities of being included in the sample. The use of equal probabilities allows the estimates of the parameters to be computed more simply. Such types of samples are often referred to as *self-weighting*. If unequal probabilities were to be assigned to the various individuals, or sets (strata) of individuals, then some type of weighting would have to be employed in a preparation of the estimates. Sampling plans employing unequal probabilities should generally be avoided except for comprehensive surveys, such as some of the projects of the National Health Survey[1] conducted by the National Center for Health Statistics.

A great variety of plans use equal probability samples. For illustrative purposes in describing various types of equal probability samples, let it be assumed that the universe consists of 8000 high school students in 10 schools of 800 each. Further, there are four grades in each school, with 200 children in each grade, divided into five classrooms with 40 students in each room. The simplicity achieved by this uniformity of distribution of the students makes it easier to illustrate the various points. From a sample of this population of 8000 students, we wish to learn what proportion is caries-free.* Let us suppose that a sample of 800 students, a 10% sampling ratio, is decided on. The choice of the sample size depends on the considerations of cost and desired accuracy of the estimate. The same number, 800, would not give equally accurate estimates for all sampling plans, since the sampling error will vary according to the way in which the sample is drawn.

Unrestricted Random Sampling

The simplest procedure that allows each of the individual elements an equal chance of being chosen is *simple* or *unrestricted random sampling*. A roster of the 8000 students (the *sampling frame*) is made, and each student is assigned a number placed on a tag. The 8000 tags are shuffled thoroughly, and 800 of these are chosen by a lottery without replacement of the tags. It is much easier to utilize tables of random numbers that are actually the results of past lotteries. In these tables, four columns of digits are employed, and the first 800 numbers between 1 and 8000 are selected. Numbers greater than 8000 are discarded as well as numbers previously selected. Each student, therefore, has a probability of 1/10 of being included in the sample.

While the estimate (mean, relative frequency) in the sample may differ from the true or universe value, on the average it is equal to this parameter. In other words, when a very large number of samples is drawn in this manner, the mean of the estimates (the expected value) is equal to the parameter, i.e., the estimate is unbiased. In spite of these properties, a random sample may, on occasion, not reflect the characteristics of the universe. This is highly unlikely except when the size of the sample is small.

The relative frequency (p) of the sample does not differ from the true or universe value (p') by more than two (more exactly, 1.96) standard errors (SE_p) more than once in 20 times. When dealing

*For simplicity, we focus here on a dichotomous scale and a relative frequency. The same discussion would apply if we were measuring some quantity x, for each individual instead of caries-free, not caries-free, e.g., blood vitamin A, blood vitamin C, etc.

with infinite universes, $SE_p = \sqrt{\dfrac{p'q'}{n}}$, where n is the sample size, p' is the relative frequency of the characteristic under consideration in the universe, and q' is the complement $(1 - p')$ of the relative frequency. When the universe is finite in size, say, consisting of M elements, then the formula becomes

$$SE_p = \sqrt{\left(\frac{p'q'}{n}\right)\left(\frac{M-n}{M-1}\right)} \cong \sqrt{\left(\frac{p'q'}{n}\right)\left(\frac{M-n}{M}\right)}$$

$$= \sqrt{\left(\frac{p'q'}{n}\right)(1-r)},$$

where r is the sampling ratio. In general, p' is unknown, and is replaced by the sample estimate, p, so that the formula becomes

$$SE_p = \sqrt{\frac{pq}{n}}\,(1-r).$$

Thus, if in the sample of 800 illustrated, 4.0% are caries-free,

$$SE_p = \sqrt{\frac{(4.0)(96.0)(0.9)}{800}} = \sqrt{0.432} = 0.66\%.$$

If $r = 0$, as for an infinite population, $SE_p = 0.69\%$. Since $2\,SE_p = 2(0.66\%) = 1.3\%$, the approximate 95% confidence range or interval for the true relative frequency is 2.7% to 5.3%. This confidence interval can be made narrower by taking a larger sample, or possibly by taking a sample of the same size and putting some restriction on the free play of chance in the selection.

The sample size to attain a given confidence interval can be calculated as in Chapter 14, except that the n will be slightly smaller if r is taken into account:

$$n = \frac{n'}{1 + \dfrac{n'}{M}},$$

where n' is the value for an infinite universe. Suppose that a simple random sample is to be drawn from a finite population of M = 10,000 children with periodontal disease, in which it is believed that the relative frequency of juvenile onset periodontitis is 10%. It is desired that the half-width of the 95% confidence interval be 1%, i.e., so that the p of a sample does not differ by more than 1% from the p' of the universe more often than 5%. The preliminary value of 10% must be used to estimate SE_p. If the universe were infinite, 1% = 1.96 SE_p = $1.96\sqrt{(10)(90)/n'}$. Solving for n', $n' = 3457$. Now, using M = 10,000, $n'/M = 0.3457$, $n = 3457/(1 + 0.3457) = 2569$, a sampling ratio of r = .2569. The sample size is about 25% smaller than when the universe is assumed to be infinite. Obviously, after the sample is taken, the sample value p must be used to estimate SE_p and establish the confidence interval on p'.

Stratified Random Sampling

It is known that caries experience is related to age (in effect, school grade level). Then, a stratification on this secondary variable should reduce the chance fluctuation. McCarthy[2] has characterized stratified random sampling:

1. The population is divided into a set of mutually exclusive and exhaustive subgroups or strata.
2. A simple random sample of elements is selected from each stratum.
3. An estimate is prepared separately for each stratum.
4. These estimates are combined in some prescribed manner to provide an estimate for the entire population.

Mainland[3] has also listed four considerations on which the decision of the choice of criteria for stratification should be based:

1. Simplicity, clarity and objectivity of the dividing lines. Potential users of the results should be able to classify them in the same way.
2. The known or presumed relative weights of the factors — their power to produce differences in outcome and thus cause variation and bias.
3. Feasibility and convenience.
4. Usefulness in the application of results. Before every investigation, the question should be asked: "By whom, for what purpose, and under what conditions, will our results probably be used?" Restrictions of conditions narrows the basis of generalization.

In our simple example, a list is prepared of the students for each grade level (2000) and 1/10 of each list is drawn by random numbers. The same sampling ratio is used for each stratum, i.e., there is proportional allocation. Each student still has a probability of 1/10 of being included in the sample. An estimate of the relative frequency is prepared separately for each stratum and a weighted average of these estimates is taken, using the known sizes of the strata as weights. The proportional allocation used ensures that the sample is self-weighting, so that the relative frequency in the total sample is directly the estimate of the true relative frequency in the population of 8000 students. Thus, the weighting of the relative frequencies for the separate strata is automatically accomplished.

The standard error of the estimate in stratified random sampling is less than that for simple or unrestricted random sampling, provided that age is indeed a relevant stratification. Even if it were not relevant, the standard error cannot, in general, be larger than that for the case of simple random sampling. For the case of proportional allocation, the SE of the relative frequency for the total sample is given approximately by $SE_p = \sqrt{\dfrac{(1-r)\Sigma n_i p_i q_i}{n^2}}$, where n_i is the sample size drawn from the ith stratum; p_i is the relative frequency in the ith stratum; $q_i = (1 - p_i)$; r is the constant sampling ratio in the various strata; and n is the total sample size. The use of this formula is not restricted to the case of strata of equal size.

The population of students is arranged by grade and school; therefore, one could take advantage of this double stratification in the sampling plan. One could take, for example, a 10% random sample of the 200 children from each grade within each school.

Sometimes, some strata are sampled more intensively than others, so that the sample would no longer be self-weighting. Thus, suppose that 3/20 of the students in the first two years of high school were sampled, but only 1/20 of the students in the second two years; the sampling ratio therefore would be different for different grades. In that case, the appropriate estimate of the parameter relative frequency would not be the relative frequency of the total sample. Rather, a weighted average of the grade specific relative frequencies according to the size of the strata in the universe must be taken. In the example chosen for illustrative purposes, the strata are equal in size, so that the weights are in the ratio of 1:1:1:1 and the weighted average becomes a simple average, $p = \Sigma p_i/4$. In general, $p = \Sigma w_i p_i$ where $w_i = M_i/M$ is the size of the ith stratum in relation to the whole population of M. Of course, the variance of p is more complicated when equal weighting is not employed.[4] The use of unequal sampling ratios might be called for when some of the strata are small and one wants a sufficient representation from such strata in order to make comparisons among strata, rather than merely obtain an overall estimate.

Cluster Sampling

Sometimes it is difficult to obtain simple random samples or stratified random samples because of the wide spatial dispersion of the
sample or complex administrative problems. In such cases, using the
illustrative example once again, it may be convenient to take all or a
portion of a classroom. There are 200 classrooms in the population
illustrated, so that a sample of 800 could be obtained by taking 1/10
of the classroom, resulting in 20 rooms with 40 students in each.
Random numbers can be utilized in the selection of classrooms. Each
student still has a 1/10 probability of being included in the sample.
Actually, the sampling frame consists of the 200 classrooms or
clusters, and the sample is, in effect, a sample of clusters. The sample
is still self-weighting, and the relative frequency of the total sample
(p) is an estimate of the true relative frequency (p').

If there is a tendency to alikeness among members of the cluster,
as there probably is, the standard error would thereby be increased as
compared to that of a simple random sample. Consequently, a sample of the indicated size (800) would generally yield a larger standard
error than a simple random sample of 800. For the case of equal
clusters, the standard error of the relative frequency (p) of the total

sample is approximately given by $SE_p = \sqrt{\dfrac{(1-r)\Sigma(p_i - p)^2}{c(c-1)}}$, where

c is the number of clusters in the sample, p_i is the relative frequency
in the ith cluster, and r is the sampling ratio (here, 1/10).

The effect of increase in the sampling error because of correlation between the members of the clusters could, of course, be compensated for by taking more clusters. Another way of reducing this
effect would be to perform the sampling in two stages, by taking
more clusters and subsampling within the clusters. For example, 40
classrooms could be selected (by random numbers) and from each
room only 20 students would be selected from a list prepared for the
room. The subsampling ratio is 20/40 or 50%. In this case, the list
does not have to be prepared for all the students, but only for those
40 classrooms selected in the first stage. Each student still has a 1/10
probability of being included in the sample. Furthermore, the sample
is still self-weighting. The formula for the standard error of p is considerably more complicated in this case.[4]

It is possible to combine cluster sampling and stratified sampling. Thus, the clusters are arranged by grade (stratum), yielding 50 clusters (classrooms) per grade. A 20% sample of classrooms could be chosen from each grade and a 50% sample of the individuals chosen from each selected cluster. Each individual still has a probability of 1/10 of being chosen and the sample is still self-weighting. The formula for the standard error of p is even more complicated.[4]

If the clusters are not of uniform size as presented in this illustrative example of classrooms, an equal probability sample, which will still be self-weighting, can be designed by adhering to constant sampling and subsampling ratios. However, the standard error formulas become exceedingly complicated.[4]

Systematic Random Sampling

If every tenth individual were selected from the complete list of the 8000 students in our illustrative example, a 10% sample would be obtained, yielding 800. The number at which the selection starts is obtained by choosing a random number between 1 and 10, say, 4. Individuals 4, 14, 24, 34, 44, 54, and so forth, are selected. If the list represents a random ordering of the individuals, then the systematic random sample is equivalent to a simple random sample. If the list is prepared by groups, such as grades, as it may be, with random ordering within the groups, then a systematic random sample corresponds to a stratified sample with proportional allocation. In some instances there may be a cyclic relation between the units sampled, in which case a systematic random sample corresponds to a cluster sample and may be much less precise than a simple random sample. In spite of this, the sample is self-weighting and the relative frequency (p) of the sample is unbiased, although not very accurate.

It may be possible to evaluate the standard error of a systematic random sample. If the ordering is known to be random, the formula for simple random sampling would apply. If the ordering is known to be stratified and random within strata, the formula for stratified sampling would apply. Unknown to the investigator, however, the ordering may be cyclic, e.g., every tenth house might turn out to be a corner house. This cyclic problem is the same difficulty encountered at times in systematic alternation in experimental design.

One way of coping with the problem of a cyclic pattern would be to choose a different random number from 1 to 10 for each group of ten individuals. This would, however, vitiate the simplicity of systematic random sampling. Another way of coping with the problem would be to pick k, say 5, random numbers between 1 and 10k, or 50 in this case. To each of these k = 5 numbers, 10k = 50 is added. We thus end up with k = 5 samples, each of which comprises a 1/10k = 1/50 = 2% sample. The total sample is the desired 10% sample. The standard error of the overall relative frequency, p, is determined from the variability of the k = 5 sample values of p among them-

selves. That is, $p = \Sigma p_i/5$; $SE_p = \sqrt{\dfrac{\Sigma (p_i - p)^2}{(5)(4)}}$.

Systematic sampling is often used in subsampling clusters, and is very useful for sampling card files. Another useful application of this method occurs when selecting areas to obtain geographical stratification, such as blocks from a certain section of the city, the blocks being numbered in a spatial order.

Oral Cavity as a Cluster

A sample of individuals corresponds to a sample of oral cavities. While the sampling unit is the oral cavity, this actually corresponds to a cluster of the units in which the dental investigator is fundamentally interested, namely, teeth. One might add that each tooth is a cluster of subunits in which the investigator may be even more interested, namely, surfaces. The individual oral cavity may be likened to an apartment house. The family in each apartment is a tooth consisting of different surfaces. These apartment houses (mouths) may not contain the same number of families (teeth). Furthermore, the families are of different sizes (number of surfaces), especially if only nondecayed surfaces are being considered. The risk of caries attack varies not only from one member of the family to another (surface to surface for a given tooth), but also from family to family (tooth to tooth). The posterior teeth are different types of families from the anterior teeth.

The investigator who wants to determine the proportion (p) of teeth that are carious in a population of teeth by taking a sample of (c) individuals, must recognize that the (n) teeth comprising the sample of teeth do not constitute an independent sample of n independent elements. Rather, there are independent clusters (oral cavities) of variable size, up to 32 in the adult dentition. This consideration of clustering is important in the preparation of the estimate (p) as well as in the determination of the sampling error of p. It is equally important in comparisons of one group of individuals (oral cavities) with another group.

If the investigator desires to determine the proportion of surfaces that are carious by taking a sample of individuals, the problem is compounded, because now there are two levels of clustering. The total number of surfaces observed in the sample by no means constitutes a sample of so many independent surfaces. Investigators who divide surfaces into different moieties for comparison carry the clustering difficulty one stage further and thereby complicate the problem even more.

If a given tooth for each individual were the focus of attention, then a random sample of individuals is, at the same time, a random sample of teeth and the clustering problem and its ramifications are eliminated. Similarly, if only a given surface on a given tooth per individual oral cavity were considered, no cluster problem arises, because a random sample of individuals is a random sample of surfaces. This focusing on a given tooth or tooth surface, however, does not yield sufficient information. It would be more realistic to focus on a series of specific teeth (or specific surfaces) *separately*, i.e., mesial of maxillary left first premolar, occlusal of mandibular first molar, and distal of maxillary left lateral incisor.

REFERENCES

1. National Center for Health Statistics: Plan and Initial Program of the Health Examination Survey. Vital and Health Statistics. PHS Pub No. 100 — Series 1 — No. 4. Pub Health Serv, Washington, U.S. Government Printing Office, May, 1962.

2. McCarthy, P. J.: Introduction to Statistical Reasoning, New York, McGraw-Hill, 1957.

3. Mainland, D. J.: Elementray Medical Statistics, 2nd ed., Philadelphia, Saunders, 1963.

4. Cochran, W. G.: Sampling Techniques, 3rd ed., New York, Wiley, 1967.

19
Reliability Studies

QUANTITATIVE DATA (MEASUREMENTS OR SCORES)

Interexaminer Reliability

In both clinical and epidemiological studies, the variability of the measurements has an important effect on the precision and power of the statistical analyses of the data generated by the study. Both precision and power will be attenuated to the extent that the variability is due to extraneous factors, e.g., interexaminer differences or measurement errors.

It is usually only during the preliminary standardization (calibration, reliability) trial that a sample of the study population is examined repeatedly by the different examiners. The analysis of the data from this preliminary study should depend on how the data from the large scale field trial will be analyzed.

Pooling Data from All Examiners

In the case where data from all examiners will be pooled in the field trial, interexaminer differences are assumed to represent just another source of random variation, provided that the subjects are randomly assigned to the examiners. The analysis of these pooled data is fairly simple, but there is some reduction in precision and power if the interexaminer differences are large.

A reliability study to determine both intra- and interexaminer consistency in caries diagnosis was performed by Slakter, Juliano, and Fischman[1] as part of a program to evaluate methods of caries prevention. Before the initial (baseline) examination and at each of the two subsequent annual examinations, the two dental examiners and recorders were trained in the examining procedures, and they all then participated in a reliability study.

On the morning of the first day of these sessions, the diagnostic criteria were determined and, following a discussion of their application, both dentists examined three or four subjects. The differences between their findings were discussed. During the next three half-day sessions, each child of a sample of 18 children (not part of the larger field trial) was examined by both examiners, for a total of six times, three by each examiner. The two dentists were the examiners in the larger field study, which was designed to have each child examined by only one examiner selected at random and then have all the resulting data pooled. The examiner effect can then be considered to be a random variable.

Table 19.1 presents the standard two-way ANOVA of the DMFS scores obtained from the third annual calibration trial of 18 subjects.[2] From this table, four *components of variance* are estimated as follows:

$$\text{Patients} = \frac{\text{Between Patients MS} - \text{Interaction MS}}{\text{Number of Examiners} \times \text{Number of Examinations}} = \frac{(A - C)}{J \times n}$$

$$= \frac{146.47 - 2.29}{2 \times 3} = 24.03.$$

$$\text{Examiners} = \frac{\text{Between Examiners MS} - \text{Interaction MS}}{\text{Number of Patients} \times \text{Number of Examinations}} = \frac{(B - C)}{N \times n}$$

$$= \frac{45.37 - 2.29}{18 \times 3} = 0.80.$$

$$\text{Interaction} = \frac{\text{Interaction MS} - \text{Error MS}}{\text{Number of Examinations}} = \frac{(C - D)}{n} = \frac{2.29 - 0.90}{3} = 0.46.$$

$$\text{Error} = \text{Error MS} = D = 0.90,$$

where J = number of examiners ($= 2$); n = number of examinations ($= 3$); and N = number of patients ($= 18$).

The estimated *intraclass correlation coefficient of reliability* is the component of variance due to patient-to-patient variation, divided by the sum of all the components of variance in the data. Thus,

$$r = \frac{24.03}{24.03 + 0.80 + 0.46 + 0.90} = \frac{24.03}{26.19} = .92.$$

TABLE 19.1
Analysis of Variance on DMFS Scores from Intra- and Interexaminer Reliability Study

Source of Variation	df	SS	MS
Between Patients	$(18-1) = 17$	2,489.96	$146.47(= A)$
Between Examiners	$(2-1) = 1$	45.37	$45.37(= B)$
Interaction	$(18-1)(2-1) = 17$	38.96	$2.29(= C)$
Error	$18 \times 2(3-1) = 72$	64.67	$0.90(= D)$
Total		107	2,638.96	

The value of r is an estimate of the population reliability coefficient, say ρ (lowercase Greek letter rho). The hypothesis that $\rho = 0$ is tested by the F-test,

$$F_{17,17} = \frac{\text{Between Patients MS}}{\text{Interaction MS}} = \frac{146.47}{2.29} = 63.96,$$

which is highly significant. It can be shown with approximately 95% confidence that the value of ρ is at least equal to 0.74, which is close to the generally accepted minimum standard of 0.75.

The component of variance due to differences between examiners can also be tested by obtaining the F ratio,

$$F_{1,17} = \frac{\text{Between Examiners MS}}{\text{Interaction MS}} = \frac{45.37}{2.29} = 19.81,$$

which is also highly significant. Nevertheless, because examiner variance accounts for only $0.80/26.19 = 3\%$ of the total variance, there would have been no problem in using the two examiners interchangeably in the field study. If the component of variance due to examiners had been both significant and larger, accounting for 10% or more of the total variance, it would have been wiser not to use the examiners interchangeably, but to consider then as separate strata in the field study. To be on the safe side, in fact, the decision was made in the Slakter, Juliano, and Fischman study to consider the examiners in this way.

Considering Each Examiner's Data
Separately and Then Pooling

In the case where the data will first be analyzed for each examiner separately and then pooled, interexaminer differences are considered to be *fixed effects*, rather than *random effects* as in the previous analysis. In this second type of analysis, the component of variance due to examiners is not used in obtaining the intraclass coefficient of correlation. Thus, the intraclass coefficient of correlation is estimated as

$$r = \frac{(A - C)}{A + (J - 1)C + J(n - 1)D}$$

$$= \frac{146.47 - 2.29}{146.47 + (2 - 1)2.29 + (2)(3 - 1)0.90} = .95.$$

This value is slightly larger than that found in the case of random examiner effects.

Comparison of Random and Fixed Effects Models

The value in the fixed effects case is larger (or smaller) than that in the random examiners case, whenever the MS for examiners is larger (or smaller) than the Interaction MS. As has been seen, the inter-examiner reliability is excellent for the current data using either method of analysis. In the random effects model, the value of ρ (which, unlike the standard Pearson product-moment correlation coefficient, does not have to be squared in order to be interpreted as a proportion of variance) can only be positive. The closer it is to 1, the more precise (reliable, interchangeable) are the measurements. In the fixed effects model, the value of ρ can be negative. A small or negative estimate suggests that an appreciable patient-examiner inter-action may be present. This can usually be remedied only by further training and calibration to assure that each examiner examines all patients consistently.

Considerations of Reliability Studies

Reliability studies should be designed, conducted, and analyzed to evaluate the relative magnitudes of the sources of variability in the measurements in the larger field study. Based on the statistical analysis, steps can be taken, consistent with the design of the study, to reduce the influence of the extraneous sources of variation.

The different components of variance which are estimated from the reliability study are often informative by themselves. The intra-class correlation coefficient is quite useful in measuring consistency by providing a single summary index of reliability.

CATEGORICAL (QUALITATIVE OR DISCRETE) DATA

When the variables under study are qualitative or categorical (e.g., the condition of a single tooth or tooth surface; the degree of inflammation of the oral mucosa), a more appropriate measure of reliability is the one based on the proportion of judgments which are in agreement. The *kappa statistic* can be used, which adjusts the observed proportion of agreement for the proportion expected if the judgments were made at random.[3]

Intraexaminer Reliability

The data on individual permanent teeth from the first reliability trial involved (N =) 27 subjects from the study described on pages 416–417. Two examiners examined each patient (n =) three times, and classified each surface and each tooth according to (k =) two categories, i.e., sound or carious. There are a total of $Nn(n - 1)/2$ pairs of intrapatient judgments by each examiner on each tooth surface.

Table 19.2 (see page 420) presents the judgments of the first examiner on the status of the occlusal surface of the maxillary right first molar. The observed proportion of agreements (P_0) is calculated from the following formula where n_{ij} is the number of judgments on patient i that were in category j:

$$P_0 = \frac{\displaystyle\sum_{i=1}^{N} \sum_{j=1}^{k} n_{ij}^2 - Nn}{Nn(n - 1)}$$

$$= \frac{(3^2 \times 12 + 0^2 \times 12 + 2^2 \times 1 + 1^2 \times 1 + 1^2 \times 2 + 2^2 \times 2 + 0^2 \times 12 + 3^2 \times 12) - (27 \times 3)}{27 \times 3 \times (3 - 1)}$$

$$= \frac{150}{162} = 0.9259.$$

Of the total of (Nn =) 81 judgments, 40 or 0.4938 stated that the occlusal surface was sound and 41 or 0.5062 noted that it was carious. The expected proportion of agreement is

$$P_e = (.4938)^2 + (.5062)^2 = .5001.$$

TABLE 19.2

Judgments by Examiner 1 on Occlusal Surface of the Maxillary Right First Molar in the First Year Reliability Study

Pattern of Judgments	Sound	Carious	Number of Children
All three sound	3	0	12
Two sound, one carious	2	1	1
One sound, two carious	1	2	2
All three carious	0	3	12
Total	40	41	27

The value of kappa (κ) is obtained from the ratio,

$$\kappa = \frac{P_o - P_e}{1 - P_e} = \frac{.9259 - .5001}{1 - .5001} = .852,$$

which indicates excellent intraexaminer reliability for examiner 1. Kappa ranges from below 0 for poorer than chance agreement, through 0 for just chance agreement, to a maximum of +1 for perfect agreement. While significances tests are available to test κ versus 0, in general, for sample sizes greater than 20, values of κ greater than 0.4 are usually statistically significant. More important, from the practical point of view, is that values of κ greater than 0.85 indicate good reliability. This value of κ (when the number of categories, κ, is equal to 2) is identical to the value of r, the intraclass correlation coefficient obtained from the one-way ANOVA, by assigning the value of 1 to all sound and 0 to all carious judgments, and by taking the df for the Between Patients MS as N (=27), rather than the usual N - 1 (=26).

Interexaminer Reliability

If these 27 patients are independently examined by the same two examiners and judgments are made on the same qualitative variables with the same (k=) 2 categories, the resulting data may be tabulated in a cross-classification table (Table 19.3).

The observed proportion of agreement between examiners is

$$P_0 = \frac{14 + 12}{27} = 0.9630,$$

TABLE 19.3
Judgments by Two Examiners of the Occlusal Surface of the Maxillary Right First Molar

	Examiner 2		
Examiner 1	Sound	Carious	Total
Sound	14	0	14
Carious	1	12	13
Total	15	12	27

while the expected proportion of agreement between examiners is

$$P_e = \frac{(14 \times 15) + (13 \times 12)}{(27)^2} = 0.5021.$$

The resulting value of kappa is

$$\kappa = \frac{P_0 - P_e}{1 - P_e} = \frac{.9630 - .5021}{1 - 0.5021} = .926,$$

indicating excellent agreement between examiners. In general, values of κ greater than $2/\sqrt{N(k-1)}$ indicate that the observed degree of agreement between examiners is statistically better than what would be predicted by chance alone.

REFERENCES

1. Slakter, M. J., Juliano, D. B., and Fischman, S. L. Estimating examiner consistency with DMFS measures, J Dent Res 55:930, 1976

2. Fleiss, J. L., Slakter, M. J., Fischman, S. L., Park, M. H., and Chilton, N. W. Inter-examiner reliability in caries trials, J Dent Res 58:604, 1979

3. Fleiss, J. L., Fischman, S. L., Chilton N. W., and Park, M. H., Reliability of discrete measurements in caries trials, Caries Research 13:23, 1979

Appendix

In this Appendix, we illustrate three common types of problems by the use of selected programs on the HP 41C,[1] namely: (1) a one-way analysis of variance; (2) an analysis of covariance; and (3) a multiple regression with two independent variables.

Many of the problems requiring tedious calculations pertain to what might be called nonorthogonal designs. The most familiar examples of these are multiple regression with two or more independent variables; the analysis of covariance where some of the variables are dummy variables and some are measured variables; and nonorthogonal analysis of variance best illustrated by a two-way model with both criteria of classification fixed and with unequal replication in the cell. While all of these problems were formerly solved by elementary procedures, the tediousness of these procedures resulted in the introduction of many approximations to the exact procedures. These three common nonorthogonal problems are illustrated by the use of program packages: (1) multiple regression illustrated in Chapter 9 of the text, using the SAS General Linear Model[2,3] and the SPSS[4] packages; (2) analysis of covariance illustrated in Chapter 10 by the Biomedical Programs, BMDP IV[5] ; and (3) the two-way layout, fixed-fixed model in the analysis of variance with unequal n_{ij}'s by the General Linear Model of SAS. In addition to the edited program output which is given for each example, annotations are made explaining the various parts of the printouts.

423

HP 41C PRINTOUTS

Analysis of Variance of Data in Table 7.8

PRINTOUT	*TEXT (Table 7.9)*
TSS = 3111.975	Total SS
TRSS = 2853.475	Between Individuals SS
ESS = 258.500	Within Individuals SS
DF1 = 19.000	Between Individuals df
DF2 = 20.000	Within Treatments df
DF3 = 39.000	Total df
TRMS = 150.183	Between Individuals MS
EMS = 12.925	Within Individuals MS
F = 11.620	$\dfrac{\text{Between Individuals MS}}{\text{Within Individuals MS}}$

Analysis of Covariance of Data in Table 10.1

PRINTOUT	*TEXT (Table 10.4)*
TSSX = 6674.9333	Total SSx
ASSX = 596.9333	Between Treatments SSx
WSSX = 6078.0000	Within Treatments SSx
TSSY = 80.9833	Total SSy
ASSY = 3.0083	Between Treatments SSy
WSSY = 77.9750	Within Treatments SSy
DF1 = 2.0000	Between Treatments df
DF2 = 57.0000	Within Treatments df
FX = 2.7990	$\dfrac{\text{Between Treatments SSx} \div 2}{\text{Within Treatments SSx} \div 57}$ (p. 227)
FY = 1.0996	$\dfrac{\text{Between Treatments SSy} \div 2}{\text{Within Treatments SSy} \div 57}$ (p. 226)
TSP = 50.5333	Total SPxy
ASP = -13.0167	Between Treatments SPxy
WSP = 63.5500	Within Treatments SPxy
TSSY. = 80.6008	Reduced Total SSy
WSSY = 77.3105	Reduced Within Treatments SSy
ASSY = 3.2902	Between Treatments Adjusted SSy*

---

*Numerator of $F_{2,56}$ before dividing by 2 (p. 235) which is Adjusted Between Treatments (Table 10.4).

PRINTOUT	*TEXT (Table 10.4)*
DF3 = 2.0000	Reduced Between Treatments df
DF4 = 56.0000	Reduced Within Treatments df
AMSY = 1.6451	Reduced Between Treatments MS*
WMSY = 1.3805	Reduced Within Treatments MS
F = 1.1917	$\dfrac{\text{Reduced Between Treatments MS}}{\text{Reduced Within Treatments MS}}$ ((p. 235)

Multiple Regression Analysis of Data in Table 9.1

PRINTOUT	*TEXT*
R^2 = 0.794187375	R^2 (p. 216)
a = 0.311562445	a (p. 211)
b = 0.983091507	b (p. 211)
c = −0.014582280	c (p. 211)

MULTIPLE LINEAR REGRESSION EDITED PRINT-OUT, SAS PROGRAM (BASED ON DATA FROM TABLE 9.1)

GENERAL LINEAR MODELS PROCEDURE

DEPENDENT VARIABLE: POST_PLQ

SOURCE	DF	SUM OF SQUARES	MEAN SQUARE	F VALUE
MODEL	2	11.74205247	5.87102623	71.39
ERROR	37	3.04293753	0.08224155	PR > F
CORRECTED TOTAL	39	14.78499000		0.0001

R-SQUARE	C.V.	STD DEV	POST_PLQ MEAN
0.794187	14.7862	0.28677788	1.93950000

Type Ia (Order of Entry: x_1, x_2)

SOURCE	DF	TYPE I SS	F VALUE	PR > F
PRE_PLAQ	1	11.67991269	142.02	0.0001
WEIGHT	1	0.06213978	0.76	0.3903

Type Ib (Order of Entry: x_2, x_1)

SOURCE	DF	TYPE I SS	F VALUE	PR > F
WEIGHT	1	0.00033586	0.00	0.9494
PRE_PLAQ	1	11.74171661	142.77	0.0001

SOURCE	DF	TYPE IV SS	F VALUE	PR > F
PRE_PLAQ	1	11.74171661	142.77	0.0001
WEIGHT	1	0.06213978	0.76	0.3903

PARAMETER	ESTIMATE	T FOR H0: PARAMETER=0	PR > ITI	STD ERROR OF ESTIMATE
INTERCEPT	0.31156244	1.10	0.2798	0.28406623
PRE_PLAQ	0.98309151	11.95	0.0001	0.08227612
WEIGHT	−0.01458228	−0.87	0.3903	0.01677592

*Numerator of $F_{2,56}$ (p. 235).

Observation	Observed Value	Predicted Value	Residual
1	2.43000000	2.58480112	-0.15480112
2	1.84000000	1.73934242	0.10065758
3	0.53000000	0.80766557	-0.27766557
4	2.02000000	1.79832791	0.22167209
5	1.89000000	1.89983321	-0.00983321
6	3.00000000	2.62191319	0.37808681
7	2.23000000	2.46494673	-0.23494673
8	2.57000000	1.93342095	0.63657905
9	1.85000000	1.74306074	0.10693926
10	2.09000000	2.37868009	-0.28868009
11	1.42000000	1.13570709	0.28429291
12	2.32000000	2.30191617	0.01808383
13	2.21000000	2.37425691	-0.16425691
14	1.00000000	1.11453854	-0.11453854
15	1.61000000	1.69602076	-0.08602076
16	1.35000000	1.50626842	-0.15626842
17	0.95000000	1.32169262	-0.37169262
18	1.20000000	1.58712733	-0.38712733
19	2.04000000	1.92203481	0.11796519
20	1.61000000	1.64676919	-0.03676919
21	1.81000000	1.83355658	-0.02355658
22	2.65000000	2.21781265	0.43218738
23	2.81000000	2.85061251	-0.04061251
24	3.33000000	2.95037989	0.37962011
25	1.27000000	1.34798922	-0.07798922
26	1.32000000	1.75646448	-0.43646448
27	1.68000000	1.92678618	-0.24578618
28	2.38000000	2.53240191	-0.15240191
29	0.86000000	0.56536853	0.29463147
30	1.82000000	1.73713083	0.08286817
31	1.71000000	1.99240644	-0.28240644
32	2.23000000	2.72977357	-0.49977357
33	2.85000000	2.45732741	0.39267259
34	1.36000000	1.34535246	0.01464754
35	2.17000000	2.49345493	-0.32345493
36	2.02000000	1.49738342	0.42261658
37	2.20000000	2.05933944	0.14066056
38	2.33000000	2.25674960	0.07324040
39	2.52000000	2.07575663	0.44424337
40	2.10000000	2.27561957	-0.17561957
Sum of Residuals			0.00000000
Sum of Squared Residuals			3.04293753
Sum of Squared Residuals – Error SS			-0.00000000

MULTIPLE LINEAR REGRESSION EDITED
PRINTOUT, SPSS PROGRAM (Based on Data from Table 9.1)

CORRELATION COEFFICIENTS

	X1	X2	Y
X1	1.00000	0.06741	0.88881
X2	0.06741	1.00000	-0.00477
Y	0.88881	-0.00477	1.00000

Notes on SAS Printout

1. SS for Model = Regression SS and does not include Intercept (see P. 218).
2. SS for Error = Reduced SS from Plane (see P. 218). Error MS = $s^2 y \cdot x_1 x_2$.
3. R-Square = R^2 (see P. 216).
4. C.V. = $s_{y \cdot x}/\bar{y}$.
5. Type Ia: SS for Preplaque = Regression on x_1 (ignoring x_2). (see Table 9.3).
6. Type Ia: SS for Weight = Regression on x_2 (beyond x_1) (see Table 9.3).
7. Type Ib: SS for Weight = Regression on x_2 (ignoring x_1) (see Table 9.3).
8. Type Ib: SS for Preplaque = Regression on x_1 (beyond x_2) (see Table 9.3).
9. Type IV: SS for Weight = Regression on x_2 (beyond x_1) (see Table 9.3).
10. Type IV: SS for Preplaque = Regression on x_1 (beyond x_2) (see Table 9.3).
11. For parameters, see p. 215.
12. For t-test on parameters, see p. 217.
13. Observed value = y.
    Predicted value = Y.
    Residual = (y − Y).

DEPENDENT VARIABLE: Y
VARIABLE(S) ENTERED ON STEP NUMBER 1: X1
                                        X2

MULTIPLE R   0.89117
R SQUARE   0.79419
ADJUSTED R SQUARE   0.78306
STANDARD ERROR   0.28678

ANALYSIS OF VARIANCE	DF	SUM OF SQAURES	MEAN SQUARE	F
REGRESSION	2.	11.74205	5.87102	71.83
RESIDUAL	37.	3.04294	0.08224	

Variables in the Equation

VARIABLE	B	BETA	STD ERROR B	F
X1	0.0930915	0.89319	0.08228	142.771
X2	-0.0145823	-0.06498	0.01678	0.756
(CONSTANT)	0.3115624			

Notes on SPSS Printout

1. Adjusted R Square = R^2 adjusted for difference in degrees of freedom in Error SS and Total SS. In rare occasions, may be negative.
2. B = b_1, b_2, and a; Beta = standardized coefficients (see P. 217); F = (B/Standard Error B)^2 (see P. 217).

ANALYSIS OF COVARIANCE EDITED PRINTOUT, BMDP IV PROGRAM (Based on Data from Table 10.1)

COVARIATE	REG. COEFF.	STD. ERR.	T-VALUE
X	0.01046	0.01507	0.69375

GROUP	N	GRP. MEAN	ADJ. GRP. MEAN	STD. ERR.
A	20.	-0.27500	-0.23666	0.26848
B	20.	-0.40000	-0.44217	0.26967
P	20.	0.12500	0.12883	0.26279

ANALYSIS OF VARIANCE

SOURCE OF VARIANCE	DF	SUM OF SQUARES	MEAN SQUARE	F	TAIL AREA PROBABILITY

EQUALITY OF ADJ.					
CELL MEANS	2	3.2902	1.6451	1.1916	0.3113
ZERO SLOPE	1	0.6644	0.6644	0.4813	0.4907
ERROR	56	77.3104	1.3805		
EQUALITY OF SLOPES	2	2.1511	1.0755	0.7728	0.4668
ERROR	54	75.1593	1.3918		

Slope Within Each Group

		A	B	P
		1	2	3
X	2	0.0555	0.0001	0.0079

T-Test Matrix for Adjusted Group Means on 56 Degrees of Freedom

		A	B	P
		1	2	3
A	1	0.0		
B	2	-0.5279	0.0	
P	3	0.9750	1.4128	0.0

Notes on BMDP IV Printout

1. For Adjusted Group Means, see P. 235.
2. For Equality of Adjusted Group Cell Means = Total Reduced SS_y - Within Treatments Reduced SS_y, see Table 10.4 and P. 235.
3. For Zero Slopes SS = Regression SS (see Table 10.4 and P. 233.
4. For Error SS = Within Treatments Reduced SS_y (see Table 10.4 and P. 233).
5. Equality of Slopes SS = SS_y around 3 parallel lines – SS_y around 3 separate lines (see Table 10.4 and P. 231).
6. For Error SS with df = 54, see Table 10.4 and P. 231.
7. For slopes within each group, see Table 10.4 and P. 230.
8. To compare two adjusted group means, see t-test matrix and P. 235 and 236.

ANALYSIS OF VARIANCE (NON-ORTHOGONAL) EDITED PRINT-OUT, SAS PROGRAM (BASED ON DATA FROM TABLE 7.17)

GENERAL LINEAR MODELS PROCEDURE

DEPENDENT VARIABLE: TIME

SOURCE	DF	SUM OF SQUARES	MEAN SQUARE	F VALUE
MODEL	7	326.91881153	46.70268736	1.65
ERROR	71	2011.03055556	28.32437402	PR > F
CORRECTED TOTAL	78	2337.94936709		0.1352

R-SQUARE	C.V.	STD DEV	TIME MEAN
0.139831	26.5767	5.32206483	20.02531646

Type Ia (Order of Entry: Solution, Method, Solution×Method)

SOURCE	DF	TYPE I SS	F VALUE	PR > F
SOLUTION	3	40.05922526	0.47	0.7069
METHOD	1	271.21414615	9.58	0.0028
SOLUTION*METHOD	3	15.64544012	0.18	0.9048

Type Ib (Order of Entry: Method, Solution, Solution×Method)

SOURCE	DF	TYPE I SS	F VALUE	PR > F
METHOD	1	273.58310365	9.66	0.0027
SOLUTION	3	37.69026777	0.44	0.7262
SOLUTION*METHOD	3	15.64544012	0.18	0.9048

SOURCE	DF	TYPE IV SS	F VALUE	PR > F
METHOD	1	264.61538647	9.34	0.0032
SOLUTION	3	34.15301897	0.40	0.7553
SOLUTION*METHOD	3	15.64544012	0.18	0.9048

Notes on SAS ANOVA Printout

1. Model SS = Regression SS = SS (Solution, Method, Solution × Method).

2. R-Square = Model SS/Corrected Total SS.

3. Type Ia
   SS for Solution ignores Method
   SS for Method adjusted for Solution
   SS for Solution × Method adjusted for Method and Solution = Adjusted Interaction.

4. Type Ib
   SS for Method ignores Solution
   SS for Solution adjusted for Method
   SS for Solution × Method adjusted for Method and Solution = Adjusted Interaction.

5. Type IV: All effects are adjusted for all other effects
    SS for Method adjusted for Solution and Solution × Method
    SS for Solution adjusted for Method and Solution × Method
    SS for Solution × Method adjusted for Method and Solution = Adjusted Interaction.

In most situations with this model, Type IV is the preferred solution.

REFERENCES

1. HP 41C Statistical Applications Handbook, Corvallis, Ore., Hewlett-Packard Company, 1979.

2. SAS User's Guide, SAS Institute, Inc., Cary, N.C., 1979.

3. Freund, Rudolph J. and Littell, Raymond C.: SAS for Linear Models: A Guide to the ANOVA and GLM Procedures. New York, McGraw-Hill, 1981.

4. Nie, N. H., Hull, C. H., Jenkins, J. G., Steinbrenner, K., and Bent, D. H.: Statistical Package for the Social Sciences, 2nd ed., New York, McGraw-Hill, 1975.

5. Dixon, W. J. and Brown, M. B.: BMDP-79, Biomedical Computer Programs, P-Series, Los Angeles, Univ. of California Press, 1979.

Index

Index